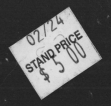

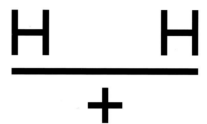

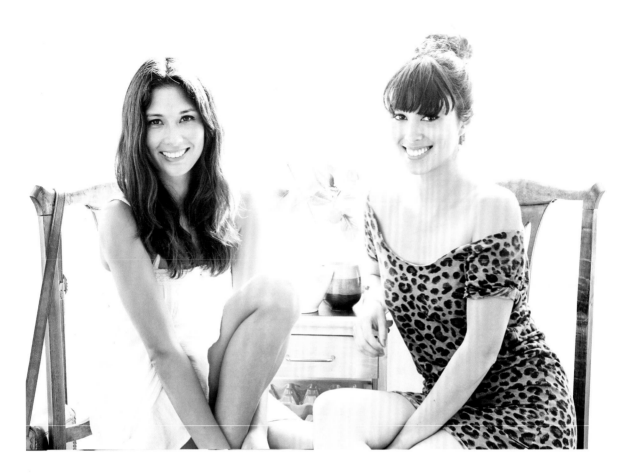

To our loved ones and all those who have inspired and supported us. For our clients who believed in a better way. And to everyone else who wants to join us on our delicious journey.

# THE ART OF EATING WELL

# HEMSLEY HEMSLEY

dear Julie
Thank you so much for your
support. long live Good Food!
Happy Cooking! love Melissa x
Jasmine
x x x

JASMINE AND MELISSA HEMSLEY

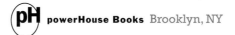

**pH** **powerHouse Books** Brooklyn, NY

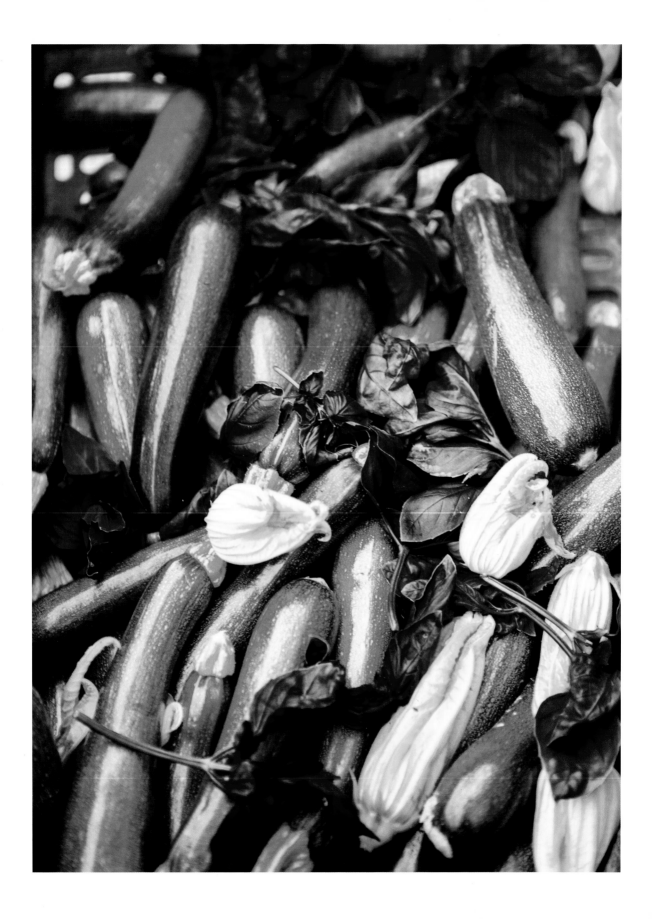

# CONTENTS

# INTRODUCTION

If you want to love what you eat AND look and feel like the best version of yourself, then this book is for you. Wellness begins from within; eating real, unprocessed, and nourishing food allows you to live a healthier, happier, and more energized life. By understanding what's good for your body, making some simple changes to your habits, and by choosing food that's both delicious and good for you, you will look better and feel amazing. This is *The Art of Eating Well.*

We've created 150 exciting and inventive recipes for every day; recipes that are easy and fun to make as well as being packed with nourishing ingredients. You don't need to be a gourmet chef, count calories, go hungry, or miss out on dessert – there is no fad dieting here. The idea is to cook and eat meals that are so delicious you'll forget that you're eating "healthy food." Many of the recipes in this book will seem familiar to you at first glance: a reworking of popular dishes from pizza and spaghetti to chocolate cake and ice cream, or traditionally "healthy" recipes like supercharged salads and nourishing veg-packed smoothies. We don't believe in depriving ourselves of treats and "comfort foods," we just make them using whole ingredients and unrefined, natural sweeteners.

Don't be put off by unusual names or worry about tracking down certain ingredients. We've included plenty of alternatives, and the stockist list on our website (www.hemsleyandhemsley.com) will help you find your local specialist store or point you in the direction of an online shop.

In amongst the recipes you'll find simple, practical tips on sourcing and preparing food and enhancing digestion. Our easy, sustainable, common sense philosophy will arm you with the knowledge and tools to take control of your food choices and begin your own journey to the art of eating well.

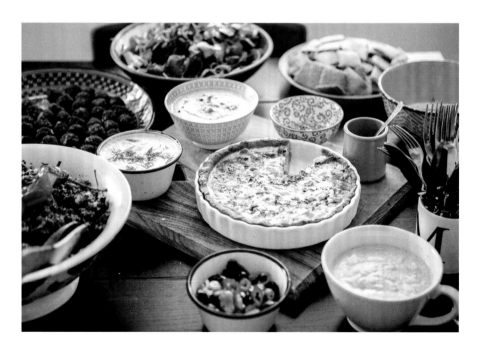

## Our food

Our society is just beginning to acknowledge the ill effects of high-sugar, high-gluten, overly processed, and chemical-laden foods in our diet. These foods have become so much a part of mainstream eating that we can be forgiven for being completely confused about what the ideal diet is.

Much of the food on offer to us is nutritionally substandard. It will keep you alive, but not necessarily in the best of health if eaten as the bulk of your diet. Natural foods are often overshadowed by commercially produced, heavily advertised "health foods," which are usually designed in a lab and are full of ingredients and chemicals that we, let alone our bodies, struggle to recognize.

The HEMSLEY+HEMSLEY way is to keep it simple and as close to nature as possible. In essence, this means we eat meat and vegetables, taking the best ingredients and foods from the plant and animal kingdoms as humans have always done. Simple food.

H+H food is free from gluten, grains, and refined sugars, and focuses on nutrient-dense, unprocessed foods, good fats, and bone broth.

We encourage you to eat organic vegetables, sustainable and ethically caught wild fish, and grass-fed naturally reared, free-range meat. We enjoy high-quality dairy and a whole range of natural fats, including butter, unrefined oils, and animal fat. This produce is better for nutrition, the environment, local economy, and, in our opinion, it really does taste better.

We avoid processed foods, refined carbohydrates and sugar, and chemical sweeteners. Instead, we stick to pseudocereals, such as quinoa and amaranth, seasonal fruit, and naturally sweet ingredients such as raw honey and maple syrup that have nutritional value.

We urge you to steer clear of food products that shout "low fat" and "no fat" as well as those promoted as "low calorie." Stay away from margarine, vegetable spreads, "sugar-free" cakes and cereal bars, along with products that claim to speed up your metabolism or contain ingredients you don't recognize. Think of these as fake foods that cause stress to the body.

Humans evolved to eat natural foods, foods that were foraged, hunted, or grown. Many of us have lost this connection to the food we eat. We believe it's important to re-establish that link.

We don't believe in dieting or that good health is as simple as "calories in, calories out"; this is not a natural way of evaluating what to eat. The answer is not to limit calories but to eat more high-quality foods and listen to our bodies. Mindful Eating.

You'll find that once your taste buds have been weaned off sugary, refined, and chemically enhanced food products, you will quickly develop a taste for fresh, unprocessed whole foods. By preparing your own meals you can be more in control of what is going into your body and feel better for it.

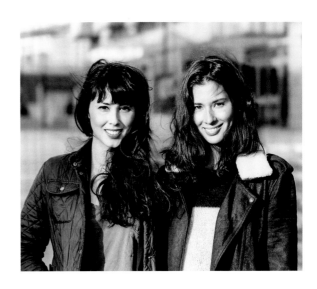

## Who we are

HEMSLEY + HEMSLEY, launched in 2010, is our family-run, bespoke food service looking after individuals and their families all over the world, including high-profile people within the music, media, fashion, beauty, health, and wellness industries.

Alongside the food delivery service, we consult for private clients, restaurants, and hotels as well as catering dinner parties and events. In 2012 we joined Vogue.co.uk as food bloggers, which allowed us to share our nourishing recipes with a wider audience.

We have been developing the H+H way of eating for almost ten years and, while it is now our business to help others overhaul their eating, it all began as a very personal journey.

Jasmine worked as a model for over 15 years, a profession that made her very aware of her food choices and health. Melissa travelled the world as a fashion brand manager and then worked in marketing for gastropubs and bars. Long hours, late nights, and trying to eat on the go were challenges for both of us.

We have always loved cooking and recognized the relationship between food and health. On the surface we thought ourselves "normal and healthy" young women. However, when we began tuning into

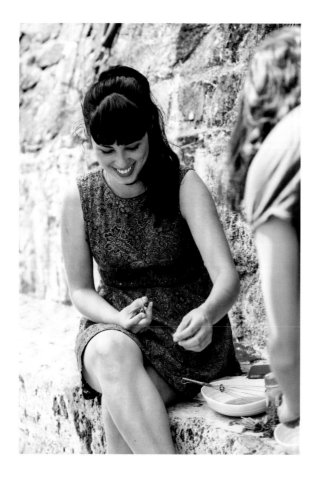

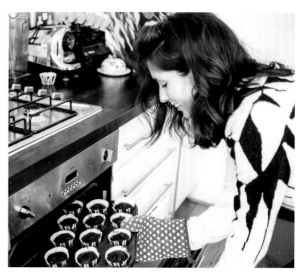

our bodies we realized that we weren't functioning at our best. We were suffering from those everyday niggles and ailments like indigestion, acid reflux, IBS, eczema, stress, and exhaustion from work. We realized that we weren't alone and that others around us were experiencing and accepting the same health problems as normal. Why were we putting up with feeling less than our best?

We researched, read, and navigated our way through the bewildering variety of food, diet options, and philosophies on offer. Through countless hours of personal study, attending talks, conferences, and lectures, and working with clients and experts in the wellness fields, we developed an approach to eating that made sense to us and made us feel great.

Friends and family noticed the dramatic change in us, loved the food we were putting on the table, and wanted to be in on the secret. At their request, we started teaching them, then their friends, and then friends of friends, how to cook a handful of our favorite everyday meals, and so, our family business HEMSLEY + HEMSLEY was born.

The third member of our team is Nick, juice master and maker of amazing stews. With 20 years working around the world as a model, actor, and photographer, he was all too familiar with eating fads in all their strangest forms: models surviving on toasted seaweed and chili flakes, red wine and jelly babies, or black coffee and egg-white omelettes washed down with protein shakes. With all these diets several things were clear: they were unsustainable, unsatisfactory, emotionally draining, and flavor was the least important factor. Nick pointed out to us that men can be as emotionally attached to food as women, particularly in a world that strives for body perfection.

Adopting the H+H way of eating, Nick was amazed by how his energy increased along with his resistance to common colds. Suddenly, daily visits to the gym were no longer a necessity. He became inspired to explore more natural, minimalistic, and traditional training methods, such as barefoot running, yoga, and body weight training, amazed at how quickly he could recover with a good mug of bone broth – no need for expensive shakes or supplements.

As self-taught cooks in an increasingly health-conscious world that is seeing a rise in allergies and autoimmune diseases, the H+H way of eating seems to resonate with many people. This cookbook is our chance to share our ethos and recipes with you. These are our easy-to-make, feel-good meals that our clients, friends, and family have adopted and loved without even realizing they were embarking on a nutritional change for the better. Our aim is simple: to get nourishing, tasty food on the table every day.

**How to use this book**

Use this book simply as a collection of delicious recipes that you know are also good for you. Jump in and start cooking the recipes right away, dipping in and out to incorporate them into your weekly routine. Or make an immediate change and read 10 Things to Do Today (below) and take control of your well-being by getting to grips with our food philosophy, understanding what's really good for you and what you should avoid. We have put together a summary of our practices on page 17 with our Twelve Golden Rules, while Our Food Philosophy (opposite) offers an in-depth guide to really understand our way of eating and how it can benefit you.

Throughout this book there are tips and tricks for ways to make better choices painlessly, in a manner that will empower you to take control of your food and enjoy it – rather than food controlling you. Turn to page 18 to find out how to overhaul and upgrade the contents of your fridge, freezer, and cupboards so you can always whip up something nutritious.

Turn to page 308 to see how a Sunday Cook Off gets you organized for the week ahead. And on page 310 you will find menus for a whole host of occasions, from work lunches to dinner parties and celebrations.

# 10 THINGS TO DO TODAY

Start with these simple changes and you'll feel better immediately.

**1** Begin your day by drinking a glass of warm water with half a lemon squeezed in, then rinse your mouth out.

**2** Before a shower, dry body brush for a minute every morning, using a soft natural bristle brush to boost and aid your circulation and the removal of toxins.

**3** Make a green smoothie (see page 284). Drink some for breakfast and save a glass for your mid-morning break.

**4** Cut down on caffeine – have one less coffee or caffeine-rich drink and replace with something refreshing and zingy (see pages 278–279).

**5** Make a shopping list and clear out your cupboards. Remove vegetable cooking oils from your kitchen and cook in butter or steam until you can introduce more of the right unprocessed fats.

**6** Take an extra 10 minutes over lunch, focus on your food not your phone/email, and chew thoroughly.

**7** Get a water filter and drink 2 quarts (half a gallon) of water throughout the day. Build up slowly and flavor it if you prefer.

**8** Move your body and sweat for 20 minutes today. Get outside and take in the sunlight and fresh air.

**9** If you feel like a snack try some nut butter on apple slices. If you get a food craving check first that you are hydrated. Drink something tangy or with bitter flavors such as ginger, lemon, or lime to bypass it. Don't go for something salty or you might have to eat something sweet afterwards and vice versa.

**10** Go to bed an hour earlier and give your eyes a rest from TV, phones, and computers as you unwind.

# OUR FOOD PHILOSOPHY

**The "better than" rule**

We are big believers in the "better than rule." This means, if you can't find what you're looking for, then choose the next best option. You can apply this to ingredients as well as choices on a restaurant menu (for more on eating out, turn to page 312). Eating real, whole food, organic or not, is always better than eating chemically processed, refined foods.

For convenience, and because no one has time to cook everything from scratch, we use some ready-made ingredients, such as coconut flour and soba noodles. Our way of eating is not restrictive and there is an increasingly large range of nutrient-dense products, which we use and discuss throughout the book, that are readily available to help make healthy eating easy to maintain; this is a long-term lifestyle choice that is wholly sustainable and enjoyable.

Nothing changes overnight, no day is the same and we cannot always be perfect in our busy lives. No one is judging you, so be kind to yourself. Make changes where you can, adopt some positive new habits and enjoy the benefits and the feeling of a better version of you.

**Eat the best food you can find**

Where your food comes from is important. Food that is not labelled organic can often be laden with toxins, pesticides, fungicides, and can be genetically modified (GM) – you do not want to be eating any of these. Similarly, foods labelled "pure," "natural," "healthy," and "whole" might not have had anything added but can still have had plenty taken away. "Fortified" means that synthetic vitamins and minerals have been added, which are not necessarily bioavailable (can be absorbed by your body) – you need to check the small print to really understand what you're putting into your body.

We always aim for home-grown, local, and naturally farmed food, including organic and biodynamic-certified produce, to ensure our food is as free as possible from chemicals and GM ingredients, especially for meat, fish and dairy. The labels "organic" and "biodynamic-certified" ensure you are buying naturally grown or reared produce so look out for these labels. It's also a good idea to support local producers who grow their produce free from pesticides, as nature intended, but don't necessarily have an organic certification. You can often get a much better price if you buy directly from the producer.

Remember that natural farming is better for the environment, as well as being better for your body. Don't see organic and naturally farmed food as elitist or specialist – before mass-production this is how all food was traditionally grown. Ask questions and use your spending power where it counts to increase the demand for naturally grown real food. In doing so you can spark change for the better for everyone. Remember it's not extreme or weird to want to eat food free from chemicals and genetic modification – it's natural!

### Rethink the way you shop

With a little research and planning you can buy the best-quality produce without breaking the bank. Buying in bulk and making your own food from scratch will free up cash to spend on the more expensive ingredients (share a food shop with a friend or two if you're struggling for space to store lots of produce). Choose cheaper cuts of meat, build up a store cupboard of good-quality ingredients over time, eat seasonally, cook double quantities and freeze half, and plan your meals for the week. You will reduce waste and make your money stretch further while improving your health. If you feel you're struggling to buy the best-quality produce, don't give up. Buy the best you can afford at that time.

### Healthy gut, happy you

The key to our philosophy is gut health and good digestion – it's not just what you eat, it's what you digest that counts. Without a healthy gut lining, your body will not be able to efficiently digest and absorb vital minerals and nutrients. So even if you are eating nourishing foods, you may not be getting all their benefits. Stomach soothing bone broths form the foundation of many of our meals along with plenty of probiotic foods.

**BONE BROTH** To help heal a damaged gut lining, you need large amounts of easily digestible substances like amino acids, gelatin, glucosamine, fats, vitamins, and minerals, all found in good-quality bone broth.

Simple to make, soothing and nourishing, bone broth is one of the oldest, most affordable homemade foods, often used as an elixir to cure ailments and nurture the sick. To get the full nutritional benefits the broth should be homemade from the bones of the healthiest animals not from stock cubes, which can include a concoction of hydrolysed protein and emulsifiers. Even the "cleanest" ready-made shop-bought stock or bouillon will not have the same benefits as homemade bone broth.

A good broth is rich in gelatin (a source of protein that helps counter the degeneration of joints) and collagen (which improves the condition of skin). Bone

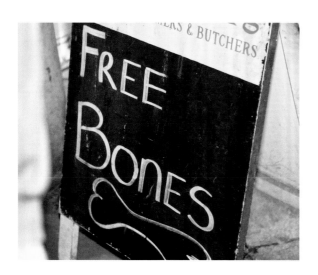

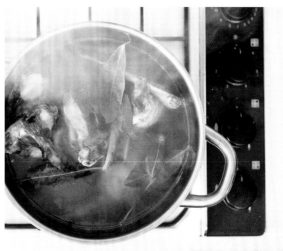

broths made with fish bones and heads provide iodine and can help strengthen the thyroid (for how to make bone broth turn to page 300).

**FERMENTED (CULTURED) AND PROBIOTIC FOODS** You may already be familiar with probiotics – also known as friendly bacteria or gut flora. They are essential to good health, enhancing immune function and improving digestion (the very name "probiotic" means "for life"). Without well-functioning gut flora, the gut becomes unprotected and malnourished. By making your own cultured foods such as sauerkraut and kimchi (pages 306 and 307), you can provide the body with a concentrated form of natural probiotics, and avoid sugary, low-quality dairy and soy-based probiotic yogurts and drinks.

These days the commercial preparation of soy has made it more of a junk food than a health food, so we advise that you avoid soy yogurts, milks, ice creams etc, which lack the health benefits that soy originally became known for. Instead, enjoy organic, traditionally fermented soy products, such as tamari and proper miso (for more info on these ingredients, see pages 18–24). Look for an unpasteurized, organic (non-GM), fermented miso and add at the end of cooking to flavor and to ensure the live bacteria is preserved.

## Meat and fish

Meat, fish, and seafood are very rich in protein, the building blocks of our body, and contain the essential vitamin B12, which is not available to our bodies in most plant foods. We choose pasture-raised, hormone- and antibiotic-free animals that have been raised on a diet that is natural to them, i.e. not grain-fed cows or corn-fed, captive chickens. When it comes to fish and seafood, we choose sustainable varieties of wild and ethically caught stock, well-regulated or organically farmed (for more on fish and seafood, turn to page 132).

Naturally raised meat naturally costs more, but we champion the less popular cuts, which make it more affordable. We love eating chicken livers, fish roe, bone broth, and bone marrow, and cooking with real fat, not only because they are all delicious and nutritious but also because these ingredients allow us to eat better quality food for less money. It is also a mindful way to eat that reduces waste and celebrates the whole animal.

We tend to eat less pork compared to other meats as it can be trickier to track down naturally reared pork products and it tends to be one of the most processed meats. Always choose unprocessed pork, free from nitrites and chemical preservatives, and make sure it is cooked through.

Although we regularly eat meat and fish, we don't have huge servings and not at every meal. Beef, lamb, and pork take the longest to digest so we tend to eat them for breakfast and lunch or stick to an early supper. The last thing you want to do is to take that steak to bed with you!

## Fats

There is a myth that fat (especially saturated fat) is bad. In reality, fat, derived from both the animal and plant kingdoms, is essential to human well-being. This nutrient-dense, nourishing food is an excellent source of energy that makes your meals satisfying and tasty.

The body needs both saturated and unsaturated fats in their most natural forms for the absorption of vitamins A, D, E, and K, slowing down the release of sugar and optimal digestion. Cholesterol is also essential to your well-being – it is vital for the communication of the nervous system and makes up all cell membranes and sex hormones. Cholesterol levels are tightly regulated by the liver, which produces the correct amount of blood cholesterol, regardless of the cholesterol content in your diet. High-quality, pasture-raised, animal-based foods not only provide an excellent source of protein, but also the fats needed for optimal brain and body health.

We keep two types of fat in the kitchen: saturated (mostly found in animal foods) and unsaturated (which includes monounsaturated fat and polyunsaturated fat mostly found in plant foods). These two kinds of fat are great not only because of their varied nutritional profiles but also because they are suitable for different types of food preparation. We use real saturated fats, such as clarified butter (ghee) and coconut oil, because they are heat stable meaning that their chemical structure is not readily altered or oxidised when used for cooking. We reserve the goodness of unrefined, unsaturated plant oils, such as extra-virgin olive oil, for drizzling over salads and vegetables and for making raw dips and dressings.

It's important that the fats you consume should be organic because toxins, pesticides, and medications are stored in the fat cells of non-organically farmed produce and will be transferred to your body as you eat them.

Please avoid trans fats and heat-treated or refined polyunsaturated fats and oils (page 12). See page 18 for more on fats and how to use them.

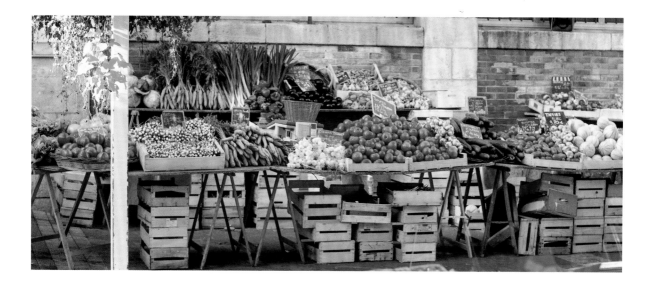

## Bad fats

Trans fats are largely artificial fats that occur when unsaturated fats are heated and chemically altered to turn them into solids in a process called hydrogenation. This process gives these fats a longer shelf life and makes foods less likely to spoil – perfect for creating long-lasting, cheap food, but very bad for us. Trans fats have been linked to cancer, heart disease, autoimmunity, and infertility.

Most margarines, butter replacements, vegetable oils, shortenings, and other fat replacements contain trans fats in some form or another and they are a staple ingredient of commercially sold pies, cakes, cookies, and general packaged foods. Steer clear and enjoy real butter instead.

Other fats to avoid are cooking oils, such as sunflower and canola oil. These usually undergo extreme pressure or heat during manufacturing, causing oxidation. By the time you've kept these oils standing in plastic bottles in a hot cupboard above the stove and then used them for frying, you may be exposing your body to a large amount of free radicals (produced by oxidation). Over time, these free radicals can cause inflammation, affecting your organs, blood vessels, and more. Stick to unrefined, cold-pressed oils on your salads and high-quality saturated fats for cooking.

## Vegetables

Vegetables are the recurring theme in our food. They take up around 60 percent, or two-thirds, of our plates at every meal and find their way into our breakfasts, cakes, crackers, and ice creams too. As you eat more of them, it's amazing how your body starts to crave the goodness from these nutrient-dense foods. Forget the target of "five a day." With these recipes, you will be eating up to ten portions a day with ease. To keep vegetables as the main event at every meal, we need to keep them interesting and varied. Eat a rainbow of vegetables and eat with the seasons to keep your taste buds excited. For added flavor and nutrition, we often cook our vegetables in bone broth (see page 300).

Vegetables are also extremely alkalizing on the body. Our body constantly maintains the blood's optimum alkaline pH level, but a diet consisting of mostly acidifying foods (lots of refined sugars, grains, processed foods, and meat, i.e. the typical western diet) makes it work much harder to maintain that natural balance. We look to remove stress on the body at every opportunity so that it can function at its best – so a diet rich in alkalizing veg is key to good health.

We aim to eat vegetables seasonally, when they are naturally at their best, are most abundant and, therefore, most affordable. Vegetables lose nutrients after being picked and the longer they've been in transit, the more nutrition is lost. Box schemes of organic seasonal fruit and vegetables delivered straight to your door are so convenient, especially when seasonal organic produce can be hard to get hold of locally.

If you cannot buy all your fruit and veg organic, then prioritize varieties where you can eat the skin (thin-skinned) e.g. apples, cucumbers, tomatoes, berries, broccoli and red peppers, as the surface is where the most pesticide residue will be found. Then if you do need to opt for conventionally grown, non-organic produce, go for thick-skinned fruits and vegetables, such as onions, garlic, bananas, and avocados, as you peel them before eating.

## Washing produce

Organic or not, always wash produce well because of handling, transporting, and possible contamination. A lot of goodness is contained in the skin so for organic root veg just scrub the earth off but don't peel. Remove tough outer leaves of anything leafy like lettuce and cabbage before you wash them.

In non-organic root vegetables, such as beets and carrots, pesticides are concentrated around the top, so chopping the top 1/2 in off helps. Even if you peel or chop off the top, the produce will still contain pesticide residue absorbed whilst growing.

You can use a homemade wash to help clean the veg and reduce the pesticide residue on the skin (turn to page 308 for our homemade wash recipes).

## Dairy

Eat full-fat dairy from organic pasture-reared animals. We source raw milk from organic grass-fed cattle – unhomogenized, preferably unpasteurized and always full-fat (as it naturally comes). As this high-quality dairy milk is hard to come by we don't drink it often, although, we do enjoy easier-to-find, good-quality cheese, butter, and yogurt (all naturally lower in lactose than milk). As a general guideline the higher the fat content, the lower the lactose content. Always choose plain (sugar-free), organic, full-fat, and probiotic (''live'') yogurt. Raw goats' and sheep's milks and milk products are also worth considering and are easier to digest thanks to their smaller fat molecules.

As well as good-quality dairy there are some deliciously creamy non-dairy options to try too, which is good news for anyone who can't eat dairy. More often than not we use dairy alternatives, such as coconut milk and coconut cream (rich in healthy fats) and even use them to make our own probiotic yogurt (page 305). Instead of cream cheese, we use avocado to make our cheesecakes and have created Mango Cashew Cream (page 49) as a tasty substitute for dairy-based yogurt, custard, and cream. Nut milks, or ''mylks'' as they are also known, offer a subtle, light, and creamy flavor. Be aware that shop-bought varieties of nut milk can come with a whole host of other added ingredients so try our quick tips on making your own (page 304).

## Sugar

Refined sugar can promote inflammation in the body. It is also the main culprit for feeding unfriendly yeast and bacteria in the gut. Sugar is easily absorbed into your system quickly releasing energy and raising the blood sugar level. The body responds by secreting a large amount of insulin from the pancreas and also producing cortisol from the adrenal glands (the classic ''fight or flight'' response). Think sugar rush followed by sugar lows.

Over time, repeated spikes and troughs in sugar levels can cause the individual to become insulin resistant, which causes an array of problems including suppression of the immune system, accelerated aging, and the increased risk of type 2 diabetes, heart disease, and cancer.

Always read food and drink labels before you buy because sugar is used in all types of foods (even savory) to make them taste better. Avoid all the many names for refined sugars and sweeteners, such as brown rice syrup, barley malt, fructose, sucrose, high-fructose corn syrup, cane juice, dextrose, mannitol, lactose, maltodextrin, sorbitol, fruit juice concentrate, the list goes on. Watch out for large amounts of natural sweeteners like dried fruits, honey, and maple syrup as too many of these can disrupt the body's balance.

Sugar is addictive because the body is hard-wired to want sweet things, which provide instant, easily accessible energy. Reduce the sugar in your diet and you'll find your sweet cravings diminish so that only small amounts of the natural sweetness of fruit and raw honey is required to satisfy you.

## Grains and potatoes

Grains, the seeds of grasses, have become a staple food source around the world, and in one form or another have found their way into the meals and snacks we consume on a daily basis (think pasta, bread, cookies, cereal, crackers, snack bars, pastries, sweets, and even drinks).

The majority of grains today are heavily hybridised and even genetically modified, and these commercial crops are heavily sprayed with chemicals – this is not what our ancestors would have consumed.

Contrary to popular belief we do not need to eat grains to survive and they offer little goodness compared to the many more nutrient-rich options out there. As you digest grains, they can cause unhealthy, quick releases of sugar and spikes in insulin levels, and some release a feel-good feeling which makes you want to eat more. These cheap calories fill you up and keep you going but by cutting them out you leave a lot more room in your diet to add more nutrient-dense foods such as meat and vegetables. Properly prepared grains are good for some individuals but for the majority avoiding them shows improvement in health.

We substitute grains with vegetables and pseudocereals (buckwheat, amaranth, quinoa), which are small, protein-filled seeds that resemble grains in looks and taste, hence the name. Importantly, pseudocereals are completely free of gluten and are rich in amino acids not found in regular grains. They are also less likely to have been heavily hybridised or subjected to industrial farming methods.

You might notice that none of our recipes call for white potatoes. We prefer not to rely on them as a staple and substitute them with other more nutrient-rich, lower-starch vegetables that do not convert so quickly into glucose when digested.

Don't worry, when we remove foods like potatoes and grains you're not missing out on carbohydrates. Other vegetables, fruits, pseudocereals, and legumes have carbohydrates too and they are the better vitamin and mineral-rich options.

## Simple food combining

There are three primary categories of food: protein, carbohydrates, and fats. Carbohydrates are divided into two categories: fruits and starches. Starches and proteins digest at different rates, so simple food combining in our day-to-day meals means we try to avoid keeping food in the stomach longer than it needs to be, which is helpful for those who suffer from poor digestion. This practice is just a general rule but we like it because it also means that we leave plenty of room on our plates for more of the mostly green, alkalizing vegetables that help our bodies to stay healthy.

Think of a plate in three parts. One part should be taken up with a protein or high-starch food, the other two parts should contain low-starch veg. This means you avoid eating protein and high-starch foods at the same time. For breakfast and lunch we enjoy one or sometimes two portions of raw low-starch veg, but for supper we prefer cooked low-starch veg for easier digestion. To help explain what we mean, we've created an illustration of simple food combining on an ideal H+H plate (opposite).

**HIGH-STARCH FOODS ARE:** tubers/root veg and fresh beans, such as beet, broad beans, Jerusalem artichokes, parsnip, peas, pumpkin, squash, and sweet potatoes; pseudocereals, such as amaranth, buckwheat and quinoa; and legumes, such as beans and lentils.

**PROTEIN FOODS ARE:** animal products, such as beef, lamb, chicken, fish, pork, and eggs.

**LOW-STARCH VEG, WHICH CAN BE EATEN WITH HIGH-STARCH OR PROTEIN FOODS, INCLUDE:** artichokes, asparagus, eggplant, broccoli, Brussels sprouts, cabbage family (including kale, dinosaur kale, and chard), carrots, cauliflower, celery root, celery, zucchini, cucumber, garlic, green beans, beet greens, fennel, kohlrabi, leeks, mushrooms, onions, bok choy, radish, red and yellow peppers, salad leaves such as endive, arugula, lettuce, and watercress, seaweeds, spinach, rutabaga, and turnips. We also include the "savory fruits" here: avocado, tomato, and cucumber.

Herbs, spices, nuts, seeds, fats, oils, dairy, our Fermented Four probiotic foods (page 305), and bone broth can be eaten with everything. Some might find it best to avoid fruit as part of a main meal, instead enjoying it as a snack between meals.

## Soaking and activating

All grains, pseudocereals, nuts, seeds, and legumes have a natural, protective layer called phytic acid (phytate) – an anti-nutrient that irritates the gut lining and prevents the absorption of certain minerals into the body. Although a small amount of phytic acid can be beneficial, we try to remove as much as is practically possible. In ancient times, these foods were usually sprouted and fermented, as well as cooked, all of which reduce the phytic acid content and increase the digestibility and nutrients available.

We recommend "activating" pseudocereals and legumes by soaking them to start germination and to reduce phytic acid before cooking. By doing this their nutrients are more available and easier to digest.

We also soak nuts and seeds to activate them. We then rinse, drain, and add the wet and softened nuts or seeds to smoothies and other recipes. To enjoy activated nuts and seeds dry, crunchy, or to make them into flour, we then dehydrate them. These dried activated nuts and seeds are known as "crispy."

Be mindful not to overdo nuts and seeds; they are nutritious but are best eaten in small amounts. If you eat them regularly or rely on them as a source of protein, then it is even more important that you prepare them properly by activating them. Also, to make the most of them, especially small seeds, you must chew them well. For more info on soaking and activating turn to page 300.

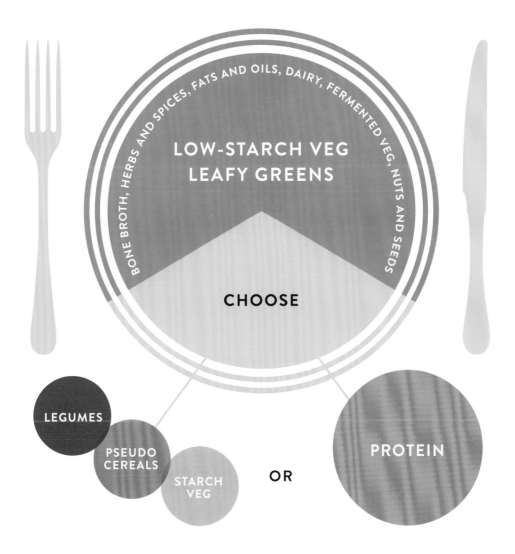

LOW-STARCH VEG
LEAFY GREENS

BONE BROTH, HERBS AND SPICES, FATS AND OILS, DAIRY, FERMENTED VEG, NUTS AND SEEDS

CHOOSE

LEGUMES

PSEUDO CEREALS

STARCH VEG

OR

PROTEIN

## Eat slowly, chew well

Not only what you eat but also the way you eat is crucial to your health. Remember, there are no teeth in your tummy so it's important to break down all foods by chewing to access their nutrition – we like the old adage of "drink your food and chew your drink."

The stomach is smaller than you might imagine – think of it as the size of two fists put together, which will give you a good indication of how much to put in it. It needs 20 percent space for digestive juices to work effectively so don't overload your plate. It takes 20 minutes for your stomach to tell your brain that it's satisfied so, if you've eaten your lunch and you're still not feeling full, wait 20 minutes then see if you're still hungry.

Aim to eat as early as you can in the evening (around 7 p.m. is ideal) in order to leave plenty of time for digestion before you sleep. If you have to eat late,

then eat a small portion and avoid beef, lamb, or pork as they take longer to digest. A soup is a good, healthy, late-night choice.

## Cooked versus raw

The benefit of cooked food is that it's partly broken down so you can access the nutrients in the food more easily, rather than having to expend more of your body's energy. Cooking carrots breaks down some of the cellulose making it easier to absorb beta-carotene, which we convert to vitamin A, while cooking tomatoes increases the lycopene content that can be absorbed by the body. For people with digestive issues, cooked food is very important (lightly or well cooked) and, if you have a thyroid disorder, then you should certainly avoid eating raw cruciferous vegetables (also known as brassicas) such as cabbage, broccoli, kale, and cauliflower) or other goitrogenic foods, such as spinach, which can have a negative impact on your condition.

Raw foods are the ultimate unprocessed foods and are packed with an abundance of goodness but only if you can properly digest them. For this reason, it's even more important to take time to chew raw foods really well before swallowing. Juices and smoothies are an excellent way to access the nutrients of raw vegetables as the grinding process helps to break down the tough cellulose walls in a similar fashion to cooking, as does fermenting raw vegetables to make sauerkraut and kimchi. Because raw foods take more effort to digest, you might find that eating raw food before 4 p.m. suits you best and that your body naturally wants more cooked food in the winter.

## Hydration

The human body is about 60 percent water, so it's important to stay properly hydrated for optimum health. It also makes sense to ensure that you're drinking, cooking, and even washing food with the purest water possible, which is why we recommend using a water filter when you can.

After sleep, your body is dehydrated and after a night of cleansing and repair it's ready to flush out toxins. Vitamin-rich lemon juice and warm water is an ideal first drink to help hydrate the body and expel these toxins (even though lemon tastes acidic it has an alkalising effect on your body).

We stick to minimal amounts of caffeine, choosing antioxidant-rich green tea and raw cacao instead of coffee and other caffeinated drinks. With the stresses of modern life, coffee is not your friend! Along with its high caffeine content, it is highly acidic and it can over-stimulate the digestive tract, aggravating health problems for people with gastrointestinal conditions like acid reflux, ulcers, and IBS. Although it may give a short energy boost, it will be followed by a low, creating a roller-coaster that places stress on your body. Slowly wean yourself off coffee, with as little or no withdrawal symptoms as possible, by mixing ground endive into your morning brew, and slowly increasing the ratio of endive to coffee. Or start by replacing one coffee at a time with herbal tea.

## Sleep

During sleep hours your body detoxifies, repairs, and rejuvenates, utilising the good things you did for it during the day and getting rid of all the bad things you shouldn't have done to it!

After waking, encourage detoxification by gently scraping your tongue of toxins and body brushing to stimulate the lymphatic system. We're fans of a gentle bedtime routine to wind down: eat supper at least three hours before you sleep, having a small snack like a mug of broth, if you need to (you will not have good-quality sleep if you are still digesting); stay away from laptops, phones, and screens or anything stimulating in the hours leading up to bed; keep hydrated during the day and during the evening, then switch to chamomile or valerian tea for a sleep aid; spray a homemade mix of lavender oil and water in your room for a relaxing environment. It's obvious, but sugar, caffeine, and alcohol and eating too late are not going to help you in your quest for a good night's sleep.

We know it's not always easy, but the earlier you go to bed the better. In an ideal world we would be in bed by 10 p.m. and wake up with the sun rise.

## Toxins

It's impossible to avoid environmental toxins, so it's even more important to live as naturally as we can in our homes. Use glass, high-grade stainless steel, stone, wood, and cast iron for storage, prep, and cooking. Look out for PTFE-free pans, avoid BPA in plastic, and never touch a microwave.

We use natural organic products like citric acid and vinegar to clean our homes. We use filtered water for drinking, cooking, soaking, and sprouting and recommend buying a water filter that removes impurities whilst restructuring and remineralising the water, as well as fitting a chlorine filter to your shower. See our Kitchen Essentials list (page 24) for more tips and ideas.

## Stress

Stress is meant to be fleeting: a surge of adrenaline, elevated heart rate, and a quickening of the senses, all designed to escape a tricky situation. It is not supposed to be the perpetual state of being that a lot of people find themselves in, living with all the pressures of modern life.

By eating regularly and healthily, and by minimizing your sugar intake, cortisol, the stress hormone involved in blood sugar regulation, is kept in check; your blood sugar levels will remain more constant and you'll avoid the roller-coaster of sugar highs and lows, mood swings, and further sugar cravings.

Rather than reaching for food when you're upset or angry, try to look for alternative ways to manage your stress levels. We find twice daily short meditations to

# TWELVE GOLDEN RULES

These "rules" are guidelines to help you change the way you eat and think about food. They provide a helpful guide as you start this new way of eating and will soon become second nature. Rules get broken so don't beat yourself up – just remember the "better than" approach means choosing the healthier alternatives and not forgetting that it is better to follow the guidelines some of the time, than not at all.

**1** Eat natural animal foods and buy the best-quality food you can find and afford (page 9). e.g seasoning your food with sea salt or Himalayan rock salt rather than table salt.

**2** Shop wisely to get more for your money. Buy local, seasonal produce and try cheaper cuts of meat and unfamiliar sustainable varieties of fish to get maximum nourishment as well as good value.

**3** Base your meals around meat and veg and eat the whole food where appropriate, e.g. the skin on the apple, the fat on the beef, the yolk in the egg.

**4** Cook with saturated fats like coconut oil, ghee, or butter and save unsaturated, unrefined plant oils for drizzling on salads. Avoid all processed fats and oils (page 12).

**5** Cook with nourishing homemade bone broth (page 300) and choose a fermented condiment such as ketchup, yogurt, or kimchi (page 306) to eat with your food for a boost of good bacteria.

**6** Avoid refined sugar and instead choose natural sugars, in small quantities, such as pure maple syrup, raw honey, and dates (page 13).

**7** Avoid gluten, wheat, and other grains because our bodies can struggle to digest them. There are many more nutrient-rich alternatives to enjoy instead (page 13).

**8** Avoid processes that harm foods, such as hydrogenation and chemical extraction. Follow processes that enhance food. Soak nuts, seeds, legumes, and pseudocereals to release nutrients and make them easier to digest (page 14).

**9** Give digestion a helping hand by practicing simple food combining (page 14). Avoid eating raw food after 4 p.m., or at all if you have poor digestion, and don't eat too much before bed.

**10** Stick to small amounts of caffeine, avoid coffee and instead choose antioxidant-rich green tea, other herbal teas, and cacao.

**11** Eat slowly, taking the time to chew and savor your food.

**12** Always enjoy what you choose to eat. Find out what works for you and don't strive to be perfect every time. Remember the most important rule of all: the "better than" rule (page 9)!

manage our stress levels work for us. Meditation can simply mean sitting somewhere quietly for 10 minutes, eyes closed, or practicing a relaxing breathing technique.

### Cooking with children

We've cooked for many of our clients' families and we don't cook special food for their children – they eat the same food ("kids food" is a very modern idea). Include children in the preparation of meals at an early age and give them simple jobs in the kitchen to get them interested in their food. You'll be surprised at what they'll put into their mouths when they feel proud of themselves for making it.

We have some great recipes that children love to help make and eat, and if you're cooking for children other than your own, just don't tell them that their rice is cauliflower, their spaghetti is zucchini or that there are black beans in their brownies! And we haven't yet found a child or grown up who wouldn't be happy with our Vanilla Maltshake on page 291.

# STOCKING YOUR KITCHEN

There is something very satisfying about decluttering your kitchen cupboards, fridge, and freezer.

We certainly don't advocate waste and throwing away good food, but just consider each product as you go through your kitchen and ask yourself, does this nourish me, is it good for me? If not, either use it up or throw it out and move forward with something that definitely will.

Here's what we keep in our kitchens – you don't need to buy them all at once, but can build up your supplies over time. And for eggs, fats, and oils in particular, try to buy organic.

**EGGS** One of the most well-rounded and nutritious foods, we love eggs. They contain protein, omega-3 fats, are high in vitamins, and have a huge dose of zinc, magnesium, calcium and dietary cholesterol. When baking, remember to use room temperature eggs. Eggs are medium in all our recipes unless stated otherwise.

## Oils and fats for cooking

We don't deep-fat fry or cook at super high temperatures, but for roasting and pan-frying, saturated fats (ghee, coconut oil, and meat dripping and duck fat) are the best fats to use. (We also enjoy quality saturated fats raw, such as coconut oil in our smoothies and butter on our banana bread.)

**BUTTER** Butter, due to milk fats, is better suited to gentle frying and for making sauces or scrambled eggs. Make sure that you buy real 100 percent butter, not a butter and plant oil spread.

**COCONUT OIL** Always go for virgin oil, which means it hasn't been overly refined or bleached. It has incredible immune-boosting properties and is antibacterial, antifungal, and antiviral. It can also help to control blood sugar levels and helps improve the body's ability to absorb minerals. Coconut oil isn't overpowering when used as a cooking oil and we love it in smoothies, while a tablespoon of it makes a quick energy and health-boosting snack.

**DRIPPING AND DUCK FAT** A great fat for cooking and, if you save it from your roasts, it's free! People have been chucking this stuff away for years thanks to "fat scare," but this traditional cooking fat is making its way back on to menus. Pour it off your roasts and into a glass container – if it's well strained it will last for 6 months in your fridge. You'll also find plenty to spare when making beef broths. Collect some up when you chill the broth.

**GHEE (CLARIFIED BUTTER)** Look for quality ghee from pasture-raised cows. This is a more neutral flavored fat and we like to use it to cook European-style dishes instead of olive oil. The rich fat from grass-fed butter, ghee is packed with antioxidants to help boost the immune system.

## Oils for drizzling

Unsaturated fats, which are liquid at room temperature, play a vital role in health and wellness but they are sensitive to heat, light, and air and easily go rancid. We use the following oils for drizzling over veg and salads because they can be bought cold pressed, keeping them in their most natural and unrefined form. Be sure to store them somewhere cool. Use them cold over, and in, food in order to preserve their nutritional profile and to avoid them becoming toxic.

**EXTRA VIRGIN OLIVE OIL (EVOO)** You will only benefit from olive oil's excellent goodness if you buy the good stuff and don't overheat it (it is monounsaturated and so can be warmed gently without compromising it). Be careful not to over whisk or over blend it as it can become bitter once it emulsifies. For Italian-style dishes, we cook with ghee or butter and then pour olive oil over the hot dish or use it to dress side dishes.

**FLAXSEED (LINSEED) OIL** Contains a high Omega-3 to Omega-6 ratio. It's very sensitive to heat so be sure to store it in the fridge for use in dressings and to drizzle over stews and soups. It has a distinct flavor that we love.

**SESAME OIL** Another antioxidant-rich oil, we use it to make mayonnaise and also add essential oils to it to make body oil. A small bottle of toasted sesame oil comes in handy for adding a potent flavor with just a few drops – delicious in dressings or drizzled over soups.

**MACADAMIA NUT OIL** is high in oleic acid and has an even better Omega-3 to Omega-6 ratio than olive oil. Its sweet, buttery, nutty flavor makes it good for mayonnaise and sauces.

## Nuts and seeds

We recommend "activating" most nuts and seeds (see the exceptions opposite) by soaking them (mostly overnight) in salted filtered water before eating. See page 300 for our methods for soaking and activating. Store nuts and seeds in a cool, dark place or in the fridge to preserve their nutrients and to help prevent them going rancid

**NUTS** High in protein, rich in energy from fats, and packed with antioxidants, vitamins, and minerals. Avoid the roasted and salted varieties (which contain refined salts and toxic oils) and always buy raw.

Our favorites include almonds, Brazil nuts, cashew nuts, hazelnuts, peanuts, walnuts, pistachios, and pine nuts. We soak all of them except for Brazil nuts, pine nuts, and pistachios. Brazil nuts are one of the highest natural sources of selenium, which is necessary for a healthy thyroid function (just be sure they were grown in Brazil as Chinese soil is devoid of selenium).

Peanuts, technically a type of bean, boast high levels of folate, which is necessary for cell building and repair. It's important to buy the best-quality peanuts because they are prone to a mould called atofloxin. Be sure not to overdo nuts, especially with peanuts.

**NUT BUTTER** Choose raw "activated" (or raw sprouted) if you can find it, but it is very expensive. Homemade nut butter is affordable and easy to make (see page 303 for our recipe), and you can make it with activated nuts. Otherwise buy an organic brand and see what works best for you either raw, dry roasted, or blanched (known as "white," which removes the skin).

**SEEDS** We like to eat a variety of seeds including hemp, chia, poppy, pumpkin, sunflower,

sesame, and flaxseeds (linseeds). Hemp seeds, or "hearts" when they are shelled, have one of the highest percentages of easily digestible protein of all nuts and seeds. Chia seeds and flaxseeds have mucilaginous properties, which means they thicken up smoothies and make great binders in baking. Chia, in particular, forms a thick gel when combined with liquid so we use it to make puddings and jams.

### Pseudocereals

These gluten-free seeds can be cooked and eaten in a similar way to grains. We recommend activating them first to reduce the phytic acid (see page 300).

**AMARANTH** An excellent source of plant-based protein, this seed is closely related to beet and quinoa as well as Swiss chard and spinach, so it's not surprising that its nutrient profile is similar to dark leafy greens. It has a nutty taste and when cooked in liquid it takes on a wonderfully sticky texture without losing its al dente bite so we love it in puddings and porridges.

**BUCKWHEAT** Ignore the misleading name, buckwheat is not a wheat! This staple food of Russia and Northern China is sold either raw or roasted, the latter often known as "kasha." In general, we use raw buckwheat in its whole "groat" (whole seed) form. It is rich in magnesium as well as flavonoids, which help vitamin C absorption and act as antioxidants. Buckwheat can also be found in flour form, which is used to make pasta and noodles (soba). Make sure to check the label specifies 100 percent buckwheat flour because wheat flour is often included

too. For anyone with digestive problems, we recommend making your own activated buckwheat flour (page 20).

**QUINOA** Highly regarded for its nutrients, quinoa is one of nature's most "complete" plant foods as it contains amino acids, enzymes, vitamins and minerals, fiber, antioxidants, and phytonutrients, all of which remain in high levels even after cooking. It's quite a recent addition to supermarket shelves after the attention it has gotten as an unrefined, high-protein, gluten-free alternative to rice and couscous. Some people can find it bitter, often because it has not been well rinsed of its coating of saponin, a gut irritant. Rinse well before and after activating. The red and black varieties have a slightly nuttier, earthy sweetness to them compared to white, and add a stunning contrast to salads.

### Legumes

Lentils and beans are legumes and a source of complex carbohydrates as well as proteins, vitamins, and minerals.

**BEANS** We like to cook our beans from scratch, which works out cheaper and means we can activate them first by soaking them overnight or longer for better digestion.

We like cannellini, black beans, butter beans, and aduki (also known as adzuki) and our favorite has to be mung beans because they are easy to sprout, delicious in salads and stir fries and are the basis of mung dahl, a regular supper for us.

We use beans in some more unusual ways too, hiding them in our BB Brownies (page 240) and blending them into soups and dips for a lovely creamy texture. If buying tinned beans, check the label because some brands add salt, which may affect the recipe.

**LENTILS** Puy (also known as French lentils) and green and brown lentils are much quicker to cook than beans – again remember to activate overnight. Red split lentils are even quicker to cook, cooking into a creamy comforting consistency in 20 minutes. They don't require soaking, making them perfect for a last-minute, cheap storecupboard supper.

## For baking

Generic gluten-free flours can be "empty" of nutrition and full of stabilizers and other funny ingredients you can't pronounce. We use the following gluten-free alternatives in our baking.

**ARROWROOT** More digestible than cornflour and other glutinous thickeners, we use just a touch of arrowroot in cooking to enhance the texture of the final product, though it can be skipped.

**BAKING SODA** We've developed our recipes around baking soda to avoid the grains sometimes found in baking powder. If you can't eat baking soda, then leave it out. In some recipes extra rise can be achieved by either adding fluffy egg whites or beating the existing one until they peak, then fold into the recipe.

**BUCKWHEAT FLOUR** The shop-bought version is a great standby but we prefer to make activated buckwheat flour by soaking and drying buckwheat groats until "crispy" and then grinding them in a strong blender to make fresh flour.

**CHESTNUT FLOUR** Made from dried, milled chestnuts, this rich, sweet flavored flour is favored by Italians in desserts.

**CHICKPEA (GRAM) FLOUR** Also known as besan flour, this is full of protein and a staple in Indian cuisine. Be sure to cook it well because it's usually made from raw chickpeas. For better digestion, mix chickpea flour batters the night before to help break down the complex starches, or look for chickpea flour made with cooked chickpeas.

**COCONUT FLOUR** Though seemingly expensive, a little goes a very long way as it expands to almost three times its size when mixed with liquid so do not be tempted to replace it as a like-for-like substitute in recipes.

**GROUND ALMONDS** Also known as almond meal. When ground, almonds make a delicious flour alternative, adding moisture to cakes and savory bakes. Ready-to-use ground almonds are usually made from blanched almonds (skin removed), so no need to soak. This highly versatile "flour" is very easy to incorporate into foods, but don't overdo it. It's also possible to buy almond flour, which is a finer version of ground almonds or, if you make nut milk regularly and have a dehydrator, it's easy to make your own (see page 304). Our recipes all use ground almonds because these are easier to find.

**FLAX FLOUR** We grind flax seeds in a strong blender to make flour. Be careful not to overblend otherwise you'll get flax butter! You can also buy ready ground to use in our

recipes. Be sure to seal and store any ground flax in the fridge to preserve their nutrients.

**SUN FLOUR** If you have a strong blender, you can grind sunflower seeds to make a flour (page 302). Use it as a direct swap for ground almonds. Sun flour is great for anyone with a tree-nut allergy or if you rely heavily on nuts in your diet. Use "crispy" activated seeds if possible (page 300).

## Natural sweeteners

We use the following natural sweeteners, packed with vitamins and minerals, and avoid addictive and empty refined sugars or toxic chemical sweeteners. Don't overdo sweet foods though, even if they are made with natural sugars – healthy treats are still treats!

**DATES AND DATE SYRUP** Look for an organic syrup without additives or preservatives.

**DRIED FRUIT** Sulphur dioxide is often used as a preservative to keep dried fruit brightly colored – natural dried apricots, for example, are dark, sticky, and sweet, not orange. We only use dried fruit that's sulphur dioxide free and some of our recipes will not work if you use the preserved types of dried fruit. Beware of freely snacking on dried fruit; it is a concentrated source of sugars. Imagine each piece of dried fruit is a fresh fruit and drink the same amount of water that's missing.

**FRESH FRUIT** Nature's sweets. As well as enjoying fruit in their natural forms, we use them to sweeten and enhance the flavor of other foods. As a readily available fresh food, fruit can be easily overdone especially if you have a sweet tooth that needs taming. If you have poor digestion, eat fruit on an empty stomach and not for dessert or in meals.

**HONEY** Raw honey, which hasn't been heat-treated or "purified," is amazing for so many reasons; it's a powerful antioxidant, antibacterial, antifungal, and full of enzymes. Rich in nutrients, including vitamins, minerals and amino acids, it reduces inflammation, numbs pain, and speeds up healing. Be aware that heating honey destroys the enzymes and ruins its health-giving properties, so save it for salad dressings and raw desserts.

**MAPLE SYRUP** Mineral-rich maple syrup is sweeter than sugar, so a little goes a long way in cooking. It is nutrient-rich and full of minerals. The grades of maple syrup, which have nothing to do with quality or nutrition, simply refer to the color of the syrup and thus its flavor. We use Grade B for its strong taste. Make sure that the syrup you buy is pure and not a blend.

**MOLASSES** Rich in zinc, this is the good stuff that is removed from sugar cane in order to make sugar white. Just like other syrups and sweeteners, be sure to read the label to ensure that you're buying a pure product.

**STEVIA** Made from the leaf of the stevia herb, stevia has a slight licorice taste and is up to 300 times as sweet as sugar but does not cause blood sugar levels to rise. It can be bought as an unprocessed green powder, but the liquid form is easiest to use. Its properties make it exciting for the health food market but we have already seen it mixed with chemically refined ingredients

so be sure to check the label for unwanted nasties. Use sparingly to enhance an existing sweetener in a recipe as too much can make food taste bitter.

## Flavor boosters

These are some of our favorite condiments to have on hand.

### APPLE CIDER VINEGAR (ACV)

Look for raw, unfiltered apple cider vinegar, also known as "with the mother." If the bottle is clear and you can see a cloudy swirl at the bottom that's the "mother," a ball of living enzymes. Most commercial ACVs are pasteurized, which detracts from their beneficial properties. Raw ACV can help promote better digestion, aid with heartburn and acid reflux, balance the inner ecosystem, help with calcium absorption, and alkalize the body. It has also been linked to reducing high blood pressure and diabetes, and helping weight loss. Use it in salad dressings and dips. It can also be used to clean vegetables (see page 308).

**BALSAMIC VINEGAR** Buy the best quality that you can afford and it will keep for years if properly stored in the cupboard. Sweet and tart, its rich flavor adds decadence to a quick salad.

### CACAO AND DARK CHOCOLATE

Quality dark chocolate and cacao are feel-good foods with plenty of antioxidants, magnesium, and good fats from the cocoa butter. The higher the cocoa percentage the better because it means less room for additives. The terms are confusing, but "cacao" tends to refer to the raw product and "cocoa" to the roasted version, but there are no strict definitions. Though raw is higher in

antioxidants, the roasted type still has benefits and can be easier to digest for some. We tend to specify "cacao" in our recipes in order to describe a less chemically processed powder, free from unwanted additives. We enjoy raw cacao, cacao nibs, good quality cocoa powder, and organic (85–90 percent cocoa solids) chocolate. Cacao is rich in caffeine so it is best eaten with plenty of fat, like its natural cocoa butter, when eaten as chocolate, or with a spoonful of coconut oil, and enjoyed well before bedtime. We like to make our own chocolate (page 270) to avoid the refined sugars found in shop-bought varieties.

**CAROB** Carob is made from the sweet pulp of a tropical tree, which is then dried, roasted, and ground. Unlike cacao, carob contains no caffeine, so it's a great alternative for those who are caffeine-sensitive. Replace cacao powder with carob in equal measures for those who need to avoid it entirely or use half and half for children. Carob is naturally sweeter than cacao, so you may like to slightly reduce the amount of sweetener used in the recipe.

**FISH SAUCE** Seek out a quality, sugar-free, additive-free version and use sparingly as it's very salty. We use one made from slowly fermented fresh wild-caught anchovies and sea salt.

**MISO** Rich in antioxidants and good bacteria, miso is made by fermenting soya beans to make a salty paste, which adds a distinct umami flavor to foods. It's a good fall back if you don't have bone broth and is delicious in dips and dressings. Try the many varieties on offer and look for unpasteurized, organic (non-GM), and traditionally fermented varieties to benefit from these health properties. If you have a gluten intolerance check ingredients and choose a bean or pure soy miso. Stir in at the end of cooking in order to retain the live bacteria.

**MUSTARD** A delicious condiment, which adds minerals as well as flavor to your meal. Mustard seeds are high in selenium and magnesium, giving it anti-inflammatory properties.

**POMEGRANATE MOLASSES**
The concentrated juice of pomegranates is full of antioxidants, vitamins, and minerals. It adds a tangy depth to stews and sauces and is great in dressings as an alternative to balsamic vinegar.

**SEA SALT AND ROCK SALT** Regular table salt is highly processed and bleached and bears little resemblance to the natural salts your body is designed for. Rather than enhancing, it leaches calcium and other minerals from our bodies. Rock and sea salt are an important part of our diet; dried in the wind and sun, the enzymes are preserved as well as the trace minerals and elements. Himalayan salt contains the same 84 trace minerals and elements found in our bodies, compared to table salt that only really contains sodium chloride. Not just a flavor enhancer, these unrefined salts support the nervous system, help to regulate blood pressure, aid digestion and support hormones, heart, and muscle function.

**TAHINI** A light or dark sesame seed paste, which is essential for hummus and the base of lots of our dressings. Dark tahini, made from unshelled seeds is more nutritious and has a coarser texture and stronger flavor than light tahini. If you find the taste too bitter, start with light tahini while your taste buds get used to it.

**TAMARI** A traditional Japanese sauce made from fermented soya beans. While similar in color and flavor to soy sauce, we prefer tamari because it is gluten-free and, thanks to the higher concentration of fermented soya beans, is thicker and richer—so remember you will need much less. Buy organic, and something to look out for, particularly with soy products, is non-GM. As well as using in Asian dishes, we add a dash to season and add depth to stews, soups, and dressings.

**VANILLA EXTRACT** This imparts a sweet, fragrant note to bakes and sweets. Don't buy the "essence," which is synthetic; buy a cold extract with no additives.

## Herbs, spices, and seasonings
Fresh herbs will always make a delicious addition to a meal but, for convenience, a stash of dried herbs and spices are a must (and good quality ones also retain nutritional value). Check out our spice mixes through the book, such as Chermoula, Southwestern, Malaysian, and Sri Lankan. They can be used to jazz up a simple soup or to flavor dips and sauces.

**BASIL** An herb with antibacterial and anti-inflammatory properties and a rich source of vitamin A, an important vitamin relating to retina health and vision.

**BLACK PEPPER** Buy whole black peppercorns and grind them fresh. Pepper has a wealth of benefits – it is antibacterial, anti-inflammatory, and aids digestion.

**CARDAMOM** Benefitting digestion, respiration, and inhibiting pathogen growth, it is delicious in both sweet and savory dishes.

**CAYENNE** A type of chili pepper, cayenne boasts antifungal properties. Great for circulation, it is said to help remove toxins from the blood, nourish the heart, and fortify overall health. You'll find it in our savory recipes, juices, and hot chocolate.

**CINNAMON** This amazing spice helps to regulate blood sugar levels whilst adding its own sweet flavor, making it great for puddings as well as savory dishes. Cinnamon has a long history in traditional medicine and is used for digestive ailments such as indigestion, gas, and bloating.

**CILANTRO/CORIANDER** High in iron, magnesium, vitamins A, C, and K, and a great cleanser. We use plenty of fresh cilantro leaves and love toasting and grinding the seeds, adding them to curries and Middle Eastern recipes.

**CUMIN** Excellent for immune support, skin disorders, and aiding digestion. Delicious sprinkled onto eggs and beet and a key flavor in our favorite spice mixes.

**DILL** With a soft sweet taste, this feathery herb is a good source of vitamins A and C and is said to have the ability to prevent bacteria overgrowth within the body. It's perfect with fish, salads, and soups.

**GARLIC** Antibacterial, antifungal, antiseptic, antiparasitic, and antiviral, we mash up a raw clove and swallow it whenever we're feeling under the weather! You'll find garlic in practically every savory dish that we make and we even use it to turn a green smoothie into a savory soup.

**GINGER** As well as its fiery flavor, ginger has incredible immune-boosting properties and is antibacterial, anti-inflammatory, and antiviral. It works well for headaches, sleepiness, indigestion, stomach upsets, nausea, and motion sickness. Don't peel it if it's organic, there is a lot of goodness to be had in the skin. Drink a freshly grated ginger tea to aid digestion or try it on a larger scale – a tangy ginger bath will help you sweat and draw out toxins.

**MINT** Mint is calming on the stomach and great for nausea, and fresh mint tea is the perfect digestive. Peppermint grows easily on windowsills so have it on hand to pop into smoothies and juices.

**ONIONS** We enjoy plenty of onions along with the rest of the allium family (leeks, scallions, chives, shallots) eating them both cooked and raw for their anti-inflammatory, antibiotic, and antiviral properties, as well as their incredible flavor. The sulphur-containing amino acids found in onions and garlic are very good at detoxifying the body from heavy metals. As our mum says, a dish can't go far wrong if you start with a base of sautéed garlic and onions.

**OREGANO** Traditionally used as a tonic for colds and stomach ailments and said to improve digestion, oregano is delicious with fish and tomatoes.

**PARSLEY** Chock-full of vitamins, particularly vitamin A in the form of beta-carotene, and C, parsley is anti-inflammatory and great for digestion, muscle stiffness, and your bones. It keeps the immune and nervous systems strong and its folic acid content is like a tonic for the heart. Delicious in savory dishes and juices.

**ROSEMARY** Anti-inflammatory, full of antioxidants, and a good source of iron and calcium, this hardy herb adds a wonderful taste and aroma to roasted veg and meats, soup, and stews.

**SAGE** Calming sage is said to help brain function and improve concentration and memory loss in aging. Delicious with roasted meats, we also love it in bean soups and it's a perfect pairing to squash.

**SUMAC** This little red berry was traditionally used as a home remedy in the Middle East thanks to its antimicrobial properties and high antioxidant content. It's delicious in dressings and different spice mixes.

**THYME** Best friends with lamb and tomatoes, thyme also has one of the highest levels of antioxidants among fresh herbs and is known to support the respiratory system. Thymol, one of the oils in thyme, has antifungal and antiseptic qualities.

**TURMERIC** The benefits of this superstar spice are endless. Anti-inflammatory, it aids in digestion and purifies the blood so we even make a tea with it. Turmeric is part of the ginger family and has been used in Ayurvedic and Chinese medicines for thousands of years to treat infections and inflammations, both inside and outside the body. Its bright color is down to the antioxidant pigments (watch your clothes and skin as it stains). We even use it to make yellow icing for our cakes.

**Seaweed (also known as sea vegetables)**
Seaweeds are rich in iodine, iron, magnesium, and calcium and contain almost all the nutrients found in the ocean, as well as the same minerals found in human blood. Seaweeds add a savory flavor that the Japanese call "umami," the fifth basic taste. Dried seaweeds expand to about ten times their initial size once soaked for ten minutes or cooked (check the packet instructions) and add a wonderful texture to dishes. Our favorites are **Arame** (a gentle sweet taste), **Dulse** (salty smoky in taste), **Kelp** (look for it in noodle form too), **Kombu** (simmer with vegetables to make dashi, a delicious Japanese soup stock), and **Wakame** (salty sweet and great stirred into soups).

**Superfoods**
No single food can maintain and promote good health. This comes from the overall benefits of a healthy diet and lifestyle. But some foods have been classed as "superfoods" because they are especially rich in health-promoting nutrients, antioxidants, and phytochemicals (bioactive plant compounds) and, therefore, pack more of a nutritional punch than others. As well as the super properties of the fats and vegetables that we have already mentioned, here are some of

the more exotic and fashionable superfoods, great in smoothies and desserts.

**ACAI** A deep purple berry from Brazil and full of antioxidants, it can be bought as frozen fruit pulp or powdered.

**BAOBAB** This powdered, nutrient-dense fruit dries naturally on the branch of the baobab tree, known as "the tree of life." It's a source of 14 essential vitamins and minerals and is particularly high in vitamin C, vitamin B6, calcium, potassium, and thiamine.

**BEE POLLEN** High in protein, enzymes, and vitamins including B complex, and is good sprinkled over smoothies and porridges.

**COCONUT** Delicious fresh coconut is not so easily available, but luckily we can buy the oil (page 18) and flour (page 20), the cream, milk, and water to use in our cooking, baking, and smoothies/drinks, and the dried and flaked meat of the coconut (shredded or chips) for granolas and breakfast bars.

**COCONUT MILK** Coconut milk is a delicious thickener in soups, curries, and smoothies, lending a creamy texture, distinct flavor, and natural sweetness. Don't buy the low-fat version as you are missing out on all of the natural goodness and taste.

**COCONUT WATER** Coconut water is full of electrolytes, vitamins, and minerals, particularly magnesium and potassium, which makes it a great pre- and post-workout drink. However, it's no substitute for water as it is full of natural sugars. Look for unpasteurized, pure coconut water with no added sugar or flavorings. You can also combine it with a good spoonful of probiotic yogurt as a milk replacement for granola.

**CREAMED COCONUT** This is coconut flesh that has been dehydrated and ground into a white paste. Solid at room temperature, chop off or grate what you need for cooking and the rest will keep in the fridge for ages. Add warm water to make coconut cream or milk. Add to curries, soups, porridges, and smoothies.

**GOJI BERRIES** Antioxidant-rich and tasty, we add these dried berries to snack bars and breakfasts for a boost or soak and plump them up for salads.

**LUCUMA** An antioxidant-rich, sweet fruit from Peru, especially good in puddings and available in powdered form.

**MACA** Mineral-rich, malty maca powder is an ancient root grown in the mountains of Peru. Maca works as an adaptogen, responding to different bodies' needs and is well noted for its ability to help increase stamina, energy, and sexual function. Packed with B vitamins and a good source of iron, it helps to restore red blood cells and aids healing and muscle repair.

### "Super" green powders
Rich in chlorophyll, vitamins, and minerals, these freeze-dried powders can be stirred into water, fresh juices, or smoothies. They don't smell too appetising but you won't taste them once mixed in. Our two favorites are **chlorella** and **spirulina**.

## KITCHEN ESSENTIALS

**BAKEWARE AND PANS** We use stainless steel, cast iron and ceramic pans, for cooking. For baking and roasting we use ceramic or lead-free enamel-lined bakeware, or line bakeware with parchment paper to avoid toxic substances such as PTFE and PFOA found in modern cookware. No aluminium cookware either, please, it's just not good for you! Try out the new generation of "green cookware" instead.

**BLENDER** We use a super-powerful blender that makes light work of nut milk and flours. If it's a toss up between buying a juicer or a blender, we say get a blender as you will get much more use out of it. Hand-held blenders are great for soups, making dips, and can be used for smoothies, if you team them with the right jug, but might not be powerful enough to blend some of the harder vegetables. Choose one that comes with a bowl attachment to make a quick job of pestos.

**CHOPPING BOARDS** Avoid plastic and choose wood and bamboo chopping boards, which are naturally antibacterial. Wash and dry well after use, use a halved lemon to deodorise them.

**DEHYDRATOR** This machine gently dries out food at a very low temperature. Great for dehydrating "activated" nuts and seeds to make them "crispy," fruit and vegetable "chips," and for making crackers and granolas. It is brilliant for turning the leftover almond pulp from making nut milk into almond flour and fermenting coconut yogurt.

**FOOD PROCESSOR** This is one of our essential appliances – grate a mountain of cauliflower or broccoli into rice in minutes. It's a lazy way of making a slaw, cakes, and cookies. Some appliances have smaller bowl inserts for easier blending of pestos, sauces, and dressings. If you don't have space, then a hand-held blender with a small bowl attachment is useful.

**GLASS CONTAINERS/DISHES WITH LIDS** The BPA in plastic used in some lunchboxes and food storage pots can leak hormone-disrupting toxins into food. By using ovenproof glass containers we also have the benefit of being able to pop them straight in the oven. If you have containers with plastic lids, try to avoid the lids touching the food.

**HOUSEHOLD CLEANING PRODUCTS** Choose plant-based natural products or make up your own cheaply using baking soda, lemon juice, and vinegar.

**JUICER** The slow grinding action of a masticating juicer (also called a cold press juicer) ensures that more of the goodness from your fruit and veg makes it into your juice. You can also use it to make nut milks and butters and the leftover pulp from carrots, beet and apples can be used in cakes and breads, etc. Centrifugal juicers have their merits too – they are faster, easier to clean, and cheaper.

**KITCHEN SCALES** We like compact digital scales for ease and for accuracy.

**KNIVES** One big, one small, and one serrated for soft foods should be all you need. Keep them sharp for safety and ease.

**MANDOLIN** Great for finely slicing fruit and vegetables quickly.

**PARCHMENT PAPER** Use unbleached, metal-free parchment paper. We're not into non-stick products as there are problems with toxins from the PTFE coating getting into food. We don't use aluminium cookware or foil either because aluminium is not good for you – beware it is toxic stuff, especially when heated.

**SALAD SPINNER** Important for making good salads – you don't want soggy leaves.

**SLOW COOKER** We can't live without it and use it for making bone broth, soups, and stews. Throw in the ingredients for a stew in the morning, then come home to an easy and satisfying supper. If you're using a slow cooker, use at least a third less liquid than the recipe says, as very little liquid evaporates during cooking.

**SPATULAS** Use a wooden one for cooking and a silicone one for scraping out a bowl.

**SPIRALIZER** Make vegetable "noodles" or "spaghetti" out of cucumber, carrot, and zucchini. Courgetti Puttanesca (page 210) is one of our favorite summer dishes. A julienne peeler is a good alternative, if storage space is an issue, and it creates finer, straighter strands.

**STAINLESS STEEL CANTEENS** Use these for carrying water, smoothies, and juices when you are on the go. Make sure you buy food-grade stainless steel so it doesn't react and double check that there are no toxins hidden in any plastic liners.

**STAINLESS STEEL INSULATED FLASK** Perfect for soups and stews, enjoy a hot lunch at work or when you're out and about by storing it in a flask. Steer clear of the microwave and, again, make sure there is no plastic liner.

**WATER FILTER** Typical tap water contains chloride, fluoride, traces of heavy metals, nitrates, pesticides, and hormones, which are all things we prefer to avoid ingesting. Filter jugs are a good starting point. We recommend a remineralising water filter that restructures the water as well as removing impurities. You can really taste the difference, so in our opinion the extra expense is well worth it.

## COOK'S NOTES

- All spoon measures are level unless otherwise stated.
- When baking, remember to use room temperature eggs. Eggs are medium and butter is unsalted unless otherwise stated.
- All recipes were tested in a fan-assisted oven. If using a conventional oven, set the temperature 100°F higher than stated in the recipes. Oven temperatures do vary so practice makes perfect.
- Pregnant women, the elderly, babies and toddlers, as well as people who are unwell should avoid recipes that contain raw or partially cooked eggs.

# BREAKFAST

PEOPLE OFTEN ASK US WHAT WE EAT FOR BREAKFAST. As the name suggests, you are "breaking" a fast and your body is looking for fuel to start the day. For us anything goes, as long as it's nourishing: a superfood packed smoothie, a thick slice of Multiseed Loaf (page 273) spread with butter and Goji Marmalade (page 48), softly scrambled eggs served with romaine lettuce and Kale Pesto (page 233) or even some leftover soup, such as our favorite, Mung Dahl (page 186).

Breakfast can be a difficult meal to navigate for those who are used to the commercial, refined versions of cereal, porridge, pancakes, pastries, and toast. These kinds of foods are either high in refined carbohydrates and sugars or contain highly processed fats, none of which are good for you and especially not at the start of your day. In these breakfasts there is often no trace of the important proteins or fruits and vegetables to give you the essential natural, rather than synthetic, vitamins and minerals.

If you've got an early start, it's best to give your appetite the chance to wake up, so avoid downing a breakfast as you rush out of the door. For an easy takeaway breakfast, a well-balanced, raw smoothie decanted into a portable flask or even a jam jar fits the bill (see pages 282–290 for recipes). Prepare some homemade Granola the night before (page 36) or make a supply of our Cranberry Quinoa Breakfast Bars and store them in the freezer ready to grab and go (page 47). A jar of granola can even be kept on your desk – just take in some homemade Nut Milk (pages 304–305) or

a pot of Coconut Yogurt (pages 305–306). We find a lot of our clients are used to skipping breakfast and even the very idea of eating early in the morning can make them feel queasy (this is often because they are suffering from poor food choices made the day before – a food hangover of sorts). For others, skipping this important meal makes them feel as if they are controlling their calorie intake and in turn their weight. The reality is that people who don't start the day off right by eating a nourishing breakfast tend to make poor food choices for the rest of the day – and so the cycle continues.

If you are not used to having breakfast, it may seem like a difficult adjustment to make. Persevere and you will soon start to notice the benefits – sustained energy, better focus and less cravings for junk foods – and you'll wonder why you never did this before.

Make your way through our breakfast recipes, but don't feel you have to limit yourself to just this chapter; any of the recipes from this book can start your day. Remember, anything goes as long as it nourishes you!

Whatever we choose to eat for breakfast, we always start the day with a glass of warm filtered water to rehydrate after sleep, often adding the juice of half a lemon to help the body cleanse and alkalize. If preparing breakfast and boiling a kettle is too much to do in the morning, try keeping a glass of water by your bed and sipping from it slowly as soon as you wake up until you walk out the door. Water is always the best option first thing in the morning rather than caffeine-laden coffee or tea.

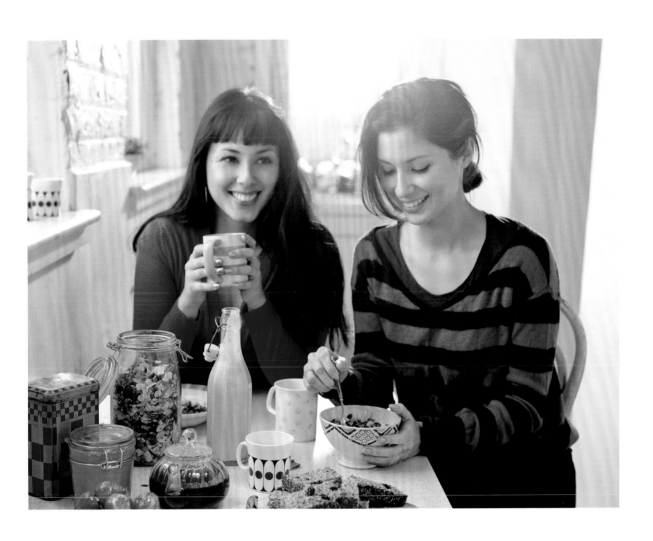

## BLUEBERRY PANCAKES WITH MANGO CASHEW CREAM

Our version of America's classic breakfast: blueberry pancakes. Unlike the usual pancake recipes, this is grain-free, gluten-free, dairy-free, and refined sugar-free!

A couple of tips: don't have too much fat in the pan – it should be lightly coated – and, secondly, these coconut flour pancakes work best on a medium heat. Remember there is no gluten to hold these fluffy pancakes together so go gentle on the cooking. Also, you'll find that the batter will thicken as it stands so just add a small dash of water to loosen the mixture up again before cooking.

You can make these into American-style thick pancakes or thin crêpes, which you can roll and fill with the blueberries and cream. Be sure to try our Mango Cashew Cream (page 49) as it adds a delicious creamy touch to the berries.

SERVES 2

6 oz blueberries

2 tbsp coconut oil or butter

2–4 tbsp warm water

2 eggs at room temperature

1–1½ tbsp maple syrup

½ tsp vanilla extract, or more if needed

2 tbsp coconut flour

¼ tsp baking soda

Mango Cashew Cream (page 49)

sea salt

**1**  Wash the blueberries and allow them to dry. Line a baking tray with baking parchment.

**2**  Melt the coconut oil or butter over a low heat in a frying pan and allow to cool.

**3**  Meanwhile, beat the water, eggs, maple syrup, vanilla, and a tiny sprinkle of salt together in a mixing bowl until light and fluffy.

**4**  Sift in the coconut flour and baking soda and blend with the melted coconut oil/butter to make a batter (don't wash up the pan yet!). Leave to sit for 5 minutes to thicken up.

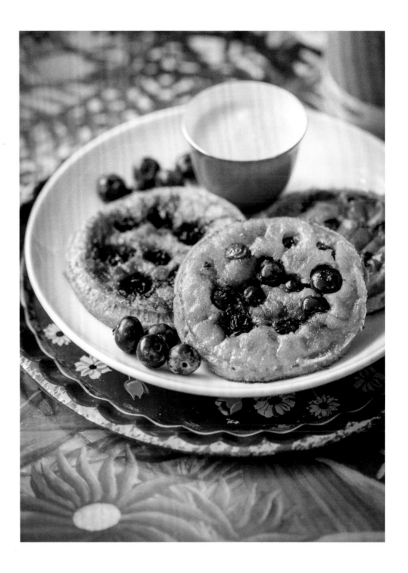

### TO MAKE AMERICAN-STYLE THICK PANCAKES

Use a spatula to redistribute any leftover coconut oil into the center of the frying pan and place a 4 in egg ring in the center. Place the pan over a medium heat and add 2 tablespoons of the batter. Push 10 blueberries into the center of the pancake.

After a couple of minutes, the bottom will have set. Carefully slide each pancake onto the prepared baking tray and remove the egg ring. Start cooking the next pancake.

Once all the pancakes are cooked (the batter should make about six), pop the baking tray in the broiler for a few minutes to finish them off. Serve with the mango cashew cream and some extra blueberries.

### TO MAKE CRÊPES

Use a spatula to redistribute any leftover coconut oil into the center of the frying pan. Place the pan over a medium heat and add 2 tablespoons of the batter. Swirl the pan to distribute.

After a couple of minutes, check if you can loosen the pancake easily – if so, it's ready to be carefully turned over.

Cook on the other side for a minute or so and then transfer to the prepared baking tray. Start on the next one.

Place a dollop of the mango cashew cream in the center of a pancake, throw over plenty of blueberries, roll up, and eat!

# ANYTIME EGGS

We love this for breakfast, brunch, lunch, or supper – all day, every day! Our version of shakshuka, eggs poached in a sauce of tomatoes and spiced with chili and cumin, is packed with plenty of greens and finished with creamy feta to make a filling dish.

Cumin and eggs are an amazing flavor combination and cumin is excellent for colds, skin complaints, immunity, and digestion. In fact, the very aroma of it activates our salivary glands, which makes this a truly mouthwatering dish.

SERVES 2

1 tbsp ghee or butter

1 onion, diced

2 large garlic cloves, diced

1 large red, orange or yellow pepper, sliced

1 tsp ground cumin

4 large tomatoes (about 1 lb), roughly chopped

1 tsp balsamic vinegar

7 oz rainbow chard, stalks finely diced and leaves sliced into ribbons – or kale, stalks discarded as they are too tough and leaves sliced into ribbons

4 eggs

a small handful of fresh cilantro and dill

a dollop of probiotic goats' yogurt or a small handful of crumbly, unpasteurized cheese such as feta

a pinch of cayenne pepper or smoked paprika

a squeeze of lemon juice

sea salt and black pepper

**OPTIONAL**

try sliced leeks, scallions, or snipped fresh chives instead of the diced onion

swap in a handful of fresh parsley, mint, or oregano for the cilantro and dill

**1**  Heat the ghee/butter in a large shallow pan with a lid over a low heat. Gently fry the onion for 5 minutes. Add the garlic, red pepper, and cumin and cook for a few minutes.

**2**  Add the chopped tomatoes, balsamic vinegar and 1½ cups water, stir, and bring to a simmer. Let everything cook down for 10 minutes to make a nice chunky sauce.

**3**  Stir in the chard or kale leaves and the diced stems and cover the pan for 5 minutes to allow them to wilt (you might need a little longer for the kale). Take the lid off, season to taste and, if needed, leave to reduce again with the lid off for a few minutes for the sauce to thicken.

**4**  Push the vegetables aside using a spatula to make four small gaps in the sauce.

**5**  Gently crack an egg into each gap and season each egg with salt and pepper. With the lid off the eggs will gently cook in about 6 minutes (for a runny yolk). If you want to give them a helping hand, then pop the lid on and keep an eye out after 4 minutes so that you catch them when the whites are just set but the yolks are runny. You could also pop the pan, uncovered, into a hot oven for a few minutes if preferred.

**6**  Scatter over the fresh herbs, a dollop of yogurt or some crumbled cheese, and finish with a sprinkling of cayenne or paprika and a squeeze of lemon juice. Serve this dish straight from the pan. Any leftovers are delicious the next day!

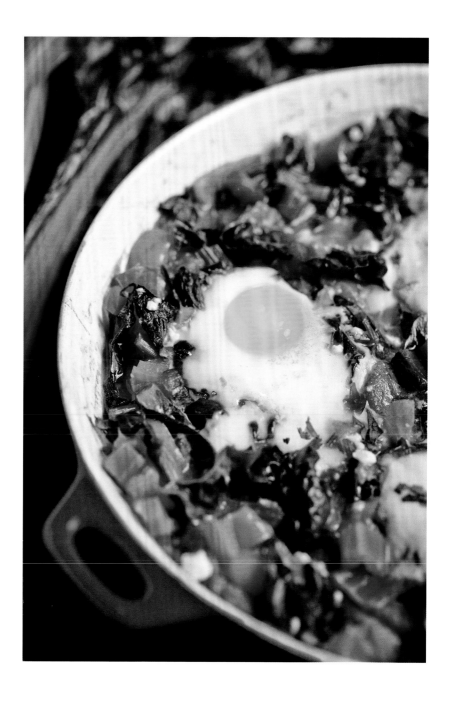

✚ **FORGET TOAST** and serve this with a side of creamy avocado instead.

✚ **MAKE A BIGGER BATCH OF SAUCE** then save it for other dishes – it's great with lamb chops, stirred into some freshly cooked quinoa, or served hot with some fried or grilled halloumi.

# BUCKWHEAT PORRIDGE AND BUCKWHEAT CREAM

An easy and versatile breakfast for a warming start to a chilly morning. Buckwheat is a gluten-free, nutritious seed rich in magnesium, one of the most important nutrients for good health. We love topping this porridge with cinnamon, an amazing spice that helps to regulate blood sugar levels. In traditional medicine, cinnamon is used for digestive ailments such as indigestion, gas, and bloating, while modern medical research has discovered its mild anti-inflammatory and anti-fungal effects.

When the porridge cools it stiffens up, so it is easy to transport to work without slopping – just mix in a little boiling water to warm through when you get there. Or you can turn this porridge into a light vanilla cream to coat a fruit salad for a decadent and colorful summer breakfast or a delicious snack.

SERVES 2–4

## FOR THE BUCKWHEAT PORRIDGE

3 ½ oz buckwheat groats (activated overnight page 300)

5 pitted dates, to sweeten (more if you prefer)

1–2 pinches of sea salt

1 tbsp coconut oil or butter

## ANY COMBINATION OF THE FOLLOWING TOPPINGS

ground cinnamon

cacao powder

cacao nibs

bee pollen

nuts or seeds (we use walnuts) (preferably "crispy" activated, page 302)

a selection of ripe, chopped fruit (we use banana, kiwi, apricots, strawberries, raspberries, and blueberries)

## FOR THE BUCKWHEAT CREAM

1 ¾ oz buckwheat groats (activated overnight page 300)

2–3 pitted dates, to sweeten (more if you prefer)

a pinch of sea salt

½ tbsp coconut oil or butter

1 tsp vanilla extract

**1** Place your soaked and rinsed groats in a food processor (for a chunkier texture) or powerful blender (for a smoother texture). Add 2 cups water and the dates and blend until smooth.

**2** Pour into a large saucepan, add the sea salt and the coconut oil or butter.

**3** Bring to boil, stirring continuously to avoid lumps. Simmer for about 5–6 minutes, stirring occasionally, to stop it sticking to the bottom of the pan.

**4** Ladle into a bowl and add your toppings to taste.

**5 To make Buckwheat Cream**, blend all the ingredients except for the vanilla extract with 2 cups water until smooth. Simmer and stir occasionally until you have a creamy consistency. Stir in the vanilla extract and check for sweetness. Serve poured over a bowl of fruit.

➕ **INSTEAD OF DATES** you could add some maple syrup or stevia. You could also add raw honey, but only once the porridge is cool enough to eat, otherwise the high heat destroys much of the honey's enzymes and nutritional value.

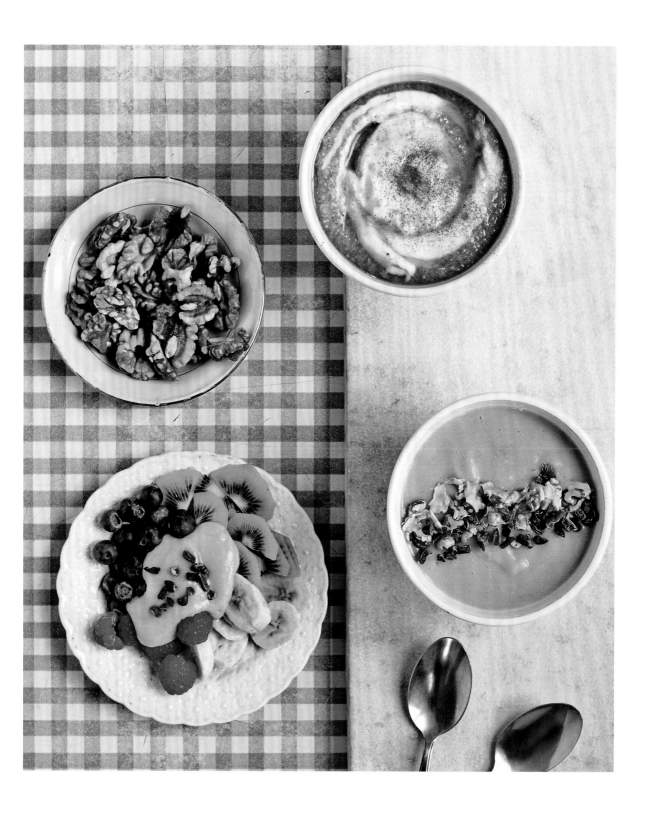

# CINNAMON AND BUCKWHEAT CRUNCH GRANOLA

Granola – the crunchy, munchy muesli. Unlike conventional granolas, this isn't a sugary-sweet way to start the day, but a satisfying breakfast with a different flavor in each mouthful. A small, nutrient-dense bowl fills you up and provides plenty of pleasure as this is one breakfast you cannot get away with not chewing! The buckwheat crunch takes a while to bake, but once combined with the extras it makes plenty of granola – at least three times the average box of cereal.

Enjoy with Almond Milk (page 304), Coconut Yogurt (page 305), or full-fat yogurt and a splash of coconut water. We like to sprinkle it onto our Acai Berry Breakfast Bowl (page 43) or pour on some hot Buckwheat Cream (page 34). It's a nice one for nibbling on too – just pack it up and carry it around like a trail mix.

**MAKES ENOUGH FOR ABOUT 15 SERVINGS**

### FOR THE BUCKWHEAT CRUNCH

18 oz buckwheat groats (activated overnight page 300)

1½ tsp sea salt

7 tbsp ground cinnamon

7 tbsp maple syrup (or raw honey if using a dehydrator)

5 tbsp chia seeds

5 tbsp coconut oil or butter, melted

### FOR THE GRANOLA EXTRAS

7 oz coconut flakes or chips

3 ½ oz pecans or hazelnuts or your choice of nuts (preferably "crispy" activated, page 302)

3 ½ oz pumpkin seeds (preferably "crispy" activated, page 302)

3 ½ oz raisins

1 ¾ oz goji berries

### OVEN METHOD

**1** Preheat the oven to fan 325°F and line 2 baking trays with baking parchment. Place the drained buckwheat in a glass or stainless steel bowl with the rest of the buckwheat crunch ingredients, stir well and leave to sit – this will help the chia to produce a gel that sticks everything together.

**2** While the mix is soaking, spread the coconut flakes out on a baking tray and toast in the oven for 8–10 minutes, turning every 3–4 minutes, until evenly toasted. Set aside to cool.

**3** Reduce the oven temperature to fan 275°F. Spread the granola mixture evenly over the prepared trays (about ½ in thick) .

**4** Bake for about 20 minutes then open the oven door to let some steam escape. Close the door and reduce the temperature to fan 225°F.

**5** Bake for a further 40 minutes then remove from the oven and, using a spatula, gently turn large sections over – it will break into large pieces.

**6** Return the granola to the oven for a final 10 minutes. Remove from the oven and leave to cool completely – the pieces will crisp up and dry out further as they cool.

**7** Mix the cooled buckwheat crunch with the granola extras, then store in a glass jar somewhere cool or in the fridge ready to serve.

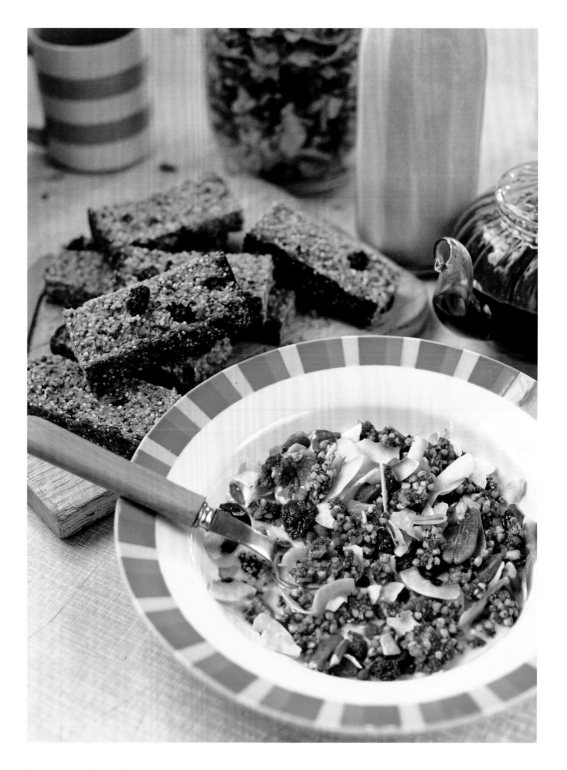

**DEHYDRATOR METHOD**
Prepare the granola ingredients as above. Distribute the mixture over dehydrator trays and spread out to ⅓ in thick. Dehydrate at 115°F for 10 hours. Break into pieces, leave to cool, and store as above.

Cranberry Quinoa Breakfast Bars (page 47) and Cinnamon and Buckwheat Crunch Granola (opposite).

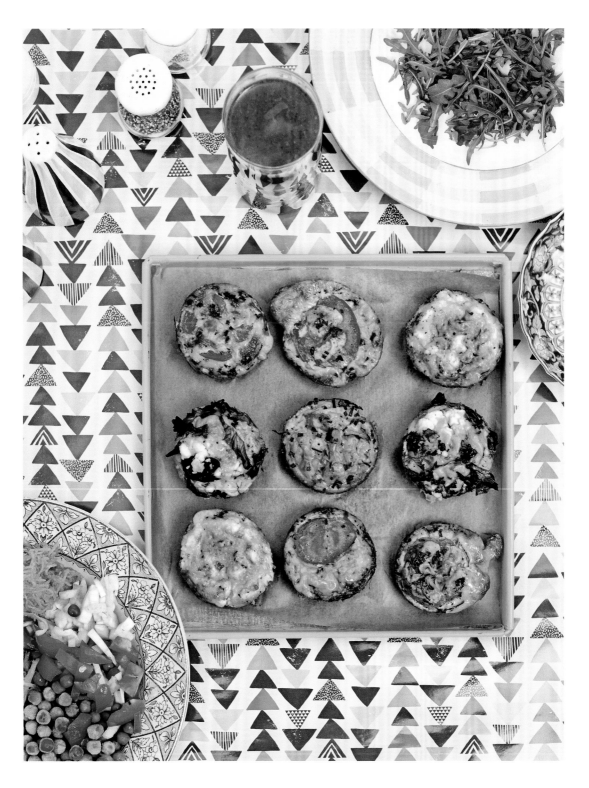

Beet Maca Smoothie (page 290) and
Muffin Frittatas (opposite).

# MUFFIN FRITTATAS

These tasty vegetable muffins are are great for packed lunches and on-the-go breakfasts. The Italian word "frittata" derives from *fritto*, to fry, and most frittata recipes call for you to fry the vegetables first. The beauty of this recipe is that we skip the frying (anything to save time) to create much fresher-tasting frittatas, made up of at least 50 percent lightly cooked, vitamin-packed vegetables. Use the coarse teeth on a grater or a mandolin to save on chopping time and avoid using tomatoes as they are often too watery. Please don't make an egg white frittata! The saturated fat in egg yolks is incredibly nutritious and good fat in every meal is important to absorb all the nutrients that are present in food.

If you're having people round for lunch, use this recipe to make up a giant frittata in a large frying pan and cut into thick wedges. Serve with a salad such as Fennel, Cucumber, and Dill Salad (page 97).

MAKES 12 MINI
FRITTATAS

8 eggs

2 large pinches of sea salt

a large pinch of black pepper

3 carrots or 3 zucchinis, roughly grated (or a mix of both)

a handful of veg – try chopped red pepper, fennel, or peas

1 onion or leek, or some scallions or fresh chives (dice, chop, or snip them finely as you won't be frying them)

1 large garlic clove, finely diced

any spices or herbs, fresh or dried (we like 1 tsp dried oregano and a small handful of fresh parsley)

a large handful of grated hard cheese, such as cheddar, gruyère or parmesan

**1**  Preheat the oven to fan 375°F. Grease a muffin tray well with a little butter/ghee or use paper cases or parchment paper.

**2**  Beat the eggs in a large bowl. Add the salt and pepper, all the grated and chopped vegetables or peas, finely chopped onion or leek, garlic, and any spices or herbs. You are looking for a ratio of around 50 percent egg to 50 percent raw veg.

**3**  Pour the mixture into the prepared muffin tray.

**4**  Bake for 12 minutes, then crumble the cheese on top and turn on the broiler. Broil for about a minute until the tops are golden brown. Alternatively, you could stir the cheese into the egg mix, not bother with the broiler, and just cook in the oven for 14 minutes.

**5**  To check if they are done, give the muffin tray a wobble – the frittatas should be just set in the middle. You can always put them back in the oven for another 1–2 minutes if you think they need cooking any longer.

**6**  Remove the frittatas from the tray and leave to cool on a wire rack. Wrap them up in baking or greaseproof paper or pop them in your lunch box for a great snack on the go.

**TRY USING FETA** instead of a hard cheese. If you do, remember to use less salt as feta is naturally very salty.

# COCONUT AMARANTH PORRIDGE AND BAKED AMARANTH PUDDING

This is the new way to enjoy porridge. We love amaranth and when combined with coconut milk it makes a wonderful breakfast. These little seeds retain just enough texture, which is why they are perfect for training your chewing technique – make sure you break down each and every one to extract their nutrition. Don't overfill your bowl – you won't need as much as usual to fill your belly and feel satisfied.

Another way to breakfast on amaranth is inspired by the old-school classic, rice pudding. We love this baked pudding as a hot or cold breakfast or 4 p.m. snack. It's wonderfully rich, so don't eat this as a dessert unless you've just had a salad or vegetables for your main course! This recipe makes plenty so we eat half and then put the rest of the dish in the freezer ready for a rainy weekend breakfast.

SERVES 8-10

## FOR AMARANTH PORRIDGE

9 oz amaranth (activated overnight page 300)

1 tin of full-fat coconut milk

2 tbsp maple syrup or raw honey

sea salt

stevia (optional)

your favorite porridge toppings, such as nuts, seeds, yogurt, and fresh or dried fruit (remembering to reduce the maple syrup or honey if using fruit)

## FOR AMARANTH PUDDING

butter, for greasing

4 eggs, beaten

18 oz amaranth (activated overnight page 300)

2 tins of full-fat coconut milk

7–8 tbsp maple syrup (we like 7, but 8 makes it more of a pudding)

1½ tbsp vanilla extract

a pinch of sea salt

2 tsp ground nutmeg

1 ½ oz butter

**1** To make the amaranth porridge, place the drained amaranth in a large saucepan with the coconut milk and a pinch of salt, cover with a lid and bring to boil. Stir and reduce to a simmer with the lid on, stirring every 5–10 minutes. Watch it doesn't catch on the bottom.

**2** After 20 minutes, the amaranth should be cooked. Add a little more liquid if you need to, or carry on simmering, lid off, to thicken the porridge.

**3** Take off the heat and stir in the maple syrup, if using, or allow to cool before drizzling with raw honey.

**4** Finish with a sprinkling of your favorite porridge toppings – we use blueberries and yogurt.

**5** **To make Amaranth Pudding**, preheat the oven to fan 350°F. Grease a 8 ½ x 10 in baking dish. Beat the eggs in a bowl, add the drained amaranth and the rest of the ingredients (except the nutmeg and butter) and mix well.

**6** Pour into the prepared baking dish and bake for 2 hours. After the first hour, remove from the oven to stir, sprinkle with the nutmeg and dot with the butter.

**7** Return to the oven for another hour or until the top has a lovely crust.

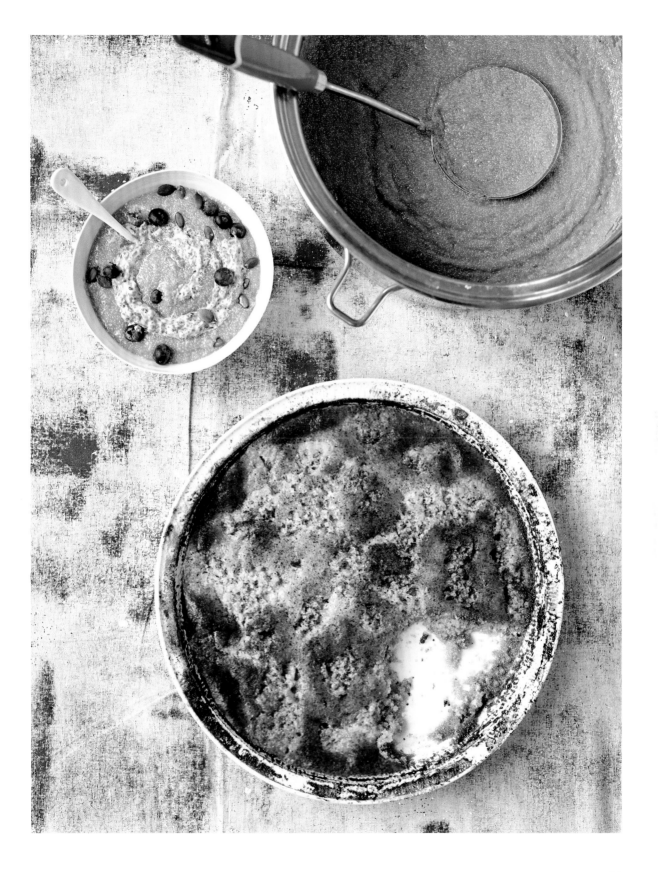

# CHIA CHAI BUTTERNUT BREAKFAST PUDDING

This is an overnight breakfast or make-ahead dessert. We've infused omega-3-rich chia seeds with our favorite rooibos chai breakfast tea and together they turn the usually savory butternut squash into a sweet start to the day. Gently heating up the pudding before layering with the Mango Cashew Cream (page 49) is our favorite way to breakfast and warm our bellies in the autumn.

This is so yummy that you'll also fancy it as a cool, creamy dessert. We love it with summer fruits, such as blackberries, grapes, figs, plums, or peaches, which are just in season as butternut comes in. In the winter months, try apple chunks, chopped clementines, or blood orange.

If you bake the butternut squash the night before, then it's ready to go in the morning. Don't forget to chew well in order to get the most goodness out of the tiny chia seeds.

SERVES 2–4

1 large butternut squash (enough to make 14 oz cooked butternut squash purée)

2 rooibos chai tea bags or 2 tsp rooibos chai tea leaves

4 tbsp white chia seeds (we used white chia to keep the pudding's bright orange color, but black also works – and is cheaper and easier to find too!)

3 tbsp coconut oil

1 tbsp raw honey

**OPTIONAL**

Coconut Yogurt (pages 305–306) and goji berries, to serve

**1**  Preheat the oven to fan 350°F and roast the butternut squash in the oven for 40–50 minutes until cooked through and tender. Scoop out 14 oz of the squash flesh and mash well. Any leftover squash can be frozen and used in a soup or smoothie.

**2**  Add the squash to a saucepan with 1 ½ cups water, the coconut oil, and the tea leaves (or the contents of the tea bags, if using). Bring to a medium simmer, then remove from the heat and leave to cool for a few minutes.

**3**  Stir in the chia seeds, continuously whisking at first to avoid lumps, then add the honey.

**4**  Leave to sit for at least 20 minutes to an hour for the chia to swell (unless you like it crunchy). Alternatively, transfer to a flask and by the time you get to work, you'll have a nice warm chia breakfast pudding.

**5**  Add the Coconut Yogurt and goji berries, if using, and enjoy.

✚ **TO MAKE A CREAMY DESSERT,** take a jar or glass and layer up the Chia Chai Butternut Breakfast Pudding with Mango Cashew Cream (page 49) and scatter 2 handfuls of seasonal fruit, such as blackberries, between the layers. Top with more fruit and enjoy.

# ACAI BERRY BREAKFAST BOWL

SERVES 2

2 tbsp freeze-dried acai berry powder

½ a frozen banana

1 small avocado

2 tbsp coconut oil

5 oz frozen berries

1 date, pitted

¾ cup coconut water or water

**OPTIONAL TOPPINGS**

hemp seeds

flaxseeds

goji berries

fresh banana slices, berries, or seasonal fruit

chia seeds

bee pollen

cacao nibs

Acai are purple berries from Brazil that are very high in antioxidants. We like to enjoy their goodness in this cool, creamy breakfast that's perfect on a hot summer's day when you are fully awake and ready for something refreshing. Savor and warm each mouthful so that you don't shock the system. Serve it in a jam jar so you can take it as breakfast on the go.

**1** Put the acai berry powder, banana, avocado, coconut oil, berries, date, and water in a food processor or blender and blend until smooth. Serve with your choice of toppings.

**+ FREEZE BANANAS** Cut bananas into chunks when they are really ripe and freeze them for easier blending.

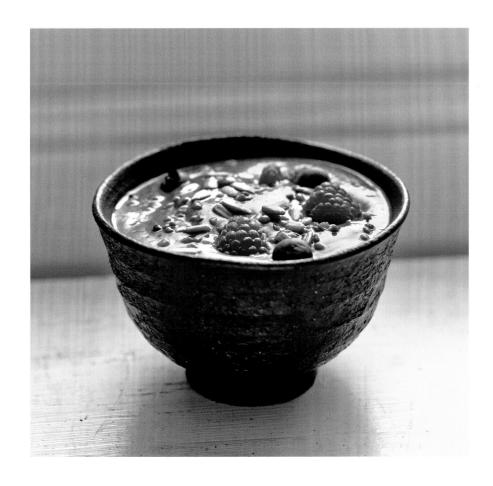

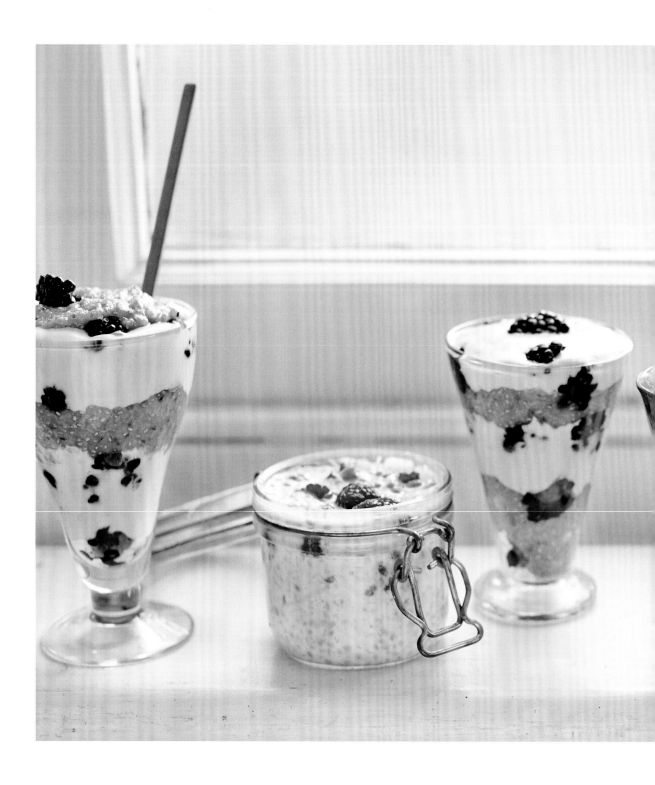

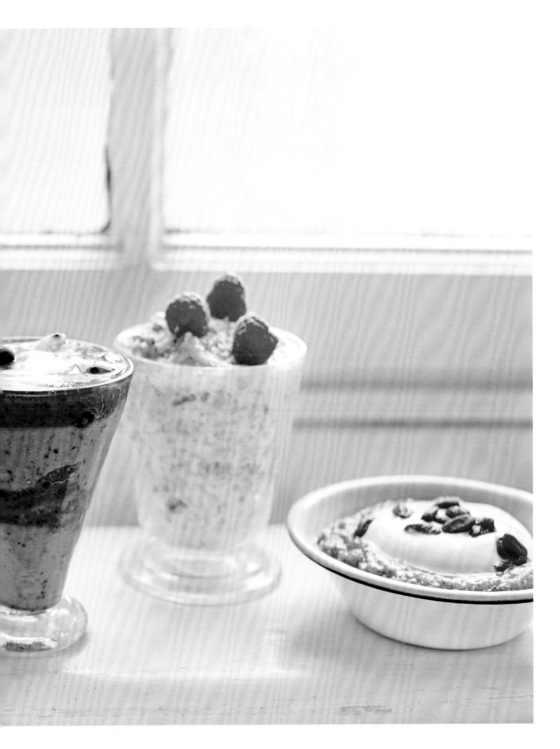

**LEFT TO RIGHT**: Chia Chai Butternut Breakfast Pudding served as a Creamy Dessert (page 42), Buckwheat Groat Bircher Muesli (page 46), Acai Berry Breakfast Bowl (page 43), Chia Chai Butternut Breakfast Pudding (page 42) topped with Coconut Yogurt (pages 305–306) and goji berries.

# BUCKWHEAT GROAT BIRCHER MUESLI

SERVES 2

A new take on the classic oat Bircher muesli. This is an overnight dish, like the original, but with the extra ingredients added in the morning. Just soak buckwheat groats and seeds overnight to activate their goodness (pages 300–302). The next morning rinse, drain, and add the rest of the ingredients and enjoy. We like it with a dollop of Instant Blueberry Chia Jam (page 48) or Goji Marmalade (page 48).

2 oz buckwheat groats (activated overnight page 300)

2–3 tbsp of your favorite seeds (try pumpkin or sunflower seeds) (preferably "crispy" activated, page 302)

4 oz full-fat probiotic natural yogurt or thick Coconut Yogurt (page 305)

¼ tsp ground cinnamon, plus extra to serve

1 tsp raw honey

1 large apple, grated with skin on

a handful of toasted shredded coconut, to serve

**OPTIONAL**

a handful of your favorite seasonal berries

**1**  In the morning, place the drained and rinsed groats in a bowl. Mix in the rest of the ingredients.

**2**  Sprinkle over the extra cinnamon, toasted shredded coconut, and/or your favorite berries, to serve.

➕ **YOU CAN ALSO DO THIS WITH SHREDDED COCONUT AND CHIA INSTEAD OF THE GROATS.** Add 1 ½ ounces shredded coconut, 2 tablespoons chia and a few tablespoons of water to all the other ingredients before you go to bed. In the morning, the chia will have absorbed the liquid and swelled to make a Bircher pudding.

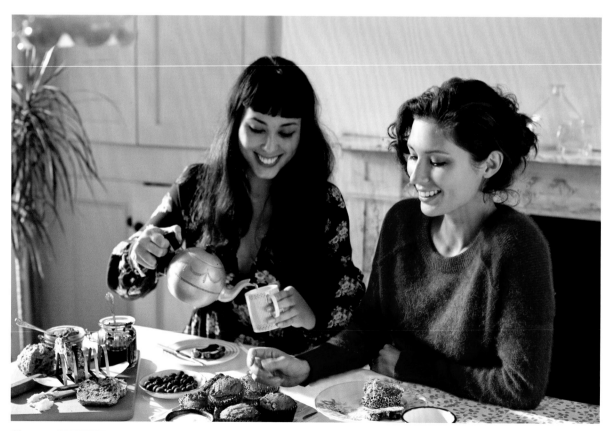

# CRANBERRY QUINOA BREAKFAST BARS

This is our easy fruit-and-seed breakfast bar (see photo on page 37). It's similar to a muesli bar thanks to the nutty crunch of protein-rich quinoa, sesame, and coconut and also has the sweet flavors of cranberries, cinnamon, and a hint of banana. Chestnut flour binds it together and gives it a moist cake texture between the crunch.

We sometimes make this recipe without the cranberries when we fancy something plain for our portable breakfast and we've also tried it with an extra banana, which makes it more of a dessert and an easier snack for kids to handle. You can also leave out the maple syrup, if you wish.

Mix the batter by hand to keep the chewy texture and make your bar last longer. Or, if you're in a rush, throw it all into a food processor to make an easy job of it. Don't forget to soak the quinoa the night before, or in the morning if you're making it that evening.

After baking, slice this into bars – large for breakfast or small for sweet snacks – freeze and defrost as needed. If we're at home, we warm a slice in the oven, spread over some almond butter and enjoy with a cup of tea.

MAKES 10 BARS OR 20 SMALL SQUARES

2 ripe bananas, about 3 oz each

9 oz quinoa (activated overnight page 300)

2 tbsp chia seeds

3 ½ oz shredded coconut

3 ½ oz chestnut flour (or 2 oz coconut flour)

1 ½ oz butter at room temperature or coconut oil, plus extra for greasing

1 ½ oz sesame seeds (or hemp seeds), plus extra for sprinkling on top

1 tbsp ground cinnamon

1 tbsp vanilla extract

½ tsp sea salt

2 tbsp maple syrup

1 ¾ oz dried cranberries (or use goji berries)

**OPTIONAL**

1 extra banana, for extra sweetness

**1** Preheat the oven to fan 350°F. Butter a 10 x 8 in baking dish (or smaller for a thicker bar).

**2** Mash the bananas by hand in a bowl, then mix in the rest of the ingredients plus ½ cup of water. Or if using a food processor, combine all of the ingredients except the cranberries plus ½ cup water and process until just blended. Stir in the cranberries with a wooden spoon.

**3** Pour the mixture into the prepared dish and spread it out evenly. Sprinkle with extra sesame seeds, if you like.

**4** Bake for 50 minutes or more until lightly golden brown on top. Remove from the oven and leave to cool before turning out and slicing into bars or squares. Freeze the bars for the week ahead!

## INSTANT BLUEBERRY CHIA JAM

A quick jam with only 3 ingredients – and it all happens like magic. No cooking required. The little chia seeds swell with the blueberries to make a wobbly jelly-like topping that looks uncannily like blackberry jam. You can add lemon juice or vanilla or both, but we like it as it is. Unlike cooked jams full of sugar, this chia jam won't last long, but it's quick and easy enough to make up little batches regularly. This lasts for at least a week in the fridge, by which time it'll all be gone!

The sweet, sharp taste of the juicy blueberries is beautiful with a creamy plain yogurt, Blueberry Pancakes (page 30), layered up with Buckwheat Groat Bircher Muesli (page 46), or smeared over a toasted and buttered slice of our Multiseed Loaf (page 273).

MAKES ONE 14 OZ JAR

6 ½ oz fresh or frozen blueberries

2 ½ tbsp chia seeds

1–2 ½ tsp raw honey (depending on your sweet tooth – we find frozen blueberries are usually less sweet)

**OPTIONAL**

½ tsp vanilla extract and a squeeze of lemon juice

**1**  Mash the berries or blend them in a food processor.

**2**  Mix in the chia seeds, 1 tbsp warm water and 1 teaspoon of the honey. Stir well to stop clumps forming or make it straight in the jar and shake to mix.

**3**  Keep the chia jam sealed in a jar in the fridge to set for at least an hour or until needed.

**4**  Taste and stir in a little more honey, if needed.

## GOJI MARMALADE

Great layered up with our Buckwheat Groat Bircher Muesli (page 46), spread over buttered Multiseed Loaf toast (page 273), or added to a cheese board as an accompaniment.

MAKES 7 OZ

2 whole unwaxed oranges

3 tbsp raw set honey (we use set honey here instead of runny honey to keep the marmalade thick)

2 ¾ oz goji berries

3 tbsp chia seeds

sea salt

**1**  Grate the zest of the 2 whole oranges using a very fine grater – you need 1 compacted teaspoon of zest.

**2**  Peel the oranges and remove any seeds, then pulse the orange flesh in a food processor or blender along with the measured zest, the honey, and a tiny pinch of salt until smooth.

**3**  Add the goji berries and chia seeds to the blended orange mix and leave to soften for about 20 minutes.

**4**  Pulse the mixture again so that there are some chunky pieces of goji remaining. You can eat this straight away spread on our buttered toast or keep it in the fridge in a sealed jar for about a week. It also freezes well.

# MANGO CASHEW CREAM

This creamy sauce, made from soaked cashews, a little dried mango and vanilla, is easily whipped up and stored in the fridge for a week. Keep these cupboard ingredients on hand for those moments when you can't get your hands on proper probiotic dairy or coconut yogurt.

You need a powerful blender to make this a very smooth cream. Soak the mango directly in your blender to save washing up. Don't forget to KEEP the water that you soaked the mango in but NOT the cashew water.

You can also make this without the mango and just add a few teaspoons more of honey, but we find the mango adds a wonderful complexity to the sweetness of this cream and hides any cashew flavor.

This goes beautifully with Buckwheat Groat Bircher Muesli (page 46) and Blueberry Pancakes (page 30) as well as Pear and Five-spice Crumble (page 250) and the Chocolate Fig Pudding (page 252).

SERVES 6–8

3 oz whole cashew nuts (preferably activated, see step 1)

1 ½ oz dried mango

¾ tsp vanilla extract

1 tbsp raw honey

sea salt

**1** Soak the cashews for 3 hours in double their volume of water with ½ tsp sea salt. Be sure to discard the soaking water and rinse before using.

**2** Soak the mango in 1 ½ cups water for an hour or more (for a thicker cream, reduce the amount of soaking water for the mango) – we like to do this directly in the blender.

**3** Blend together the mango and the water it has been soaking in, the cashews, vanilla, raw honey, and a tiny pinch of salt until smooth. Add a little more water if you find the mixture too thick.

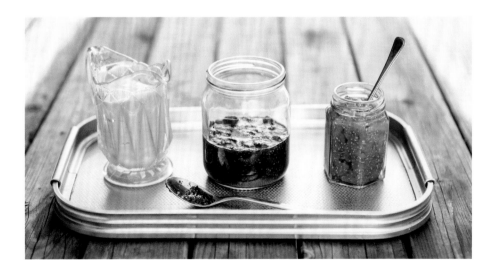

# SOUPS

**N**UTRIENT-RICH BONE BROTH IS AT THE HEART OF WHAT WE DO. Full of flavor and deeply nourishing, broth, also known as stock, made from meat and fish bones has been used as a cure-all remedy across cultures and, in our opinion, is the secret to a great-tasting soup.

Homemade soups offer a big dose of nourishment in every mouthful and are an inexpensive food, particularly if you use local, seasonal vegetables, which are always better value. The HEMSLEY + HEMSLEY Soup Service delivers delicious, nutrient-rich soups to help reset and fortify the body. We have numerous soup recipes (many of our favorites are here) inspired by the seasonal produce that arrives in our veg box deliveries. A well-cooked soup, packed with vegetables, removes much of the burden from your digestive system, allowing your body to direct its energy wherever it is needed most (hence chicken soup being a traditional food for the sick).

Soup is a regular meal for us. It's one of the most convenient ways to enjoy hot food on the go and at your desk, sipped straight from an insulated flask. It also makes a great late-night supper because your body can digest soup easily and quickly before you go to sleep. Just remember that you still need to take time while eating your soup, so don't gulp it down and flood your stomach.

No fancy knife skills needed here, just roughly chop the veg and simmer in the bone broth, along with an unlimited combination of herbs and spices. Cook large batches of soup at a time as they freeze and reheat brilliantly. Soups can be blended until silky smooth or left chunky. Always make sure that your soup is cool enough to eat before drizzling with a good quality flaxseed or extra-virgin olive oil to preserve the nutrients. Soups are a great way of using up leftover vegetables, meat, and pseudocereals – nothing beats the end-of-the-week-fridge-pot-luck soup!

Make a simple soup special enough to serve to guests by adding an array of toppings, such as toasted nuts and seeds, grated Parmesan, crumbled goats' cheese, or even broken Carrot and Flax Crackers as croutons (page 121). Drizzle over some homemade pesto, dressing, or sauce, such as our Kale Pesto (page 233), Brazil Nut Cream (page 54), or Chimichurri Sauce (page 158) for a decorative swirl of contrasting color, taste, and texture, or finish with a spoonful of any one of our dips (from pages 231–235), a lime wedge, a sprinkle of chopped fresh chives, a dash of smoked paprika or lemon zest – the list is endless.

One of our favorite meals is a salad and soup combination. We heat up a bowl of soup, then top it with our Quicker-than-toast Zucchini Salad on page 84 or any salad leaves we have in the fridge. The hot and cold complement each other and the textures of the crunchy salad mixed with a hot, smooth soup works beautifully – it's a great way of enjoying raw food in winter.

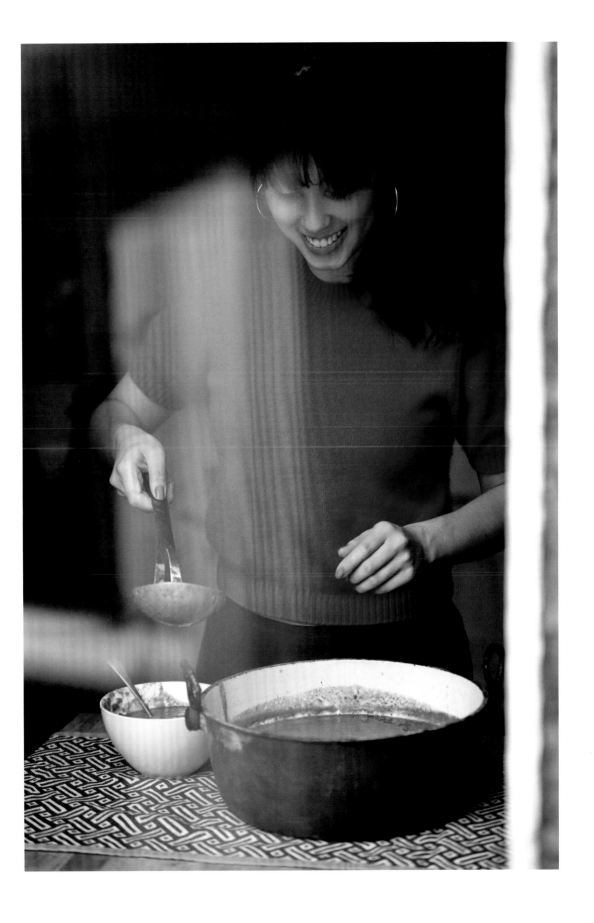

# WATERCRESS SOUP WITH BRAZIL NUT CREAM

Watercress is bursting with vital nutrients and minerals and it's one of the best things to eat before exercise as its abundance of iron helps red blood cells carry oxygen to the body's tissues for energy. The natural fats in the Brazil nuts, olive oil, butter, and homemade bone broth make this a nourishing and satisfying meal – definitely no need to fill up on bread with this soup.

Brazil nuts don't need activating so this is a quick pesto to pull together, but you'll need a strong blender to get it smooth. As an alternative, you could also drizzle the soup with a little flaxseed oil or extra virgin olive oil and add a squeeze of lemon and a grind of black pepper if you prefer.

SERVES 3

### FOR THE WATERCRESS SOUP

2 tsp ghee or coconut oil

1 large onion, roughly chopped

2 garlic cloves, roughly diced, or a small handful of wild garlic if you can get it (our favorite)

5 oz celery root, peeled of all the knobbly bits and any green parts, roughly diced

1 quart bone broth (page 300) or vegetable stock

14 oz watercress, stalks and leaves (give it a good wash)

sea salt and black pepper (being careful with the pepper as watercress is already quite peppery)

fresh or ground nutmeg, to garnish (optional)

### FOR THE BRAZIL NUT CREAM

16 Brazil nuts

2 tbsp lemon juice, about ½ large lemon

2 tbsp extra virgin olive oil

2 pinches of sea salt

2 pinches of black pepper

**1** Heat the ghee or coconut oil in a large saucepan with a lid over a low heat and gently fry the onion and garlic for about 5 minutes until softened but not brown.

**2** Turn up the heat to medium and add the celery root, stirring to coat with the ghee or oil.

**3** Add the bone broth, and salt and pepper to taste.

**4** Put the lid on and leave to simmer for about 15–20 minutes, or until the celery root is tender. Turn off the heat.

**5** Meanwhile, blend the ingredients for the Brazil nut cream in a blender with 4 tablespoons of warm water. Season to taste and transfer to a small jug or bowl to serve — add more water if needed to get a smoother consistency.

**6** Without washing the blender, pour in the celery root soup base and add the watercress. If the blender is small, then do this in batches. Alternatively, carefully blend the soup together in the saucepan using a hand-held blender. Add more liquid if you want to adjust the consistency and blend for longer if you'd like a really smooth soup.

**7** Season to taste and ladle into bowls. Drizzle with the Brazil nut cream and top with a sprinkle of freshly grated or ground nutmeg, if desired.

✛ **INSTEAD OF BRAZIL NUTS** you could use a handful of cashew nuts (preferably activated page 302).

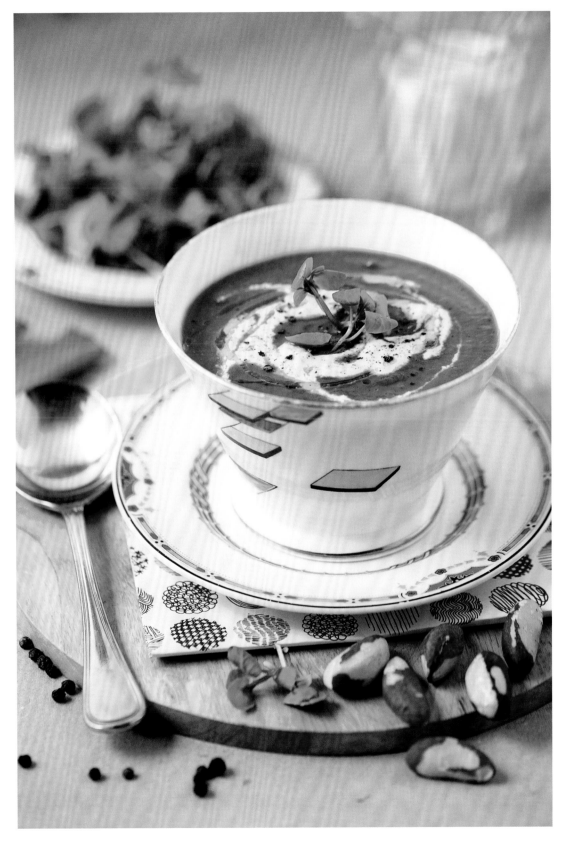

# CHICKEN TINOLA

Introducing Chicken Tinola, a favorite dish of the Philippines and a taste of our childhood. This soup of poached chicken, and plenty of onions, garlic, and ginger is great for restoring one's health — the homemade chicken broth is key, so make sure you have a batch ready to go. You can then save the carcass or bones from the poached chicken for your next batch of broth. Serve with a squeeze of lemon juice for an immune-boosting dish that is flavorsome, soothing, and warming.

SERVES 6

### FOR THE CHICKEN TINOLA

2 tbsp ghee or coconut oil

3 large onions, diced

8 garlic cloves, diced

a thumb-sized piece of fresh root ginger (about 1 ½ oz) – unpeeled if organic – finely diced or grated

1 large chicken or 6 large chicken thighs

6 large carrots, chopped into medium chunks

2 quarts (half a gallon) bone broth (page 300) or water

3 large zucchinis, chopped into medium chunks

1 large green or white cabbage, shredded

sea salt and white or black pepper

### FOR THE TAMARI LEMON DRESSING

4 tbsp tamari

4 tbsp lemon juice

a large pinch of white pepper (or black)

**1** Heat the ghee or coconut oil in a large saucepan (large enough to fit a whole chicken, if using) over a medium heat and gently sauté the onion, garlic, and ginger until soft and translucent, but not browned.

**2** Add the chicken and carrot to the pan and pour over the bone broth to cover. Bring to the boil, then reduce the heat immediately and simmer for 30 minutes or until the chicken is cooked through.

**3** Remove the cooked chicken from the pan and add the zucchini. Simmer for 10 minutes. Meanwhile, shred the chicken into large pieces using a knife and fork, return to the pan and season.

**4** Stir through the shredded cabbage and turn off the heat.

**5** Mix the ingredients for the tamari lemon dressing together in a small bowl. Serve alongside the tinola and let everyone add a teaspoon or so to taste.

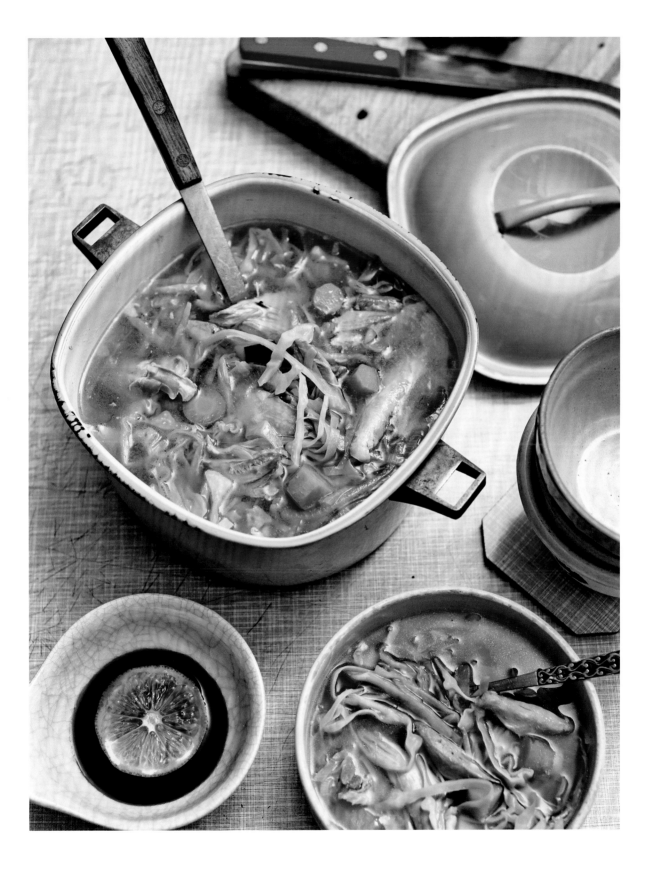

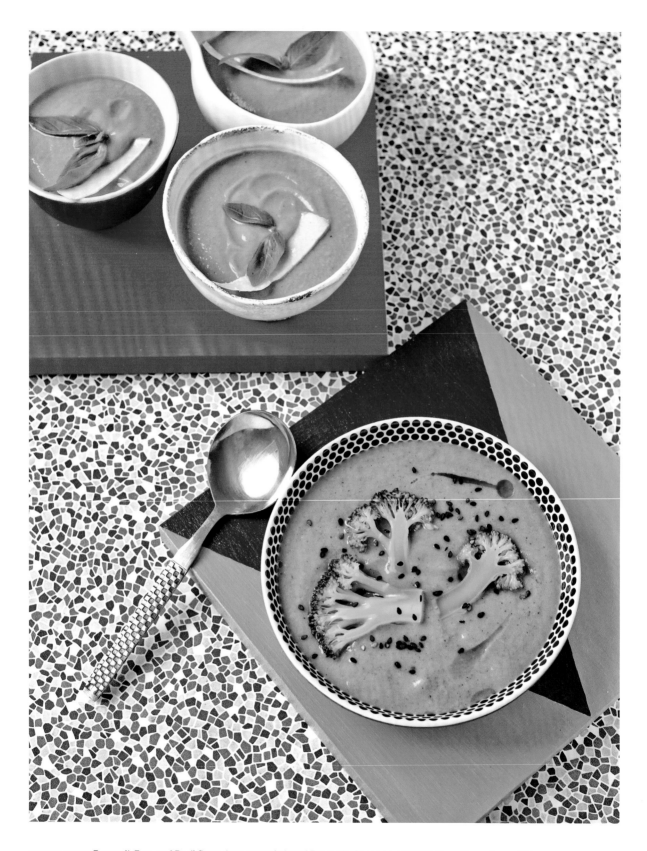

**LEFT TO RIGHT:** Broccoli, Pea, and Basil Soup (see opposite) and Broccoli, Ginger, and White Bean Soup (page 60).

## BROCCOLI, PEA, AND BASIL SOUP

A pea soup is delicious but very sweet and starchy by itself, so the added green goodness of broccoli balances it out. This soup is a great way of using up the less popular broccoli stalks – after enjoying the florets for stir-fries and roast dinners, we freeze the stalks, ready to make a big batch of soup like this. With plenty of garlic and basil, it tastes like a comforting bowl of pesto, so much so that we were inspired to make a thick version to top bruschetta with (page 115).

For a creamier soup with a ginger and cayenne kick, try our other favorite broccoli soup (page 60).

SERVES 6

2 tbsp ghee

2 large onions, roughly chopped

2 garlic cloves, diced

3 celery sticks, roughly chopped

a large pinch of dried oregano

2 ¾ oz fresh basil (pull the leaves from the stalks and roughly chop the stalks)

3 ⅓ lb broccoli, slice the stalks and roughly chop the florets

6 cups bone broth (page 300) or vegetable stock

18 oz frozen peas

juice of 1 lemon

extra virgin olive oil or flaxseed oil, to serve

a little parmesan

sea salt and black pepper

**1**  Heat the ghee in a saucepan with a lid over a low heat and gently fry the onion for 10 minutes until soft, stirring occasionally.

**2**  Add the garlic, celery, oregano, and chopped basil stalks and stir.

**3**  Add the broccoli, broth, and a large pinch of salt and pepper and stir.

**4**  Bring to a medium simmer, pop the lid on, and simmer gently for 10–15 minutes until the broccoli stalks and florets are just tender (you don't want to overcook the broccoli).

**5**  Remove from the heat and add the peas, basil leaves, and half the lemon juice.

**6**  Blend the soup (in batches if needs be), adding a little more liquid if it's too thick. Check for seasoning and finish with an extra squeeze of lemon juice if needed.

**7**  Serve each bowl with a drizzle of extra virgin olive oil or flaxseed oil and a shaving of parmesan.

## BROCCOLI, GINGER, AND WHITE BEAN SOUP

Easy to digest and warming, we use a stainless steel flask to keep this soup piping hot for a meal on the go. It keeps our internal fire stoked with plenty of vegetables, spices, and herbs. Broccoli stalks are not as pretty as the flowery tops, but with just as much nutrition, it makes sense to save them and blend them into a tasty soup full of antioxidants. If you don't have any bone broth on hand, then use some quality miso (we always have some traditionally fermented miso paste handy in our fridge).

Soup and bread go hand-in-hand, but we steer clear of improperly prepared grains and the refined gluten-free loaf alternatives. Instead, we make our soup into a more hearty meal by blending in some cooked white beans. You could also use celery root or, for a creamy taste, whip in a few soaked cashews or almonds.

SERVES 4

1 tbsp coconut oil

2 large onions, roughly chopped

5 garlic cloves, diced

a large piece of fresh root ginger (about 5 ⅔ oz) – unpeeled if organic – roughly chopped

a small pinch of cayenne pepper

1 ⅓ lb broccoli, slice the stalks and roughly chop the florets

1 quart bone broth (page 300) or vegetable stock

1 tin (9 oz drained weight) of cannellini, navy, or butter beans (soak and boil your own page 300)

4 large handfuls of fresh cilantro

juice of 2 small limes or 1 large lemon

2–3 tbsp tamari or 2–3 large pinches of sea salt

black pepper, to taste

flaxseed oil

**1**  Heat the coconut oil in a large saucepan over a low heat and gently fry the onion, garlic, ginger, and cayenne pepper for 5 minutes.

**2**  Add the broccoli stalks and the broth. Bring to boil, then reduce the heat immediately and simmer on a medium heat for 8 minutes.

**3**  Add the broccoli florets, beans, and cilantro. After 5 minutes cooking, use a knife to pierce the broccoli. If tender, then turn the heat off and leave to cool slightly before you start blending. If you want to keep some whole broccoli florets for serving on top of your soup, remove them now.

**4**  Add the fresh lime or lemon juice, the tamari or sea salt, and pepper and blend. Taste and check for seasoning.

**5**  Serve with a drizzle of flaxseed oil and add more cayenne, if you dare!

# RIBOLLITA WITH PARSLEY LEMON OIL

Ribollita is a traditional peasant dish from Italy that's bulked out with potatoes and bread. Our ribollita-inspired soup is satisfying without being heavy and has received the approval of our Italian family friends. This is even better the next day and you can make it in advance without the leafy greens. To serve, reheat the ribollita, adding the greens at the end. In the summer, add some chopped zucchinis or in the winter, a little turnip or celery root – it's a great dish for using up leftover bits and bobs of veg. We like to accompany this soup with a little bowl of parsley lemon oil for a bit of a zing.

SERVES 4

**FOR THE RIBOLLITA**

2 tins of cooked cannellini beans (drained weight 18 oz) or 18 oz homecooked beans (dried weight 7 oz, activated overnight see page 300)

2 tsp ghee

2 large onions, diced

2 celery sticks, diced

1 bay leaf

3 garlic cloves, diced

2 large carrots, diced

½ tsp dried oregano

½ tsp dried basil

¼ tsp fennel seeds

¼ tsp chili flakes

3 ⅓ cup bone broth (page 300) or vegetable stock

1 tin of tomatoes (or in the summer, use 6 large tomatoes)

7 oz cabbage, dinosaur kale, or kale (stalks removed), sliced in half and then into ribbons

sea salt and black pepper

a large handful of grated parmesan, to serve

a parmesan rind to flavor the broth (optional)

**FOR THE PARSLEY LEMON OIL**

a large handful of fresh parsley, finely chopped

5 tbsp extra virgin olive oil

juice of 1 lemon

sea salt and black pepper

**1** Drain the beans and rinse them.

**2** Heat the ghee in a large saucepan with a lid over a low heat and gently sauté the onion, celery, and bay leaf for 8 minutes until softened.

**3** Add the garlic, carrots, oregano, basil, fennel seeds, chili flakes, bone broth, and parmesan rind, if using, to the pan. Bring just to boil, then reduce the heat immediately and simmer, covered, for 8 minutes.

**4** Meanwhile, make the parsley lemon oil. Whisk the chopped parsley in a bowl with the extra virgin olive oil, lemon, and some seasoning. Set aside.

**5** Add the tomatoes and rinsed and drained beans to the pan and continue to simmer for a further 8 minutes, stirring occasionally.

**6** Stir through the dinosaur kale, cabbage, or kale (kale will need a few minutes longer and should be sliced very finely) and cook for a further 5 minutes, tasting for seasoning.

**7** Scoop out the parmesan rind and discard, if using. Ladle the soup into bowls, scatter over the freshly grated parmesan, and drizzle over the parsley lemon oil.

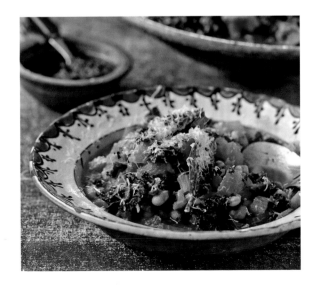

## ROASTED TOMATO AND BUTTERNUT SQUASH SOUP

Everyone loves a tomato soup, but as a main meal people often find they need bread to give it substance. We prefer to fill up on veggies, so butternut squash provides the perfect blend for a thick, smooth soup, simmered with fresh rosemary, lots of garlic, and plenty of bone broth.

The sweet squash also helps to counteract the acidity that you can find in tomato-heavy dishes and adds a sweetness that only usually comes with long, slow cooking (or added sugar!). Cooking tomatoes enhances their nutritional value by increasing the lycopene content that can be absorbed by the body. Lycopene is an antioxidant (a fighter of free radical damage in the body) and has been shown to improve the skin's ability to protect against harmful UV rays. Out of tomato season, use tinned tomatoes or, even better, passata.

This soup is popular with children and, since its sweet, creamy taste is also gentle on the taste buds first thing in the morning, we love to eat it for breakfast.

**SERVES 6**

6 ½ lb butternut squash (you can use different squashes, but make sure there is at least one butternut for sweetness)

2 ⅔ lb fresh tomatoes or passata or 3 tins of chopped or plum tomatoes

3 large onions, roughly chopped

1 garlic bulb

2 tbsp ghee or coconut oil

4 tsp of fresh rosemary leaves or 2 tsp dried rosemary

6 cups bone broth (page 300) or vegetable stock (more or less depending on how thick you like your soups)

extra virgin olive oil or flaxseed oil, to drizzle

sea salt and black pepper

**OPTIONAL**

parmesan shavings and extra finely chopped rosemary leaves, to garnish

**1**  Preheat the oven to fan 425°F.

**2**  Halve the squash and fresh tomatoes, if using, and lay on one or two baking trays, flesh side up. Add the onion and the garlic bulb. Bake in the oven for 30–45 minutes until the squash is tender.

**3**  Gently heat the ghee or coconut oil in a large saucepan and fry the rosemary for a few minutes. If you're using tinned tomatoes or passata, add them now and let the tomato sauce simmer for 20 minutes.

**4**  Add the roasted onions, roasted fresh tomatoes, if using, and any juices to the saucepan. Scoop out the squash flesh, squeeze 6 cloves of roasted garlic out of their skins (you can use the remaining roasted garlic in sauces or dressings), and add to the pan too.

**5**  Cover with broth, starting with just over 4 cups, turn up the heat and bring to a medium simmer. Simmer with the lid on for 20 minutes to let the flavors combine, adding more bone broth if it seems too thick. Blend until smooth and season to taste.

**6**  Drizzle each bowl with extra virgin olive oil or flaxseed oil and add a few parmesan shavings and some finely chopped fresh rosemary leaves.

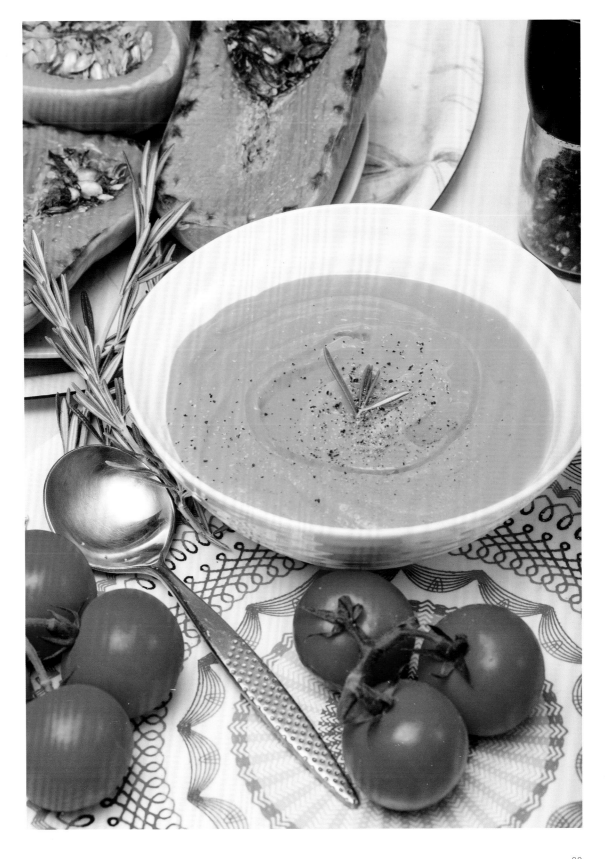

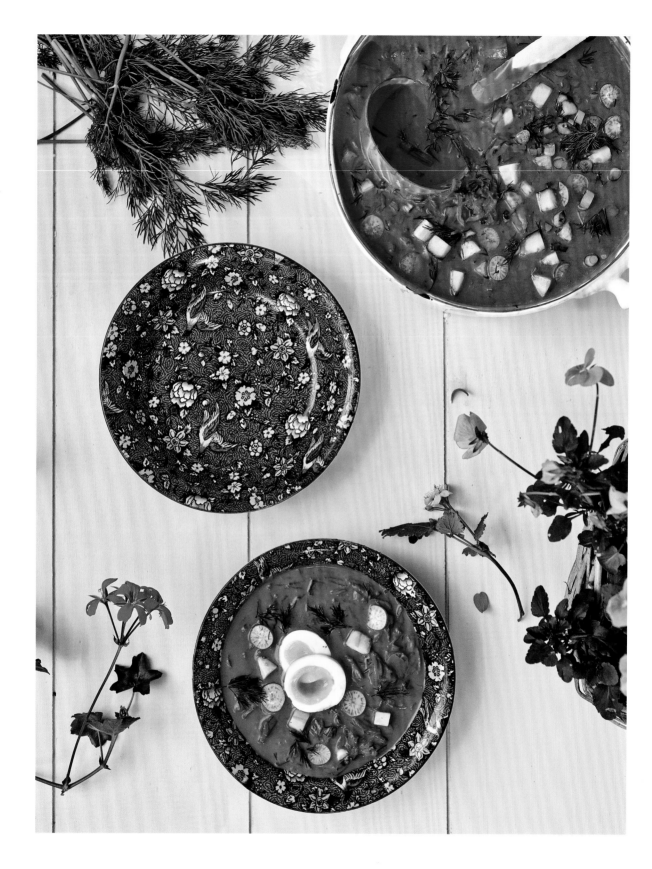

# CHILLED PINK BEET SOUP

We love pink soup! The traditional Polish dish Chlodnik is, for us, the true taste of summer. Our easy version is one that our Filipino family has grown very fond of – so much so that we're dedicating this recipe to our Auntie Angelina who, after trying this creamy and refreshing soup, requests it at every family get together.

Look for young beets with their long stalks and the leaves still attached – if you can't get hold of any, then chard is a great substitute. The traditional recipe has sauerkraut juice in it – a great way to use up any of the juice leftover from our homemade Sauerkraut (page 306) and to enjoy some probiotics – just add a few tablespoons to taste. We recommend you wear an apron to make this and a bib or napkin to eat it!

SERVES 8

6 beets (roughly 1 ½ lb), washed

18 oz full-fat probiotic natural yogurt

3½ tbsp lemon juice

2½ tsp sea salt

1 large cucumber, peeled and diced into ¾ in cubes

6 radishes, halved lengthways and finely sliced

6 scallions, finely sliced

a large handful of fresh dill, chopped, plus extra to garnish

4 garlic cloves, diced

### OPTIONAL

2–3 hard-boiled eggs, chopped

**1** Remove the leaves and stalks from the beet and chop fairly coarsely. Discard the knobbly tops of the beets and use washing-up gloves to peel and grate them (we use a food processor for ease).

**2** Place the grated beet in a saucepan with 1 ⅓ cup water. Bring to boil, then reduce the heat immediately and simmer for 5 minutes. Add the beet stalks and leaves for the last 2 minutes. Remove from the heat and leave to cool.

**3** Combine the yogurt and ⅔ cup water with the lemon juice and 2 teaspoons of salt in a large bowl, whisking to a smooth consistency.

**4** Add all the chopped vegetables, plus the dill, garlic, grated beet, chopped stalks and leaves, and the cooking liquid and mix thoroughly.

**5** Taste for seasoning, adding more salt and lemon juice, if you prefer.

**6** Enjoy straight away or, for an even better flavor, refrigerate, covered, for at least 4–6 hours or overnight.

**7** Serve cool or at room temperature, garnished with plenty more fresh dill and the optional chopped hard-boiled eggs.

# VIETNAMESE CHICKEN PHO WITH ZUCCHINI NOODLES

So much more than a soup, a really good pho or noodle soup can change your day. The key to all soups, both for flavor and sustenance, is a nourishing bone broth and you can really taste the difference here. Star anise, cloves, cinnamon, and fish sauce are essential ingredients in this soup. If you love Asian flavors, then stock up on these store cupboard favorites, which you can make use of all year round in many other sweet and savory dishes.

Zucchini noodles replace refined rice noodles and, as well as chicken, we like to use prawns and leftover shredded beef – or simply drop in an egg. A good pinch of dried seaweed, such as wakame, can be added for extra nutrients during the last 6–8 minutes of the cooking time, or add fresh or rehydrated seaweed at the end.

SERVES 4

## FOR THE PHO

2 quarts (half a gallon) bone broth (page 300) or vegetable stock

1 cinnamon stick or ¼ tsp ground cinnamon

2 large onions, finely diced

a thumb-sized piece of fresh root ginger (about 1 ½ oz) – unpeeled if organic – finely diced or grated

2 garlic cloves, finely diced or grated

2 tbsp fish sauce

4 whole cloves

2 star anise

grated zest of 1 unwaxed lime or lemon (avoid the bitter white pith)

4 chicken thighs, skin on

4 zucchinis

5 oz green beans, halved

sea salt

## TO SERVE

2 tbsp peanuts (preferably "crispy" activated, page 302)

1 red chili, finely sliced

2 limes, quartered

1 tbsp fresh mint leaves, roughly chopped

1 tbsp fresh basil leaves or Thai basil if you can get it, roughly chopped

2 handfuls of fresh cilantro, roughly chopped

a handful of radishes, sliced

2 scallions, sliced

a little bowl of tamari

5 oz bean sprouts

**1** In a large dry pan, toast the peanuts over a gentle heat for a minute until golden, giving the pan a shake to make sure they are golden all over, then set aside the peanuts.

**2** In the same pan, add the broth, cinnamon, onion, fresh ginger, garlic, a pinch of salt, fish sauce, cloves, star anise, and lime or lemon zest. Bring to a medium simmer.

**3** Add the chicken thighs, reduce the heat to a low simmer and gently cook for 25–30 minutes to let the flavors infuse into the chicken.

**4** Meanwhile, use a spiralizer or julienne peeler to make the zucchini noodles. Or use a regular vegetable peeler to slice the zucchinis lengthways into very wide pappardelle-style ribbons. You might want to cut the long strands in half to make them easier to eat.

**5** Roughly chop the toasted peanuts or crush them with the back of a knife. Arrange the peanuts, chili, lime wedges, mint, basil, half the cilantro, radishes, and scallions in separate dishes as accompaniments to the pho, along with the bowl of tamari.

**6** Once the chicken is cooked through, remove to a plate to cool, then shred using two forks.

**7** Strain the broth and taste for flavor. Return to the pan with the halved green beans and simmer for about 3 minutes.

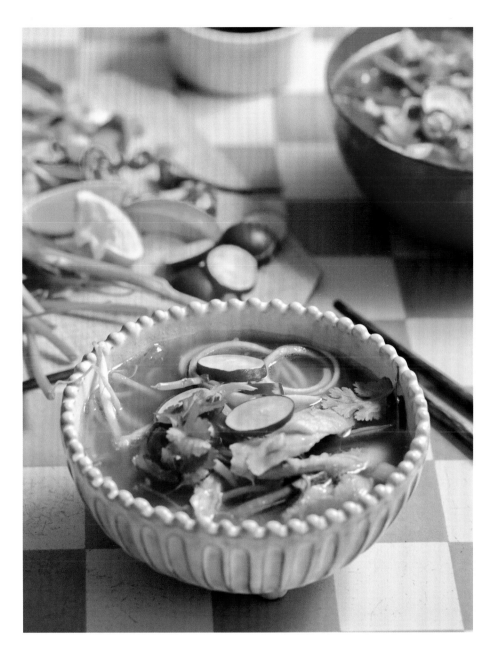

**8** Add the shredded chicken to warm through along with the zucchini noodles and the rest of the cilantro.

**9** Divide the pho among 4 bowls, top each with a small handful of bean sprouts and a lime wedge, and let everyone help themselves to the rest of the accompaniments.

**+ FOR A VERY QUICK PRAWN VERSION** skip step 3 and 6, then, after you strain the broth, add 12 oz raw peeled prawns (or 14 oz prawns with shells on) and simmer for a minute, then add the green beans and simmer for a further 3 minutes.

# KELP POT NOODLE

**SERVES 1**

Here's an instant hot dish to see you through working week lunches – no microwave needed. If it's a comforting bowl of goodness that you're after, then all you need is 10 minutes to throw any leftover veggies or coleslaw, shredded chicken or cooked quinoa into a heatproof jar before you leave for work or do it the night before. Come lunchtime, just add boiling water and wait 5 minutes for the magic to happen.

### FOR THE BASIC KELP POT NOODLE

1 ¼ oz kelp noodles

a pinch of dried dulse or other seaweed/sea vegetable (see page 23 for our favorites)

½ tsp grated fresh root ginger (unpeeled if organic)

1 tbsp chopped fresh cilantro or mint

a squeeze of lemon or lime juice

2 tsp unpasteurized miso paste

plus your choice of steamed veg, such as green beans, broccoli, and cabbage, and raw veg, such as sliced mushrooms, peppers, bok choy, scallion, grated carrot, and zucchini

### OPTIONAL

a few tablespoons of cooked quinoa, a chopped soft-boiled egg, or shredded chicken

**1** Rinse the kelp noodles and drain.

**2** Add everything to the heatproof jar with the miso. Keep refrigerated until ready to eat.

**3** Five minutes before you want to eat, boil the kettle. Let the water cool for a few minutes before filling the jar, leaving ¾ in from the top empty. Stir and leave to steep for 5 minutes with the lid on loosely. Stir again before diving in.

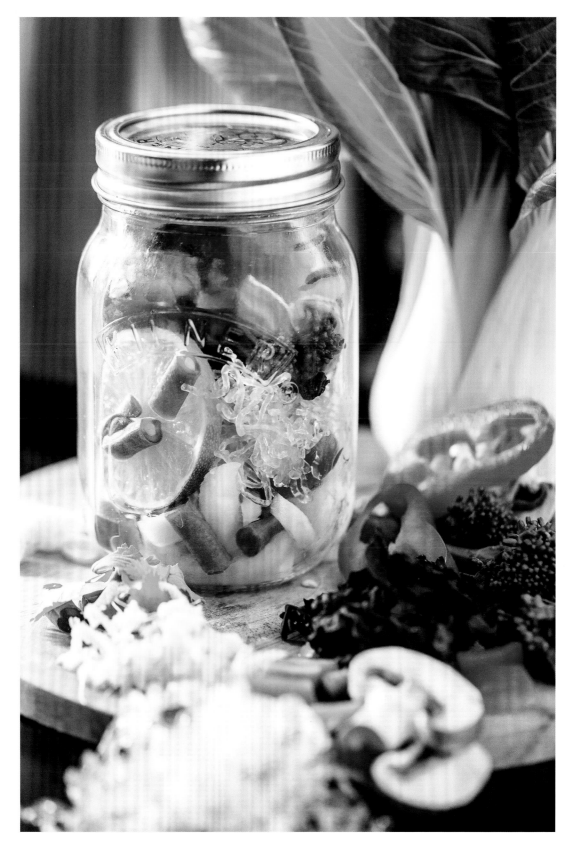

# NO-COOK COCONUT SOUP

This is one of our favorite soups because it's just so easy to make. Similar in many ways to our Go To Green Smoothie on page 284, both are essentially quick, savory smoothies enjoyed as chilled soups.

Rich and aromatic, this soup is sweet, spicy, sour, salty, and full of nutrients, with good fats from the coconut and avocado, probiotics from the fermented miso paste, and immune-boosting lime, garlic, onion, and ginger. Chilled or warmed, it's perfect for hot and cold days alike and with a strong blender it only takes a few minutes to make. This would be a great starter to a dinner party or a quick no-cook lunch.

SERVES 2

## FOR THE SOUP

1 tin of full-fat coconut milk

2 ¾ oz tomatoes, roughly chopped

½ an avocado

1 garlic clove

a thumb-sized piece of fresh root ginger (about 1 ½ oz) – unpeeled if organic – roughly chopped

3 tbsp unpasteurized miso paste

½ tsp sea salt

juice of 1 lime or lemon

¼ small onion or 2 spring onions

a tiny pinch of cayenne pepper

½ handful of fresh cilantro or a little mint or Thai basil

## TO SERVE

a tiny pinch of cayenne pepper or to taste

finely chopped fresh cilantro

**1** Blend all the soup ingredients together, adding a little water if you like it thinner.

**2** Serve chilled or, on a cold day, warm gently on the stove top and stir in the miso just before serving to preserve the probiotic benefits.

**3** Finish with a pinch of cayenne pepper and a sprinkling of chopped cilantro.

✛ **IF YOU'RE USING A HAND BLENDER** roughly chop the avocado and garlic clove before blending them with the rest of the soup ingredients.

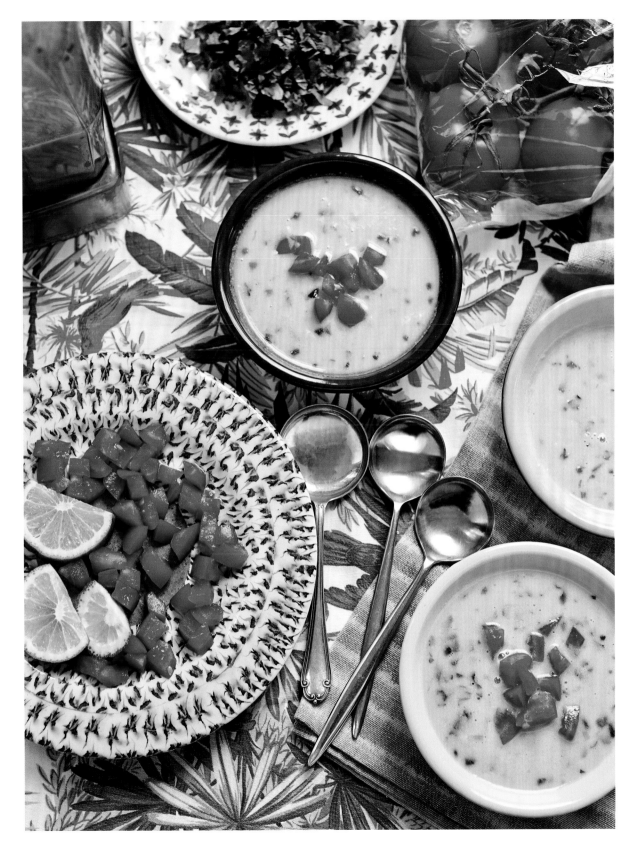

# SALADS

**S**ALAD ADDS A SPLASH OF GREEN AND A PALATE-CLEANSING FRESHNESS TO ANY DISH BUT CAN ALSO BE A COMPLETE MEAL. In this chapter we're talking about more than just a bowl of leaves. These are satisfying and nutrient-rich plates of food with a myriad of flavors and textures, often mixing both raw and cooked ingredients.

Think about creating a salad like you would any other nourishing meal. You need a good balance of seasonal vegetables, plenty of good fats, plus some protein or starch to satisfy.

In keeping with simple food combining (see page 14), we've created starch- or protein-based salads in order to avoid mixing these food groups for better digestion and to ensure more space on your plate is dedicated to lots of green veg. Start with a base of low-starch green vegetables like broccoli, green beans, kale, and salad leaves, then top with pseudocereals or high-starch veg, such as roasted beets. Alternatively, for a protein-rich salad, add some leftover roast chicken, fish, or sliced steak. We prefer eating raw food earlier in the day so in the evenings try a dish of sautéed veg for a warm salad experience in the evenings.

The perfect partner to a salad is a rich and zingy dressing, which can transform the plainest plate into a mouth-watering affair. Complete your salad with a drizzle of lemon juice and extra virgin olive oil or one of our dressings or dips (pages 228–235).

Along with an oil-based dressing, a sprinkle of crunchy nuts and seeds can add quality fats to help absorb fat-soluble vitamins found in meat and vegetables, while topping your salad with a probiotic side like Kimchi or Sauerkraut (pages 307–308 and 306–307) will further aid digestion.

As well as creating fresh flavors and textures, salads are even more enticing when they look visually vibrant. After all, your body starts preparing for digestion the moment it sees and smells food so give it something beautiful to look at and eat a rainbow of colors. Experiment with textures: grate, spiralise, chop, slice, and dice your vegetables.

Add fresh or dried fruits to a salad for a sweet and sour contrast. Try enzyme-rich pineapple and papaya (including the radishy tasting black papaya seeds), a handful of sliced peaches and apples, or a scattering of dried cranberries. (Note: for those with poor digestion, you will find it more beneficial to eat fruit separately). Prioritize organic, thin-skinned fruit and veg when shopping. Organic vegetables are free from chemical sprays and are always grown in soil so expect some mud, grit, and the odd bug (if a bug is living on your lettuce, then it's a really good sign that it is free from toxic pesticides).

With the above in mind, it's worth having a good salad spinner to drain washed leaves – soggy leaves are a menace and will dilute the flavors of your dressing. Avoid pre-washed, pre-packed bags of salad, if possible, because they are often washed in a solution of chlorine, which is far from natural or good for you. If bagged salad is your only option, then seek out organic or choose unwashed or packs washed in spring water. See page 12 for more on organic produce.

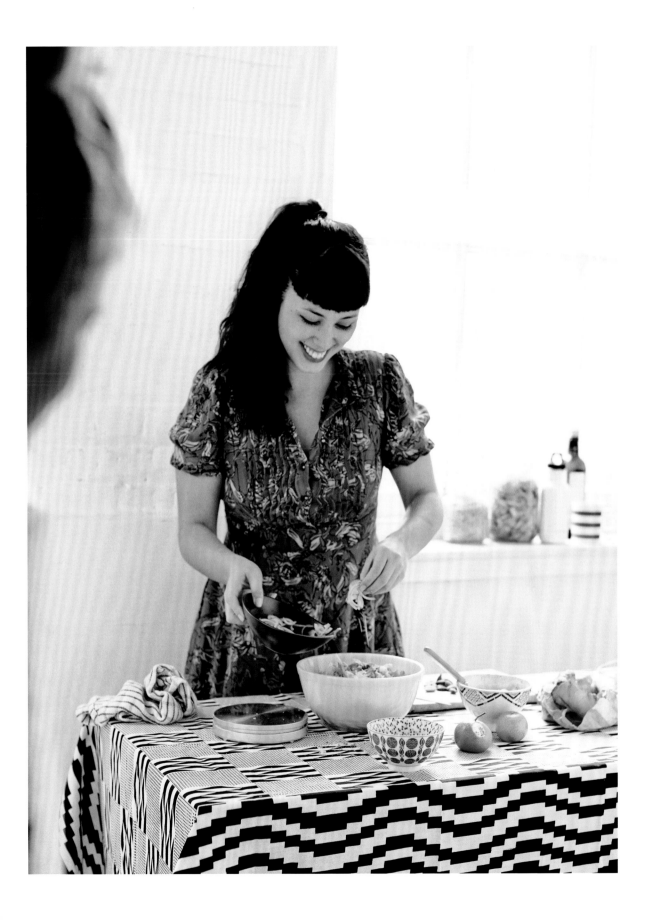

# SUPERFOOD SALAD WITH MISO TAHINI DRESSING

SERVES 2

As the name suggests, this salad is packed with a number of tasty superfoods: seaweed, onion, broccoli, asparagus, and the Asian wonder shiitake. Rich in B vitamins and protein, shiitake mushrooms are also a great source of iron, helping to improve the circulation of oxygen through the blood. Eat them regularly to strengthen your immune system. This health-boosting mushroom lends a "meaty" bite to our crunchy salad.

## FOR THE SALAD

2 tbsp dried arame seaweed or other sea vegetables like dried dulse (see page 23 for our favorites)

1 tbsp furikake (a mix of sesame seeds and dried seaweed) or 1 tbsp black and white sesame seeds

1 tbsp coconut oil

6 large shiitake mushrooms, cut into slices about ¼ in thick (don't wash them, just brush the dirt off with a kitchen towel) or use 9 oz other mushrooms

10 ½ oz asparagus (once you snap off the woody ends you'll be left with approximately 7 oz)

7 oz purple sprouting broccoli (or use Tenderstem or normal broccoli)

7 oz green beans

1 head of endive (the red/purple colored ones add a splash of color)

½ small red onion, thinly sliced or 2 scallions, sliced on the angle

1 red chili, finely sliced

a handful of chopped fresh cilantro

½ handful of chopped fresh mint

## FOR THE MISO TAHINI DRESSING

1 tbsp tahini

1 tbsp sweet white miso paste

1½ tbsp lemon or lime juice

1 tbsp sesame oil (not toasted)

a small piece of fresh root ginger (about 1 ½ oz, unpeeled if organic), finely grated

a pinch of sea salt or ¼ tsp tamari, to taste

**1** Soak the arame in water for about 8–10 minutes, or according to the packet instructions. Drain and rinse.

**2** Dry fry the furikake or sesame seeds in a large frying pan for a minute until toasted, then set them aside.

**3** In the same pan, heat the coconut oil over a medium heat, then fry the sliced mushrooms, in batches, for a minute on each side until browned. Avoid overcrowding the pan otherwise they tend to steam. Remove and set aside.

**4** Using the same frying pan, add the asparagus, broccoli, green beans, and about 2 tablespoons of water or just enough to cover the bottom of the pan. Cover and steam for 2 minutes until al dente, then remove, rinse with cold water, and drain.

**5** To make the dressing, mix all the ingredients together with 2 tablespoons of water and blend until smooth and creamy, whisking with a fork (using a little hot water if the tahini is really thick).

**6** Slice the end off the endive and then slice the leaves into ribbons. Arrange with the cooked vegetables, the arame seaweed, onion, and chili in a serving dish and add the chopped herbs. Dress with the miso tahini dressing and scatter over the toasted furikake or seeds.

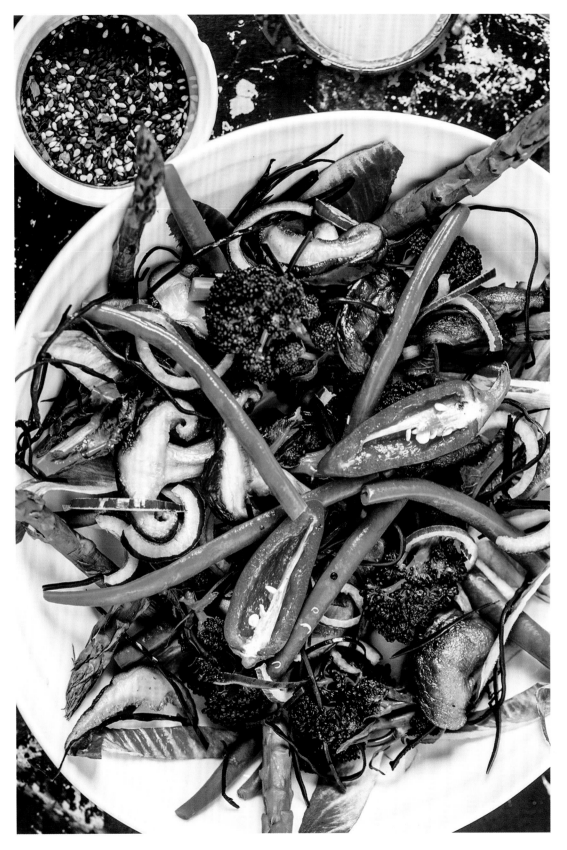

# PAPAYA, HALLOUMI, AND WATERCRESS SALAD

The perfect, speedy summer salad. It's nutrient-dense and encompasses all the five discernable flavors: bitter, sweet, sour, spicy, and salty. Perfect for a day when you feel in need of something fresh and zingy to awaken sluggish taste buds.

Papaya has three very powerful antioxidants – vitamins C, E, and A – but best of all it contains papain, an enzyme that helps digest proteins. We buy the long, large variety of papaya found in local grocery stores; it's ripe when the skin is yellow, smells fragrant, and looks almost bruised, yielding a little when you press it. Papaya helps to cleanse and soothe the digestive tract, calming indigestion and gas and restoring balance to your intestinal bacteria. You'll notice that we use watercress in any meal we can, and here its peppery, fresh flavors are the perfect accompaniment to salty, caramelized halloumi and the sweet papaya.

SERVES 4

## FOR THE SALAD

4 large handfuls of watercress

a container of cherry or baby plum tomatoes, halved

1 red onion, finely sliced

2 large avocados, flesh scooped out and sliced

a handful of pine nuts or pumpkin or sunflower seeds (preferably "crispy" activated, pages 300–302)

½ a large papaya

1 tsp ghee

9 oz pack of halloumi, sliced ½ in thick (seek out 100 percent sheep or goats' milk varieties of halloumi for a better flavor)

sea salt and black pepper

## FOR THE DRESSING

4 tbsp extra virgin olive oil

a squeeze of raw runny honey

1½ tbsp apple cider vinegar or lime or lemon juice

**1** Snip the watercress into bite-sized pieces and arrange it over a large, flat serving dish.

**2** Scatter the tomatoes, onion, and avocado over the bed of watercress and sprinkle over a touch of sea salt (not too much as the halloumi is salty).

**3** Toast the pine nuts in a dry frying pan, then set aside.

**4** Halve the papaya and scoop out the seeds (you can keep the seeds to add to smoothies or salad dressings – they taste like radishes so use sparingly). Using a large spoon, scoop out thick slivers of the papaya flesh and pile onto the salad. If you're struggling to make it look nice, then try slicing or cubing the fruit.

**5** Heat the ghee to a high temperature in a large frying pan and fry the halloumi slices in batches for about a minute on each side until each piece takes on a golden brown color – keep your eye on them, too long and they toughen up. Lay the hot halloumi across the salad.

**6** Sprinkle over the toasted pine nuts, drizzle with the olive oil, honey, vinegar, or citrus juice and a good grinding of black pepper, then tuck in while the halloumi is still hot.

+ **HAVING A BARBECUE?**
Cook the halloumi on the grill outside as you throw the rest of this salad together.

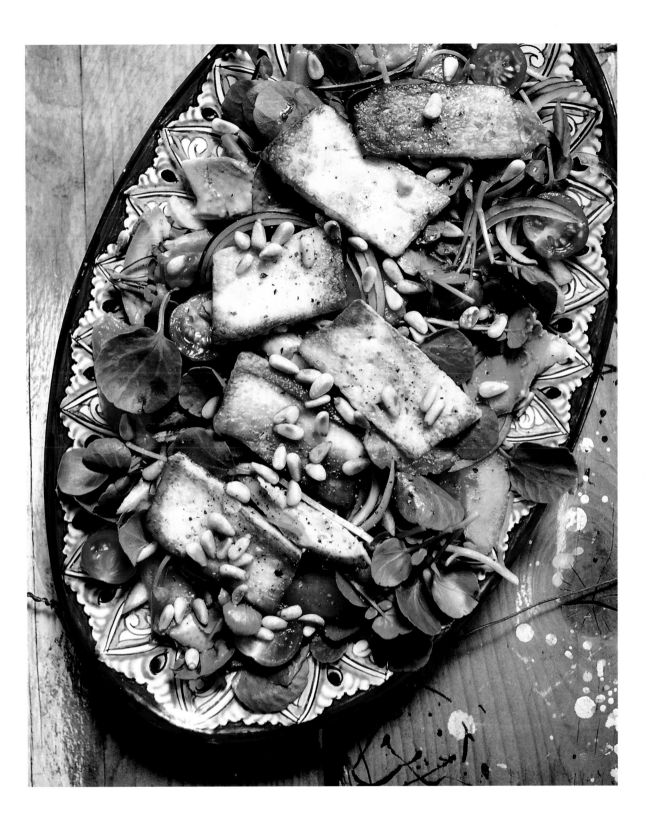

# SUMMER LIME COLESLAW

A simple tricolor coleslaw. Use a sharp knife or, quicker yet, a food processor. Red cabbage is a tasty show stopper of a vegetable that doesn't break the bank, so it's a favorite to serve to guests. That brilliant deep color is evidence of its antioxidants and its bitter flavor works well with the sweet and sharp of carrot and lime, the aniseed from the fennel, and the rich crunch from the peanuts. Fennel cleanses the liver and colon and the lime dressing is full of vitamin C, so together with the rest of the vegetables you have a wonderfully alkalizing salad for the body.

Add some homemade Ginger Poppy Seed Mayonnaise (page 88) if you want a satisfying main course or serve with some grilled fish or our Pablo's Chicken (page 166).

This is the perfect barbecue offering and if you want to make it in advance, just toss with the lime juice to keep the veg fresh, then save the sesame oil, salt, and pepper until 10 minutes before serving to keep everything crisp and crunchy.

**SERVES 4 AS A SIDE**

**FOR THE COLESLAW**

½ a large red cabbage, about 14 oz

1 small fennel bulb with fresh fronds (the delicate leaves)

2 medium carrots, julienned

1 celery stick, finely sliced

2 scallions, sliced

a handful of fresh cilantro, roughly chopped

2 tbsp peanuts, almonds, or pumpkin seeds (preferably "crispy" activated, page 300), roughly chopped

**FOR THE LIME DRESSING**

grated zest and juice of 1 unwaxed lime or lemon (avoid the bitter white pith)

1½ tbsp sesame oil (not toasted) or extra virgin olive oil

sea salt and black pepper

**1**  Finely shred the red cabbage using a knife or food processor. Finely chop the fronds of the fennel bulb and thinly slice the stalks and bulb with a knife or mandolin.

**2**  Combine the cabbage and fennel in a large mixing bowl with the carrot, celery, scallion, and cilantro.

**3**  Shake all the dressing ingredients together in a jam jar, then use your hands to mix it into the coleslaw.

**4**  Toast the peanuts in a dry frying pan for a few minutes until toasted, then scatter over the top of the coleslaw and serve.

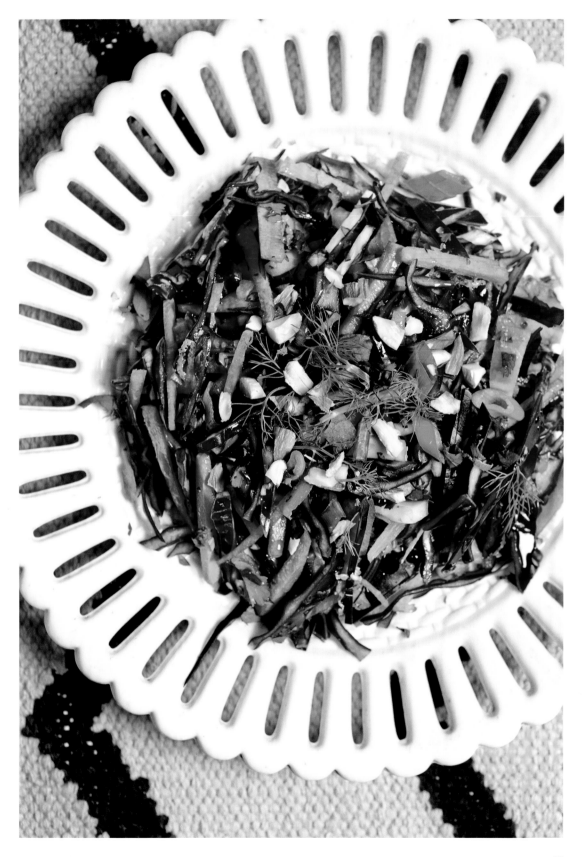

# PUY LENTIL, BEET, AND APPLE SALAD

This autumn salad with plenty of flavor, color, and crunch is equally good served warm on a platter or packed cold in your lunchbox. Add the cooked lentils to the dressing while they are still hot so the lentils absorb the sweet mustard dressing as they cool.

You could substitute green or brown lentils here, but we highly recommend that you seek out puy lentils, also known as French green lentils, as they have a wonderful texture and nutty flavor – a tasty base to showcase the other ingredients.

**SERVES 4**

### FOR THE SALAD

7 ¾ oz puy lentils (French green lentils, activated overnight page 300)

2 cups bone broth (page 300) or vegetable stock

1 bay leaf

4 small raw beets (2 purple and 2 golden if you can)

2 heads of radicchio

1 tsp fresh thyme or lemon thyme or ½ tsp dried thyme

1 large green apple

14 oz seasonal leaves, such as watercress, arugula, or lamb's lettuce

2 tbsp dried cranberries

a small handful of pecans or walnuts (preferably "crispy" activated, page 300), roughly chopped

1 small red onion, finely diced

a large handful of fresh parsley, roughly chopped

### FOR THE MUSTARD DRESSING

2 tsp mustard (we use wholegrain)

4 tbsp apple cider vinegar

¾ cup extra virgin olive oil

2 tsp raw runny honey

1 garlic clove, diced

sea salt and black pepper

**1**  Cook the puy lentils in a pan with the broth and the bay leaf for 12–15 minutes until tender.

**2**  Meanwhile, prepare the dressing by whisking everything together in a bowl or shaking vigorously in a jam jar. Set aside until needed.

**3**  Peel the raw beets then use a sharp knife or mandolin to slice the raw beets (beet juice stains so watch your clothes). Slice the radicchio ends, leaving the bright leaves whole, then set aside.

**4**  When the puy lentils are cooked, immediately drain them and add to a bowl with the dressing and the fresh thyme. Give them a good stir to coat and leave them to cool for 10 minutes.

**5**  Last of all, core, halve, and slice the apple. If you're making this ahead, dip the apple slices in lemon juice to prevent browning.

**6**  On a large serving platter, lay out the seasonal leaves. Add the cranberries, nuts, apple, beets, onion, and fresh parsley to the bowl of warm lentils, mix to combine, and pile it on top of the leaves.

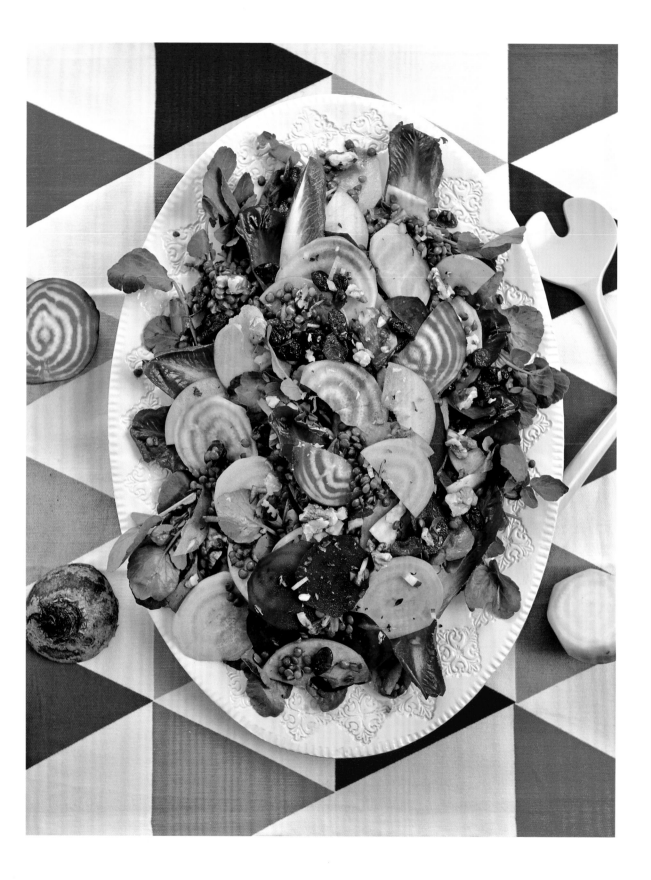

# QUICKER-THAN-TOAST ZUCCHINI SALAD

This is one of the first recipes we teach clients because, as the name suggests, it makes a fast, energy-boosting snack. Get this into you before reaching for the cookies at 4 p.m. and you might well find that you can pass on that daily sugar fix. It makes a great side salad for absolutely everything and also makes a wonderful starter.

To give this raw, alkalizing salad a tasty finish, throw on some "popped" pumpkin seeds for warmth and a mouthwatering aroma. Just before you whip out your grater and zucchini, start toasting a handful of seeds in a dry frying pan until golden and "popped." As you sprinkle them over the dish you'll hear a "snap, crackle, and sizzle."

SERVES 1 AS A SIDE

a handful of pumpkin seeds (preferably "crispy" activated, pages 300–302)

1 zucchini

2 tbsp extra virgin olive oil

2 tsp balsamic vinegar

sea salt and black pepper

**1**  Toast the pumpkin seeds in a dry frying pan over a medium heat, shaking the pan every minute or so until the seeds are golden and start to puff up and jump around the pan.

**2**  Meanwhile, wash the zucchini, wipe it dry, hold onto the stalk end, and grate into a pile on a plate.

**3**  Top the zucchini with your seeds and drizzle over the extra virgin olive oil and vinegar and sprinkle with salt and pepper. Et voilà!

**IF YOU REALLY NEED TO SAVE A PRECIOUS MINUTE**, or are making this fresh at work, make up a batch of toasted seeds and keep in a jar somewhere cool ready to finish off any salad at the drop of a hat.

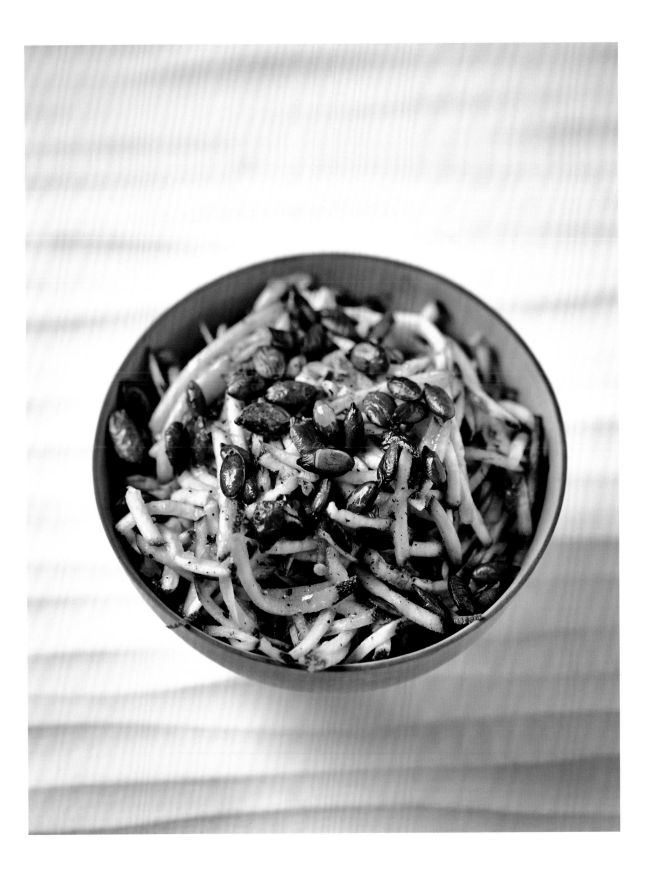

# CARROT, RADISH, AND SEAWEED SALAD WITH SWEET MISO DRESSING

We love the speed and crunchy texture of this salad. Seaweed (sea vegetables) are rich in calcium, magnesium, phosphorus, iron, and potassium (see page 23 for more on them). You can buy fresh seaweed or rehydrate the dried versions.

This goes perfectly with the Sea Bream Teriyaki (page 155) or Chicken Adobo (page 170). Or steam up some quinoa or simmer some buckwheat noodles and stir through the salad. The delicious sweet miso dressing keeps well in the fridge; any spare can be spooned over fried eggplants or stir-fried greens.

**SERVES 2 AS A SIDE**

**FOR THE SALAD**

a small handful of fresh seaweed or 2 tsp dried seaweed

2 large carrots

2 tbsp black or white sesame seeds or furikake (a mix of sesame seeds and dried seaweed)

6 pink radishes, sliced

2 scallions, sliced on the angle

a handful of fresh cilantro, roughly chopped

**FOR THE SWEET MISO DRESSING**

1 tbsp lime or lemon juice

½ tsp tamari or sea salt

3 tbsp sesame oil (not toasted) or extra virgin olive oil

½ tsp toasted sesame oil

½ tsp raw runny honey

½ tsp apple cider vinegar

1 tsp sweet white miso paste

1 red chili, finely chopped

**1** If using fresh seaweed, follow the instructions (it usually needs rinsing a few times). If using dried, follow the packet instructions, soaking the seaweed in water for the required time. Drain and rinse.

**2** Meanwhile, whisk or blend all the dressing ingredients together.

**3** Use a spiralizer or julienne peeler to create thin, noodle-like strands of carrot. Or use a regular vegetable peeler to slice the carrots lengthways into wide ribbons, which you can then slice in half. You might want to cut the long spiralized strands in half to make them easier to eat.

**4** Gently toast the sesame seeds in a dry pan until fragrant.

**5** Put the seaweed, carrot, radishes, and scallion in a serving bowl. Use your hands to mix the dressing into the salad. Top with the toasted sesame seeds and cilantro.

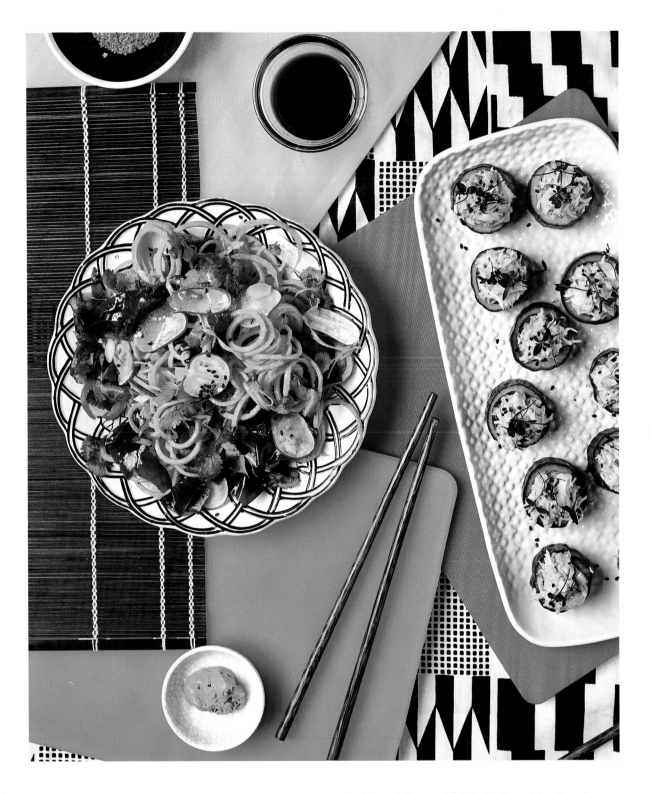

**LEFT TO RIGHT**: Carrot, Radish, and Seaweed Salad with Sweet Miso Dressing (opposite) and Cucumber Maki Crab Rolls (page 180).

87

# BROCCOLI SLAW WITH GINGER POPPY SEED MAYONNAISE

A superfood slaw – broccoli, goji berries, apple cider vinegar, ginger, and poppy seeds. Make sure that you chew the crunchy poppy seeds well to get the nutrients. If you're feeling cold or run down, then lightly steam the broccoli first and fold everything through for a warm salad that's easier to digest. Add more ginger for an extra kick. This makes a very tasty side dish to our Sea Bream Teriyaki (page 155) or just add some cooked, shredded chicken or buckwheat noodles.

SERVES 2

### FOR THE SLAW

1 large head of broccoli, about 12 oz

½ red onion, finely sliced

1 tbsp apple cider vinegar

2 tbsp goji berries

2 tbsp almonds (preferably "crispy" activated, page 300), roughly chopped

### FOR THE GINGER POPPY SEED MAYONNAISE

1 egg yolk (use the egg white in our Flower Power Pizza page 194)

¾ cup sesame oil (not toasted) or macadamia oil

½ tbsp apple cider vinegar

1 tsp raw runny honey

½ a thumb-sized piece of fresh root ginger (about 3/4 oz) – unpeeled if organic – grated finely and added with any juices

1 tbsp poppy seeds

a pinch of sea salt

**1**  Soak the red onion slices in the vinegar for 15–20 minutes to cure (you can reserve the soaking juices for adding to salads, including this one if you'd like a bit more tang).

**2**  Soak the goji berries in a little warm water for about 10 minutes so they plump up.

**3**  To make the mayonnaise, whisk the egg yolk and then, drop by drop, whisk in the sesame oil stopping when the dressing goes very thick. Stir in the apple cider vinegar. You can then start pouring a slow, steady stream of the remaining oil into the mayonnaise, while continuing to whisk. When all of the oil has been added, mix in the rest of the ingredients and taste for seasoning.

**4**  Grate the broccoli using the slicing attachment of a food processor or the coarse side of a hand-held grater (you can grate the whole broccoli or just the head, saving the stem for juicing or soups).

**5**  In a large bowl, combine the broccoli, cured onion, soaked goji berries, and chopped almonds.

**6**  Pour the poppy seed mayonnaise over the broccoli mixture and stir to combine.

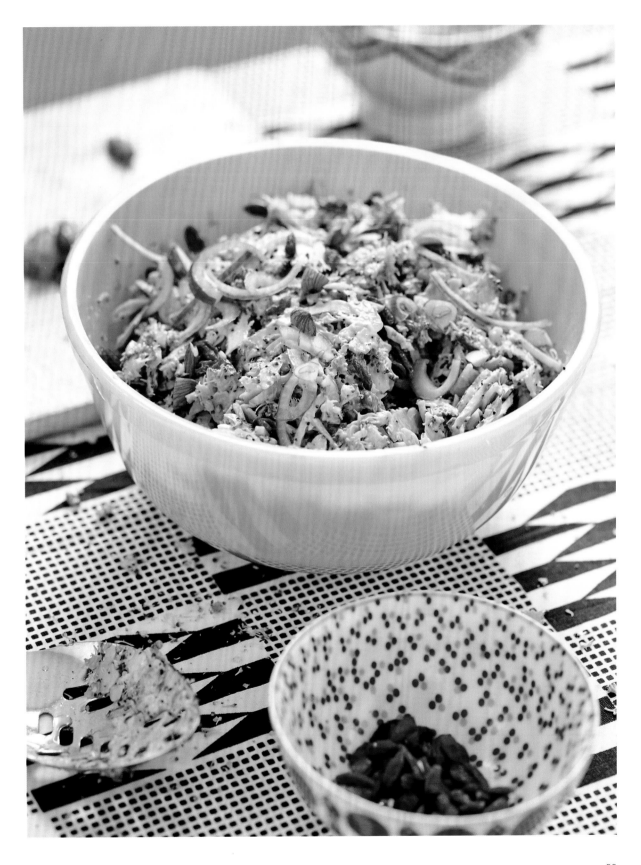

# PEA, PEACH, AND GOATS' CHEESE SALAD

This mix of hot caramelized zucchinis with soft, ripe, flat peaches and sweet, tender fresh peas, crunchy lettuce and strong, creamy cheese aims to please.

Don't worry about trying to get these exact ingredients: good frozen peas, the usual green zucchinis and regular tennis ball-shaped peaches will do. We are particularly fond of butter lettuce though – also known as Bibb lettuce – but substitute with any salad leaves you can find. If you can't find goats' cheese, use slivers of a hard cheese like pecorino or Parmesan, or a pesto such as Brazil Nut Pesto (page 198). Or blend up a handful of soaked and rinsed cashews with a garlic clove, sea salt, and a little water to make a cashew and garlic "cream cheese" and spoon that over. If you're a halloumi lover, grill a few slices and serve immediately with the peach salad for a twist on our Papaya, Halloumi, and Watercress Salad (page 78).

Peaches continue to soften and get juicier after picking, but they stop developing flavor and sweetness so a soft peach is not necessarily a ripe peach. Scent strength is a very good guide to flavor and sweetness so smell and touch your fruit.

SERVES 2

## FOR THE SALAD

1 head butter lettuce, a.k.a. Boston or Bibb lettuce, or use any tender lettuce

4 ¼ oz fresh peas in their pods (or 2 oz frozen peas)

1 tsp ghee

2 medium zucchinis, any color (we used yellow), sliced ½ in thick

3 large ripe peaches (we used flat ones), sliced into eighths

3 ¼ - 4 ¼ oz per person of unpasteurized goats' cheese (we love fromage Cathare)

12 fresh mint leaves, torn

¼ red onion, very finely sliced

## FOR THE DRESSING

4 tbsp extra virgin olive oil

1 tbsp balsamic vinegar

sea salt and black pepper

**1** Carefully wash the lettuce leaves and leave to dry. If the leaves are large, tear them into smaller pieces. Shell the peas or if using frozen peas, leave to defrost in some cold water, then drain.

**2** Heat the ghee in a pan over a medium heat, then add a single layer of zucchini slices. Don't let them touch otherwise they will steam rather than fry. Fry each side for 1 minute until lightly browned. Set aside.

**3** Arrange the lettuce over serving plates and distribute the zucchini slices, peach wedges, peas and goats' cheese on top.

**4** Scatter with the torn mint and red onion slithers.

**5** Drizzle with the olive oil and balsamic. Finish with a sprinkle of sea salt and black pepper, or to taste.

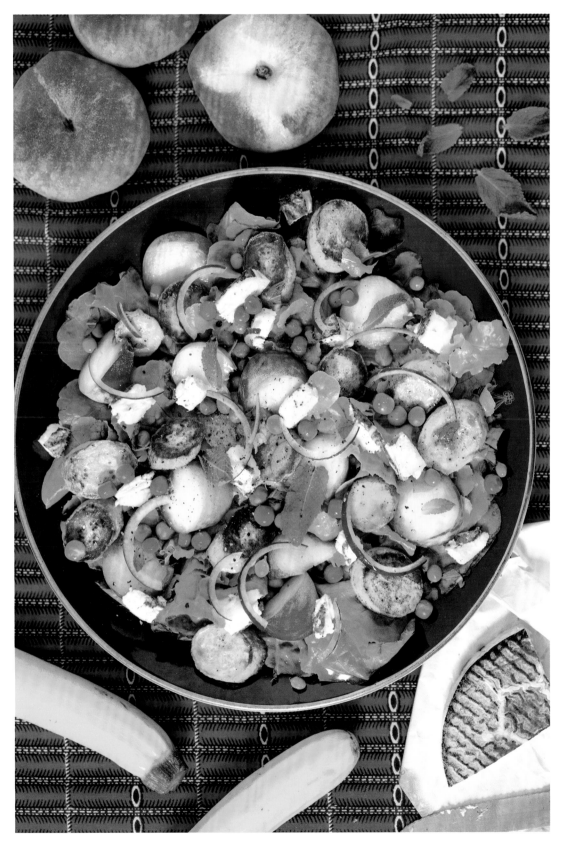

## ROASTED BONE MARROW WITH WATERCRESS SALAD

Bone marrow, fought over across the dinner table when we were growing up, has fallen out of favor, only making a slight resurgence in popularity on the menus of more fancy restaurants. This nourishing staple, which Queen Victoria reputedly ate every day, is pure decadence at an affordable price. Rich in nutrition and flavor and cheap to buy – what could be better? You can get the bones cut to any length you want – we find 3 in is ideal and allows easy access to the goodness inside. Ask your butcher for pieces cut from the center of the leg bone, where the ratio of marrow to bone is highest.

The classic pairing for this is parsley, shallots, and capers – salty, bitter, and sharp flavors that prepare your gastric juices to digest and absorb every morsel. We're often lazy, so as long as we have a bit of watercress and lemon juice with it, we're happy.

For dinner parties, you can place a big serving board full of the bone marrow on the table so that everyone can gather round and help themselves. It's a real statement piece. Adding a few side dishes also makes this more of a main meal. Try Roasted Vegetables (page 192), Kale Caesar Salad (page 94), Summer Lime Coleslaw (page 80), and Fennel, Cucumber, and Dill Salad (page 97) with some toasted Flax Sandwich Bread (page 272) or Multiseed Loaf (page 273).

SERVES 4 AS A STARTER

8–10 center-cut rose veal or beef marrow bones, 3 in long, about 3 1/3 lb total

4 handfuls salad leaves, such as watercress

2–3 tbsp capers

a little sliced onion

juice of 1 lemon

sea salt and black pepper

**1** Preheat the oven to fan 455°F.

**2** Place the bones, wider cut side down, into a roasting pan or tray lined with parchment paper. Roast the bones for about 15–20 minutes, depending on the thickness of the bones, until the marrow is soft and begins to separate from the bone, but catch it before it begins to melt.

**3** Meanwhile, prepare a light salad, making sure you have some sour, bitter, and salty accompaniments, like capers, sprinkled through it. A little sliced onion works well in the salad too. Dress with lemon juice and season.

**4** Season the marrow bones with sea salt and eat with the salad. (Don't forget to save the bones to make broth.)

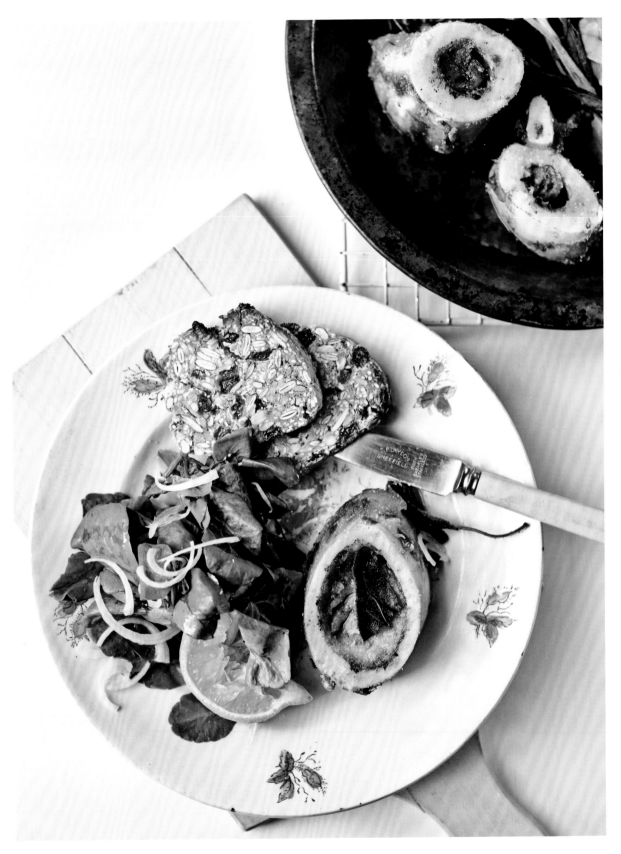

# KALE CAESAR SALAD

A go-to side salad or, for a main meal, add shredded cooked chicken, prawns, or flaked fish. Dress the kale an hour in advance to let the leaves soften in the salt, lemon, and oil and allow the flavors to marinate (delicious after 2 days). This is a great packed lunch and an excellent way to eat more kale. Forget kale chips – this salad is incredibly delectable.

Don't be afraid of raw egg yolks. Buy quality eggs, which are full of nutrients and eat them fresh.

SERVES 4 AS A SIDE

**FOR THE SALAD**

7 oz kale

a handful of walnuts (preferably "crispy" activated, page 300)

1 tbsp ghee

1–2 slices of Flax Sandwich Bread (page 272) or Multiseed Loaf (page 273), chopped into chunks

Parmesan shavings, to garnish

**FOR THE CAESAR DRESSING**

zest and juice of ½ an unwaxed lemon (avoid the bitter white pith)

1 small garlic clove

1 tsp Dijon mustard

1 ¾ oz parmesan cheese, grated

1 egg yolk

4 anchovy fillets

4 tbsp extra virgin olive oil

**1**  Remove the stalks from the kale, then stack the leaves, roll into a cylinder and slice into thin ribbons.

**2**  Blend all the Caesar dressing ingredients together, except for the extra virgin olive oil, in a food processor or blender. As you blend, slowly add the extra virgin olive oil so it emulsifies. Taste for seasoning.

**3**  Toss the kale pieces with the dressing using your hands and leave to marinate for an hour. If you've only got a few minutes, rub the dressing into the leaves and mix well.

**4**  Toast the walnuts in a dry pan for 30 seconds until lightly golden, then set aside.

**5**  In the same pan, heat the ghee and fry the chunks of bread until crispy, shaking the pan to fry all sides.

**6**  Pile the kale onto a plate and serve with the croutons, toasted walnuts, and a few more parmesan shavings.

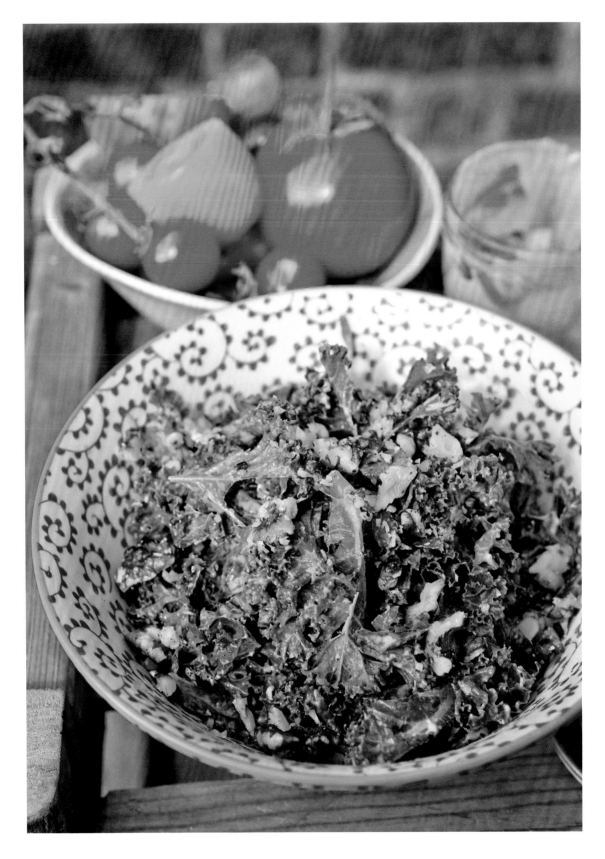

# RED CABBAGE, BACON, AND APPLE SALAD

This coleslaw uses many of our favorite autumnal ingredients – red cabbage, apple, pecans, and cranberries. With its deep rich color, it's a feast for the eyes! Like most of our favorite salads, this is made of both cooked and raw ingredients, which suits cooler weather, but if you want to eat this in the evening, then we recommend lightly sautéing the cabbage and the apple along with the other ingredients and serving the salad warm for better digestion. You can also swap the bacon for some mushroom slices fried in butter and garlic. The French-style vinaigrette is quick to make, will keep for a week in the fridge, and is perfect on any green salad.

SERVES 4

## FOR THE SALAD

½ a large red cabbage, about 14 oz

4 rindless unsmoked bacon rashers, chopped into pancetta-like cubes

1 tsp ghee

1 small red onion, sliced

1 crunchy red apple, diced into ¾ in cubes

2 tbsp roughly chopped pecans or walnuts (preferably "crispy" activated, page 300)

1 tbsp dried cranberries

## FOR THE MUSTARD DRESSING

5 tbsp extra virgin olive oil

1 tbsp mustard (we use wholegrain mustard)

2½ tbsp apple cider vinegar

¾ tsp sea salt

¾ tsp black pepper

1 tsp raw runny honey

**1**  Finely shred the red cabbage using a knife, mandolin, or food processor and place in a large mixing bowl.

**2**  Shake all the dressing ingredients together in a jam jar and drizzle over the red cabbage.

**3**  Heat the ghee in a pan over a medium/high heat and fry the bacon until crispy then set aside.

**4**  Using the same pan, sauté the onion in the bacon fat for a few minutes (along with the apple if you like), then add the pecans or walnuts for 30 seconds to warm through, before transferring everything to the mixing bowl, remembering to scrape out any delicious caramelized bits.

**5**  Add the cranberries and crispy bacon, toss everything to combine and serve.

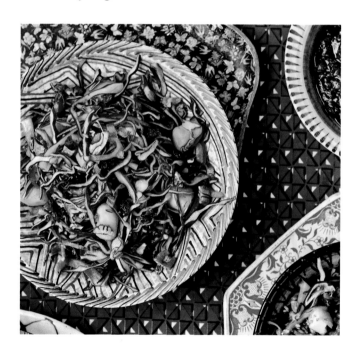

# FENNEL, CUCUMBER, AND DILL SALAD

A salad inspired by a love for the clean, refreshing taste of fennel and dill. Serve with a soft-boiled egg, smoked fish, or feta cheese. This very simple dressing will suit any salad and is as easy as pie to make.

SERVES 2 AS A SIDE

**FOR THE SALAD**

1 fennel bulb

½ large cucumber

1 large avocado, halved and sliced

1 tbsp chopped fresh dill

1 tbsp snipped fresh chives or 1 scallion, sliced

1 tbsp poppy seeds (optional)

**FOR THE DRESSING**

1 tbsp lemon juice or apple cider vinegar

2 tbsp extra virgin olive oil

1 tsp raw runny honey

sea salt and black pepper

**1**  Using a mandolin or very sharp knife, finely slice the fennel, keeping the feathery fronds and chopping them up. Halve the cucumber lengthways and very thinly slice on the angle, then add everything to a big serving bowl.

**2**  Add the sliced avocado, chopped dill, and the chives or spring onion.

**3**  Whisk the dressing ingredients together, pour over the salad, and mix well with your hands. Top with the poppy seeds, if using.

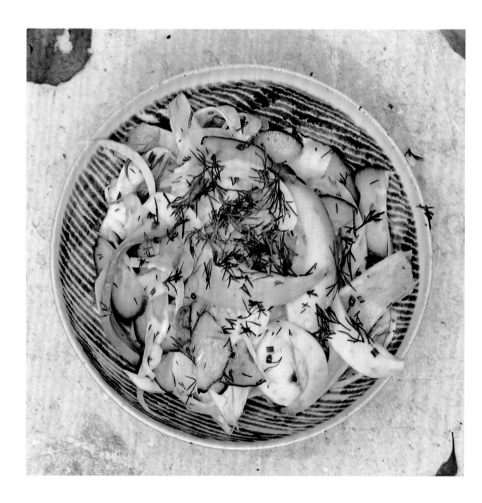

# SIDES AND SNACKS

**T**HIS CHAPTER IS ALL ABOUT THOSE LITTLE EXTRAS – THE DELICIOUS DISHES THAT FIT IN AND AROUND OUR MEALS. We've gathered together a variety of side dishes to complement a main or add a fresh lease of life to leftovers, as well as our favorite snack recipes to boost energy levels and sustain you until the next meal.

Our vegetable-based side dishes like our Garlic Lemon Green Beans (page 113), are so tasty in their own right you won't mind eating all that extra veg. We don't rely on potato, pasta, and grains to accompany our mains and fill us up. Instead, we've made tasty and nutritious versions of popular sides so, if you think you might miss your pasta and potatoes, try our Cauliflower Mash (page 104), Cauliflower and Broccoli Rices (page 102 and 170), Courgetti (page 140), and Baked Zucchini Fries (page 110), which all pair perfectly with protein or high-starch dishes.

We're big fans of a mezze and in the summer months we put together platters using four or five sides to make a feast. Keeping an assortment of them in the fridge works like a pick 'n' mix, creating lunches and suppers with a bit of this and a bit of that. Alternatively, adding a portion of meat, fish, egg, legumes, or pseudocereals to any of these sides makes a meal.

Having the right snacks on hand at all times is essential, as your resolve can be tested with every shop, café, and vending machine you pass. The colorful offerings call out to you just as your tummy realizes it's been two hours since lunch and another two hours until dinner.

Hydration should be your first line of defense when your mind turns to snacking, followed by a pick-me-up that won't make you crash an hour or so later. Rather than reaching for chips or the cookie packet, opt for a snack made from real, whole foods containing a good amount of fat and/or protein for sustenance and satisfaction. Our Tahini Bliss Balls (page 124) are the ultimate snack, being nourishing, not too sweet, but also easily transportable. Freeze a batch ready to pull a few out in the morning for the day ahead.

See pages 308–310 to find out how we get ahead and stock up on snacks as part of our Sunday Cook Off, as well as for some lunchbox ideas to team with your snacks. We know only too well that trying to eat properly while travelling or working late can be extremely difficult without good snacks on hand, so see page 313 for tips on what to pack when you travel. Let these recipes become your go-tos. The secret is to always be prepared for a "snack attack"!

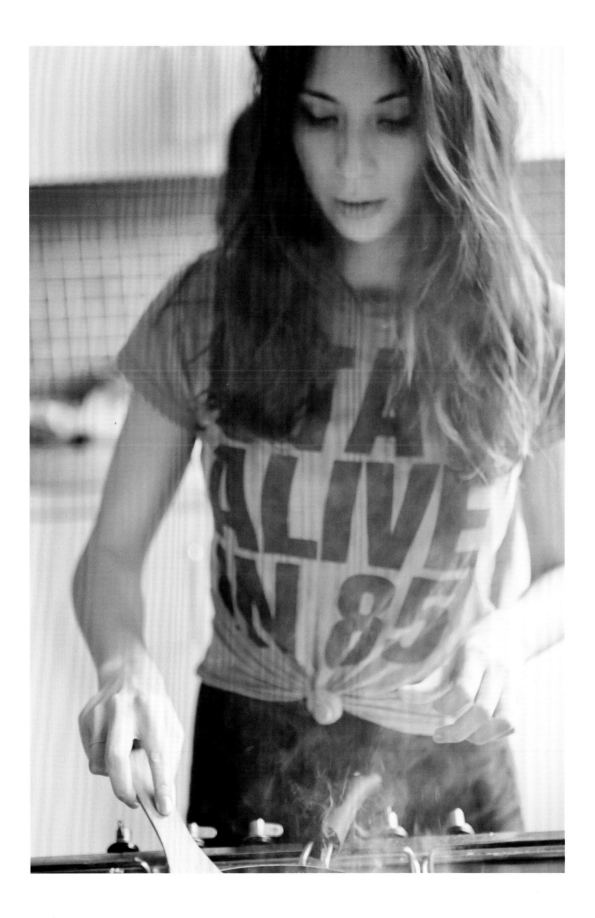

# CAULIFLOWER RICE AND PILAF-STYLE CAULIFLOWER RICE

This 100-percent vegetable alternative to rice only takes 10 minutes from start to finish. Cauliflower contains several beneficial phytochemicals and especially high levels of vitamin C, which is missing in the dry grains of brown or white rice. Sometimes we like our cauliflower rice plain, sometimes we cook it with some coconut milk or, for us, the ultimate would be this aromatically scented cauliflower pilaf rice.

SERVES 2

**FOR THE CAULIFLOWER RICE**

1 cauliflower

1 tsp ghee or coconut oil

2 tbsp bone broth (page 300) or water

sea salt and black pepper

**FOR THE PILAF-STYLE CAULIFLOWER RICE**

1 cauliflower

1 tbsp pistachios or flaked almonds

1 tsp ghee or coconut oil

1 medium onion, finely chopped

1 tsp ground turmeric

2 dried bay leaves

3 cardamom pods, crushed

1 tbsp raisins

2 tbsp bone broth (page 300) or water

1 tsp lemon juice

sea salt and black pepper

**+ MAKING A BIGGER BATCH?** You can make cauli rice by hand but a food processor really helps!

**1 To make Cauliflower Rice**, remove the cauliflower leaves and the tough end of the stalk. Use a food processor or the coarse teeth on a grater to grate the cauliflower into rice-sized pieces.

**2** Add the ghee or coconut oil to a pan with the grated cauliflower, the broth or water, and turmeric, if using, and stir to mix.

**3** Cook over a medium heat, lid on, to let the grated cauliflower steam for 4–6 minutes until tender. After a few minutes, check to make sure that there is still enough water on the bottom of the pan to stop it catching. Once the cauliflower is tender, season to taste and serve.

**4 To make Pilaf-style Cauliflower Rice**, grate the cauliflower into rice-sized pieces as in step 1. Gently toast the pistachios or flaked almonds in a dry pan for a minute, then set aside.

**5** In the same pan, turn up the heat, add the ghee or coconut oil, and fry the onion, turmeric, bay leaves, and crushed cardamom pods for 8 minutes or until the onion is soft and translucent. Stir occasionally to prevent the onion sticking.

**6** Add the grated cauliflower, raisins, and broth or water to the pan, stir, and cover the pan to let the cauliflower steam for 4–6 minutes until tender as above.

**7** Once the cauliflower is tender, season to taste and stir through the lemon juice to serve (you could remove the cardamom or keep it in).

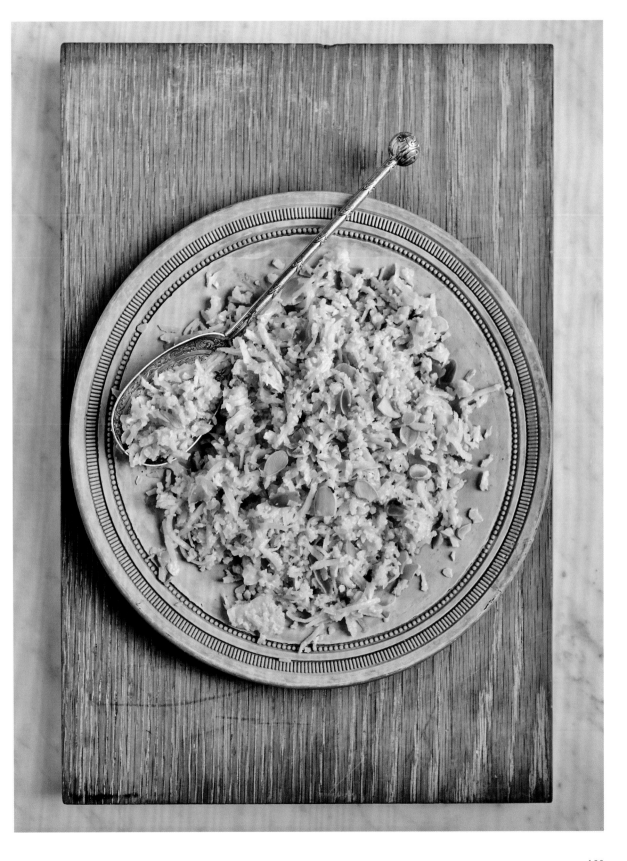

# CAULIFLOWER MASH

A low-carb, pure veg accompaniment that food combines well and goes with everything – this is one recipe everyone should master. It's as easy as pie to make – no peeling, 8 minutes to steam, and then pulse a few times before serving. You can make this without the garlic by the way, but we find that the garlic gives an even better texture without an overpowering flavor, since the cloves are steamed. For a more pronounced garlic flavor, fold in some gently fried garlic.

Treat this like any other mash and add your favorite twists like mustard and cheese – see some other suggestions below. We like it with roast lamb, Osso Bucco Beef Shin (page 160), and, of course, it's great for topping a Shepherd's Pie (page 164) or a Fish Pie (page 156).

SERVES 4

2 cauliflowers, outer leaves removed

just under an ounce butter

4 whole garlic cloves, peeled

sea salt and black pepper

**THERE ARE LOTS OF POSSIBLE VARIATIONS FOR THIS MASH.** Stir though Mustard Leek Sauce (page 139) or some chopped scallion, a handful of stilton, feta, or grated mature cheddar, a teaspoonful of strong English mustard or wasabi paste, or add fresh thyme or rosemary, a dusting of nutmeg, plenty of freshly grated black pepper, or some crushed sautéed garlic.

**1** Remove the tough parts of the stalk then roughly chop the cauliflower into 2 in chunks. Place the butter in the bottom of a large pan with 4 tablespoons water and top with the cauliflower and garlic cloves.

**2** Cover the pan and steam over a medium heat for around 8 minutes, or until the cauliflower is tender when tested with a knife. Check on it to make sure the cauliflower has enough water to steam in, and add a splash more if needed – allow any excess water to evaporate.

**3** Remove the pan from the heat and purée or blend the cauliflower with a hand-held blender or food processor until smooth and creamy or roughly textured, if you wish.

**4** Stir in any of the variations (see opposite) and season with salt and pepper to taste.

**5** If it's too sloppy or wet, reheat in a pan, over a low heat, to allow some moisture to evaporate.

# MUSHROOM, ROSEMARY, AND ARAME SAUTÉ

Seaweeds are delicious in all types of cuisine, not just Asian dishes. They are rich in iodine, which is often lacking in our diet. We keep several dried types on hand and since they only take 10 minutes to rehydrate, we can add them into any dish at the end.

This is a simple side dish that focuses on arame, one of our favorites. The little black strands add a sweet, delicate flavor to meals along with their many nutrients. We team the seaweed with a light sauté of mushroom, carrot, onion, and rosemary, with a pop of color and sweetness from the peas. For a more substantial dish, just add some cooked quinoa or top with a piece of fish and leave out the peas for better food combining. A nice introductory dish for anyone trying sea veg for the first time.

SERVES 2

2 tbsp dried arame

1 tbsp ghee or butter

1 leek or onion, diced

1 tsp fresh rosemary or
    2 tsp dried rosemary

5 oz chestnut, portobello
    or shiitake mushrooms,
    diced

1 large carrot, diced

a large handful of frozen
    peas

1 tbsp lemon juice

a handful of fresh parsley,
    finely chopped

sea salt and black pepper

**1** Soak the arame in water, following the packet instructions (about 8–10 minutes). Drain and rinse.

**2** Meanwhile, heat the ghee or butter in a pan over a medium heat and fry the leek or onion and rosemary for 5 minutes until softened. Add the mushrooms, stir and fry for a few minutes.

**3** Add the carrot, stir and cook for a few minutes, until the carrots are just tender. Add the peas and stir through until they defrost.

**4** Chop up the arame and add this to the mix. Season and add the lemon juice and fresh parsley.

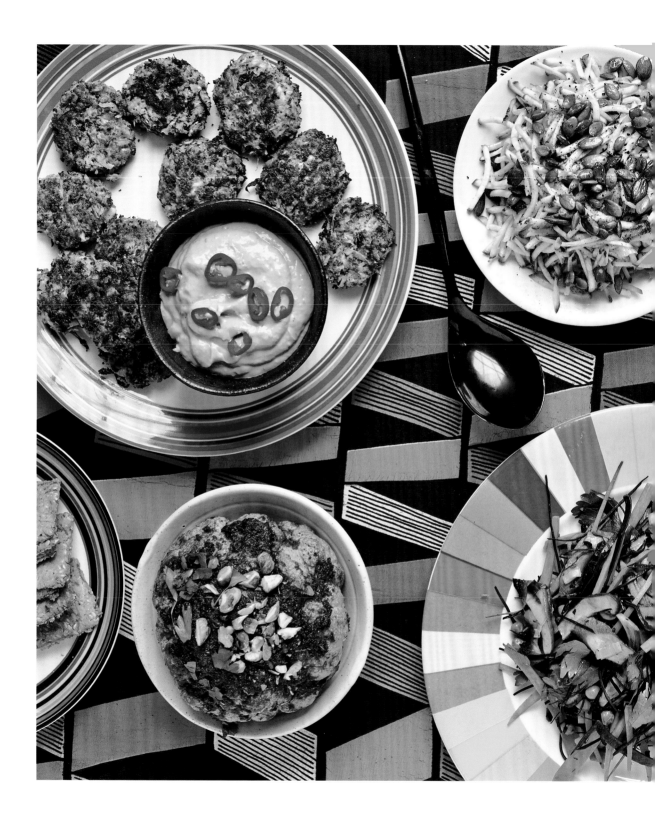

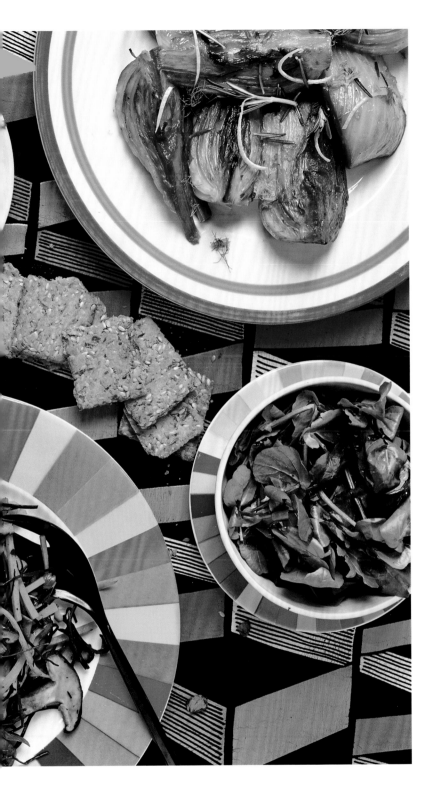

**LEFT TO RIGHT:** Baked Broccoli Fritters with Spicy Avocado Dip (page 126), Whole Roasted Cauliflower (page 108), Quicker-than-toast Zucchini Salad (page 84), Mushroom, Rosemary, and Arame Sauté (page 105), Carrot and Flax Crackers (page 121), Braised Fennel with Lemon and Rosemary (page 109), watercress salad.

## WHOLE ROASTED CAULIFLOWER

As you can see from our recipes, we're big fans of the humble cauli. If you can get a romanesco, roast it in the same way (it tastes like a cross between a broccoli and a cauliflower and cooks in half the time).

This nice, easy side dish for a roast or vegetable mezze is also delicious with our Malaysian and Southwestern Spice Mixes (pages 212 and 119).

SERVES 4

a handful of pistachios

2 tbsp ghee or coconut oil

1 large cauliflower, outer leaves removed

1 tsp ground cumin

1 tsp smoked sweet paprika

1 tsp ground sumac

1 tsp dried thyme or oregano or 2 tsp fresh thyme or oregano

2 garlic cloves, grated

drizzle of extra virgin olive oil, to serve

juice of ½ lemon

a handful of fresh parsley, roughly chopped, to serve

sea salt

**1** Preheat the oven to fan 350°F.

**2** Toast the pistachios in a dry pan for a minute, then crush them with a rolling pin or chop with a sharp knife and set aside.

**3** In the same pan, gently melt 1 tablespoon of the ghee or coconut oil.

**4** Sit the cauliflower on a baking tray. Pour over the melted ghee or coconut oil, sprinkle over a good amount of sea salt and roast in the oven for 35 minutes.

**5** Melt the remaining tablespoon of ghee or coconut oil and stir in the spices, herbs, and garlic. Remove the cauliflower from the oven and reduce the oven temperature to fan 160°C. Pour over the flavored ghee or coconut oil.

**6** Roast the cauliflower for another 10 minutes. Serve whole, drizzled with extra virgin olive oil. Squeeze over the lemon, then scatter with parsley and a little more salt and top with the pistachios.

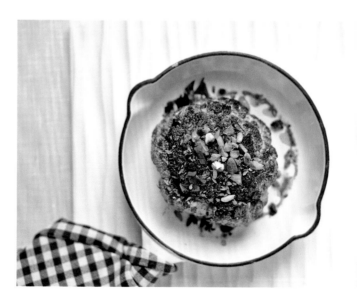

## BRAISED FENNEL WITH LEMON AND ROSEMARY

We like these braised fennel quarters chopped into salads and quinoa risottos. They make a beautiful side to most dishes, especially fish or to accompany a roast dinner. This method gives the lightly aniseed-flavored fennel sweet, caramelized edges, while keeping it tender and juicy. The rosemary and lemon can be swapped for any other herbs and flavors – try fresh oregano and orange zest in the summer.

SERVES 4

2 large fennel bulbs

2 tbsp ghee or butter

2 tsp fresh rosemary leaves or 1 tsp dried rosemary

zest and juice of ½ an unwaxed lemon (use a zester or sharp knife to create thin strands of zest)

2 garlic cloves, diced

1 ⅓ cup bone broth (page 300) or water

sea salt and black pepper

**1** Prepare the fennel by chopping off any fronds at the top (the delicate green leaves) and save these for garnishing at the end. Slice each fennel in half from top to bottom, then in half again so you have quarters.

**2** Heat the ghee in a pan wide enough that it can fit all the fennel in one layer.

**3** Add the fennel and brown it for a minute on the first side then, using tongs, turn over, brown the other side, then remove and set aside.

**4** Add the rosemary, lemon zest, seasoning and garlic to the pan and cook for a minute, stirring and scraping up any bits of caramelized fennel.

**5** Return the fennel back to the pan, add the broth or water, cover with a lid, and bring the heat up to a medium simmer. Cook for 40–50 minutes until the fennel is tender.

**6** Taste for seasoning, then squeeze over some lemon juice and scatter with the fennel fronds.

# BAKED ZUCCHINI FRIES

Got a craving for fries? Make these in 20 minutes and eat them hot and crispy. Vary the flavorings and enjoy with Probiotic Ketchup (page 306) or dips like Spicy Avocado Dip (page 126), Ginger Poppy Seed Mayonnaise (page 88), or our favorite, Sun-Dried Tomato and Jalapeño Yogurt Dip (page 231).

SERVES 2

2 large zucchinis

1 ¾ oz ground almonds

1 oz parmesan, grated

some herbs and spices (we like ½ tsp dried oregano and a small pinch cayenne pepper)

1 egg

sea salt

**1** Preheat the oven to fan 425°F.

**2** Slice the ends off the zucchinis, halve them and slice each half lengthways. Slice each length into French-fry style strips. You want your zucchini fries to be slightly larger than normal French fry size. Season them with sea salt.

**3** Mix the ground almonds, grated parmesan, and your chosen herbs and spices in a bowl.

**4** Beat the egg, dip each zucchini piece into the egg, then into the herb-and-spice mix to coat evenly.

**5** Lay the zucchini fries in a single layer on a baking sheet and bake for 10 minutes until golden brown.

**6** Enjoy them hot and crispy.

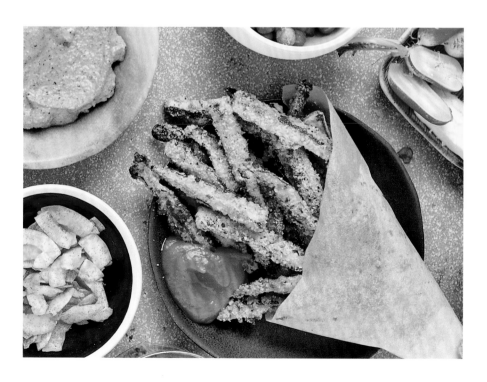

# CANNELLINI BEAN MASH

A quick store cupboard mash up (you can also make it with butter beans), this is a really easy side dish when you're short of time. Blend if you like a smooth mash, but we prefer it chunky with a few beans whole. This is wonderfully filling and satisfying, so we have it with just some veg and a dressing or try with our Puttanesca sauce (page 210) and some Tenderstem broccoli. The mash also works well to soak up any leftover juices from stews. Just remember to avoid teaming it with meat or fish, which will be harder to digest alongside it.

SERVES 2

2 tsp ghee

1 garlic clove, diced

½ tsp dried rosemary or thyme or 1 tsp fresh rosemary or thyme

2 tins of cooked cannellini beans (drained weight 18 oz) or 18 oz homecooked beans (dried weight 7 oz, activated overnight see page 300)

2 tsp lemon juice

sea salt and black pepper

**1** Heat the ghee in a pan over a low heat and gently fry the garlic and herbs for 2 minutes.

**2** Meanwhile, drain the beans and rinse.

**3** Add the beans and 6 tablespoons water to the pan and stir to combine for 2 minutes over a high heat.

**4** Add some seasoning and lemon juice and turn off the heat.

**5** Use a vegetable masher to roughly mash the beans or blend it up with a little more water if you want it smooth.

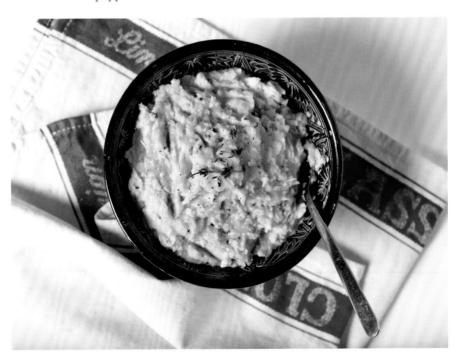

# TOASTED COCONUT GREEN BEANS

A super-quick side and great eaten hot or cold. We like to cook the green beans until just tender, but retaining bite. These flavors work well with broccoli or greens like kale or chard.

SERVES 2

7 oz green beans

a small handful of coconut flakes/chips

1 tsp coconut oil or ghee

2 scallions, sliced on the angle

1 red chili, deseeded

zest and juice of ½ an unwaxed lime (avoid the bitter white pith)

a small handful of chopped fresh herbs, such as cilantro, mint, or Thai basil

sea salt and black pepper

**1** Steam the green beans in a pan with 3 tablespoons water, lid on, for about 5 minutes until just tender.

**2** Meanwhile, toast the coconut flakes for a few minutes in a dry pan until just golden and fragrant, stirring to keep them moving, then set aside.

**3** In the same pan, heat up the coconut oil or ghee and stir through the scallions and fresh red chili for just 30 seconds, season, then turn off the heat.

**4** Drain the green beans and toss in the pan of scallions and chili to coat. Season to taste.

**5** Serve scattered with the lime zest, toasted coconut flakes, fresh herbs and squeeze over the lime juice.

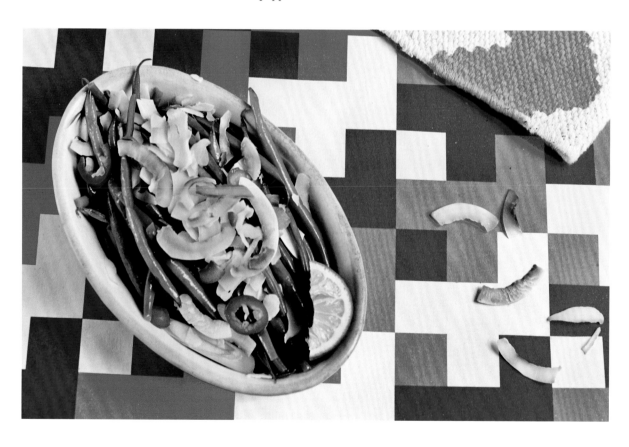

# GARLIC LEMON GREEN BEANS

We have a friend who could eat these green beans for breakfast, lunch, and dinner. We've combined the beans here with the winning combo of lemon, butter, and garlic – and lots of freshly cracked black pepper too. This is a much-loved side to any savory dish, hot or cold – but if it's taking center stage, then throw on some parsley and toasted nuts. In the summer, the recipe also works well with runner beans, making use of the bounty that appears in our seasonal veg boxes.

SERVES 2

7 oz green beans

1 tbsp ghee or butter

1 garlic clove, diced

zest and juice of ½ an unwaxed lemon (avoid the bitter white pith)

sea salt and black pepper

**OPTIONAL**

a handful of fresh parsley, chopped and 1 tbsp toasted, crushed nuts, like hazelnuts or flaked almonds

**1**  Steam the green beans in a pan, lid on, with 3 tablespoons water for 5 minutes or until just tender.

**2**  Meanwhile, heat the ghee or butter in a separate pan over a low heat. Add the garlic and stir for 1 minute (don't let the garlic catch or burn), then add the lemon zest and juice and fresh parsley, if using.

**3**  Drain the green beans, then quickly toss through the pan to coat and season to taste.

**4**  Serve immediately and top with chopped parsley and nuts, if desired.

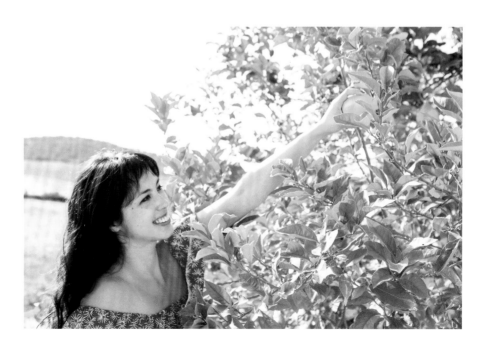

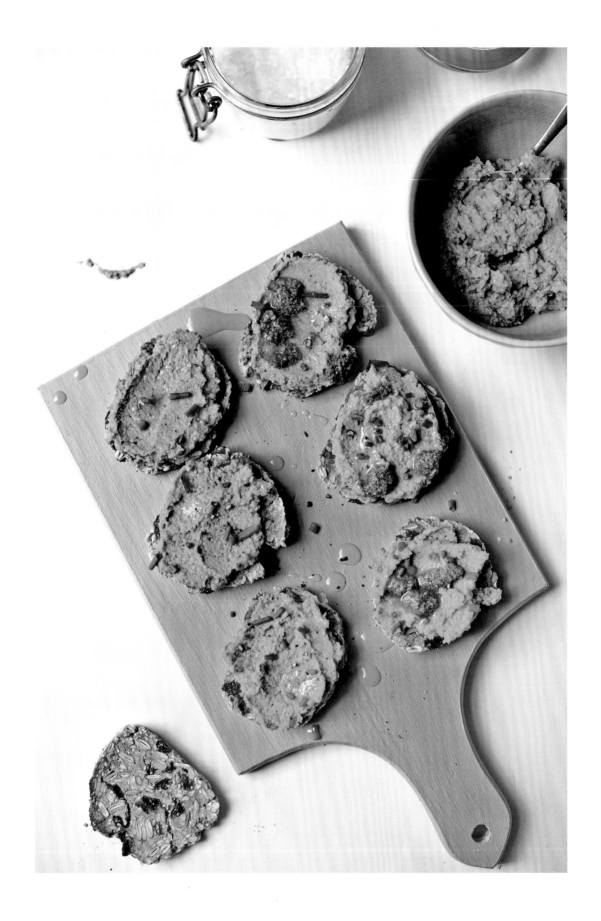

# PEA, MINT, AND BROCCOLI MASH

Peas are sweet and delicious, which means they're good at masking other veggies. So just like our Broccoli, Pea, and Basil Soup (page 59) we've sneaked in the goodness of broccoli, complete with stalks, and mashed them up together.

We love hot, mushy peas and comforting creamy mash, but don't forget that as well as a side dish or base, this recipe also works cold as a filling dip or bruschetta-style topping – try with our toasted Multiseed Loaf (page 273) or Flax Sandwich Bread (page 272).

Rather than topping with herbs, finish with a drizzle of any of our pestos for extra flair.

SERVES 4

1 garlic clove, diced

1 head of broccoli, about 10 ½ oz, cut into florets and stalks finely chopped

12 oz frozen peas

juice of ½ lemon

2 tbsp extra virgin olive oil

1 tbsp snipped fresh chives

a small handful of fresh mint leaves

sea salt and black pepper

OPTIONAL

pesto of choice, to drizzle

**1** Steam the garlic and broccoli in a pan with 4 tablespoons of water, lid on, for 5 minutes until tender. Check on it to make sure the broccoli has enough water to stop it catching on the bottom of the pan and add a splash more if needed.

**2** Turn off the heat, drain and stir through the peas, then cover and leave to sit for 5 minutes for the peas to defrost in the residual heat.

**3** Add the garlic, broccoli, peas, and all the remaining ingredients to a food processor or blender, saving a few chives to garnish, and blend until creamy.

**4** Check for seasoning and serve hot as a mash with snipped chives or pesto on top or cool and enjoy as a dip or on toasted bread.

# APPLE CHEDDAR BUCKWHEAT MUFFINS

These simple, gluten-free savory muffins make a delicious mid-morning snack or side to a flask of soup at work. The sweet apple and onions complement the tang of the mature cheddar. Add your favorite herbs such as sage or rosemary and a good grind of black pepper.

MAKES 8 MUFFINS

**FOR THE BATTER**

butter, for greasing

2 eggs

5 oz buckwheat flour

4 tbsp arrowroot

1 tsp baking soda

1 tsp sea salt

4 tbsp lemon juice

**FOR THE FLAVORINGS**

1 onion, finely sliced

1 large or 2 small apples, skin on, cut into 1 in chunks (not too small otherwise they disintergrate)

1 tbsp favorite herbs e.g. fresh sage or rosemary or black pepper, to taste

2 ¾ oz mature cheddar, cubed

**1** Preheat the oven to fan 350°F. Line a muffin tray with paper cases and grease the cases with a little melted butter.

**2** Whisk the eggs in a bowl, then add the rest of the batter ingredients and 3 tablespoons water, whisking well to combine.

**3** Stir the sliced onion, apple chunks, herbs, black pepper, if using, and the cheddar into the buckwheat batter, then spoon into the paper cases.

**4** Bake in the oven for 20–25 minutes until nicely browned. Remove the cooked muffins from the tray and leave to cool slightly on a wire rack.

**5** Enjoy warm or store any cooled leftovers in a sealed container in the fridge for up to a week. Warm again in the oven before serving.

**+ PLAY AROUND WITH FLAVORS** Try adding 2 ¾ oz of goats' cheese instead of cheddar, along with chopped fresh parsley and chili, to taste, plus the chopped apple. Or try some caramelized garlic cloves and cooked squash taken from the Caramelized Garlic Tart on page 202 along with some tarragon and yogurt.

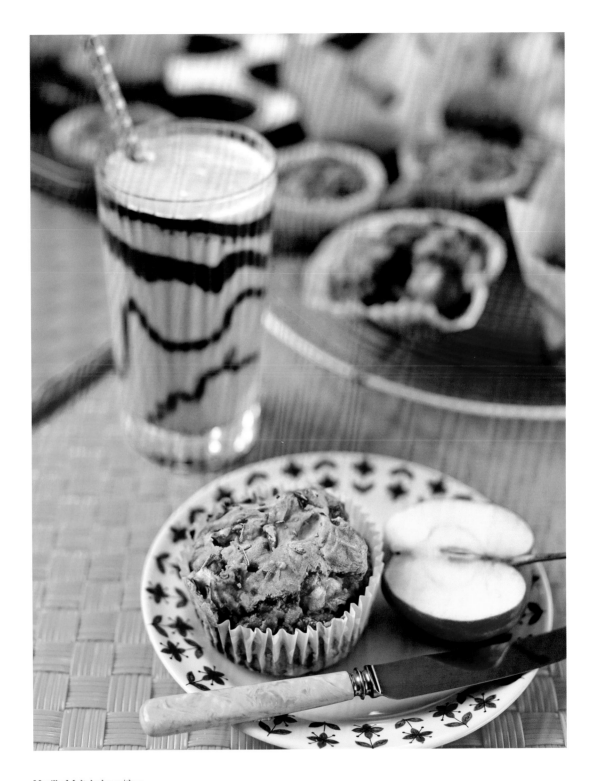

Vanilla Maltshake with a
Chocolate Swirl (page 291) and
Apple and Cheddar Buckwheat
Muffins (opposite).

# FALAFEL AND ITALIAN VEG BALLS

We like to make the most of the food we buy, so we turn the carrot and beet pulp from our juicer into delicious veg balls. We season the pulp with herbs and spices, add an egg to bind, roll into balls, and bake them for the perfect snack. When juicing, run the carrots and/or beets through first so that you can collect the pulp easily – a bit of apple is nice too, but celery will be too stringy and fibrous to eat. Pop the pulp into glass containers with lids kept in your freezer and when you have enough, make up a batch of these veg balls. Our favorite two varieties are Italian with parmesan, or falafel flavored with cumin and coriander. For the falafel, you can also shape the balls around small cubes of feta.

**MAKES 12 BALLS OF EACH TYPE**

### FOR THE BASIC BALLS

14 oz carrot and/or beet pulp leftover from juicing – it's the equivalent of 2 ¼ lb fresh veg

4 scallions or ½ small onion, finely chopped

2 garlic cloves, finely grated or diced

a large handful of fresh parsley, finely chopped

a tiny pinch of cayenne

½ tsp baking soda

½ tsp lemon juice

1 egg

sea salt and black pepper

### FOR THE FALAFEL BALLS

1½ tsp ground cumin

½ tsp ground coriander

4 tbsp black or white sesame seeds, or a mix of both, to decorate

### FOR THE ITALIAN BALLS

2 oz parmesan, finely grated

2 tbsp fresh basil, finely chopped or 1 tbsp dried basil

2 tsp dried oregano

**1**  Preheat the oven to fan 375°F and line a baking tray with baking parchment. Depending on how good your juicer is at extracting the juice, give the pulp one last good squeeze to get any excess liquid out (don't forget to drink it!).

**2**  Mix together the pulp, onion, garlic, parsley, cayenne pepper, baking soda, lemon juice, and egg in a bowl with your hands and taste for seasoning, then adjust with more salt and pepper if you like.

**3**  Divide the mixture between two bowls. Add the spices for the falafel to one bowl and the parmesan and herbs to the other, then mix well with your hands.

**4**  Shape the two mixtures into 24 bite-sized balls, using about 1 tablespoon of mixture per ball, and place on the prepared tray. For the falafel balls, roll in the sesame seeds first.

**5**  Bake for 12–15 minutes. The balls are delicious hot or cold served with a dip or oil.

✚ **DELICIOUS** with Mung Bean Hummus (page 232), to serve

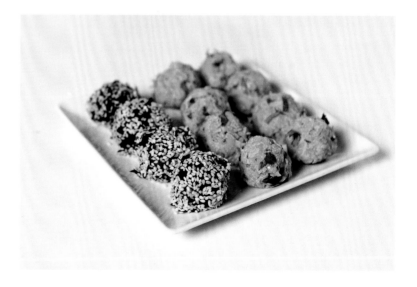

# SOUTH-WESTERN SPICED NUTS

These are a great snack to keep in your bag, on your desk, or to have ready when friends come over. Keep in a tightly sealed jar in the fridge, ready to snack on. We soak the nuts to activate then coat in buttery spices and dry them overnight in a dehydrator until "crispy." If you already have a batch of "crispy" activated nuts and want to save time, or you only have raw nuts and no dehydrator, you can use an oven for this recipe but be aware that oven-baked nuts will no longer be raw.

The southwestern flavors make a winning spice mix, but play around with your own flavor combinations, too – try fresh herbs like rosemary or add a touch of cinnamon or turmeric. You can also make a spicy seed mix using sunflower, pumpkin, and hemp seeds.

MAKES 14 OZ NUTS

3 ½ oz each of almonds, peanuts, walnuts, and cashew nuts (almonds, peanuts, and walnuts preferably activated overnight, cashew nuts preferably activated for 3 hours, page 302, and wet or crispy)

**FOR THE SOUTHWESTERN SPICE MIX**

2 tbsp butter or ghee

1½ tbsp maple syrup

2 tsp sea salt

1 tsp smoked hot paprika or ¾ tsp smoked sweet paprika with ¼ tsp cayenne pepper

2 tsp ground cumin

**1** Melt the butter or ghee and maple syrup in a large frying pan. Remove from the heat and add the salt and spices and stir.

**2** Add the activated nuts and stir to coat in the spices.

**DEHYDRATOR METHOD**

**3** If you're using "wet" activated nuts, spread them in a thin layer on a dehydrator tray and dehydrate for 12–24 hours at 115°F until crispy.

**OVEN METHOD**

**4** If you're using "crispy" activated nuts, or raw nuts, and don't have a dehydrator, preheat the oven to fan 350°F and line a tray with baking parchment.

**5** Bake in the oven for 10 minutes, shaking the pan halfway through, and being careful not to let them burn.

**6** Remove from the oven and leave to cool for a few minutes to crisp up before serving. Leave to cool completely before storing.

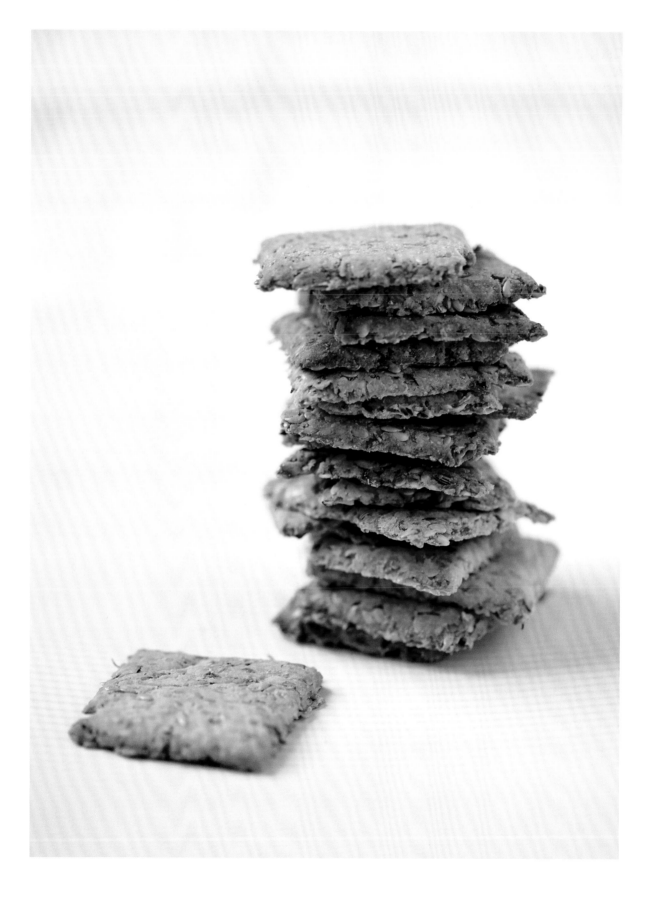

## CARROT AND FLAX CRACKERS

Crunchy crackers of goodness! It's all in the title – a blend of almond, flaxseed, and carrot with some herbs and spices, rolled out and baked into crackers. We bake a batch at least every other week, leaving them to crisp in our dehydrator overnight or popping in the oven for 12 minutes. Keep them in the fridge, ready for a salty, crunchy snack. It's also one of our favorite recipes for using up the leftover carrot pulp from our juicer – although finely grated carrot works well too. Experiment with your favorite flavors or leave them plain to accompany some good cheese and our Goji Marmalade (page 48). Also delicious with Spicy Avocado Dip (page 126), Lemon Parsley Cashew Dip (page 233), Mung Bean Hummus (page 232), or spread them with our Baked Chicken Liver Mousse (page 168) and serve with a salad.

MAKES 30 CRACKERS

3 ½ oz ground almonds or Sun Flour (page 302)

2 oz carrot pulp (leftover from juicing) or grated carrot, about 1 carrot (use the fine teeth on the grater)

just over 3 oz whole flaxseed

1 tsp garlic powder or finely grated fresh garlic

1 tbsp herbs or spices, such as fennel seeds, herbes de Provence, or fresh or dried thyme or rosemary

½ tsp sea salt

**CRUMBS AND BROKEN CRACKERS** can be sprinkled on salads for a crunchy topping.

1  Preheat the oven to fan 350°F, if using.

2  In a large bowl, combine all the ingredients with your hands to make a dough, but don't overmix otherwise it becomes too moist.

3  Bring the dough together into a ball and roll it between 2 sheets of baking parchment to a 1/8 in thickness. When rolling out, try and roll into a neat rectangle with straight edges as this will make it easier to snap off good-sized, evenly baked crackers.

4  Keeping the top layer of baking parchment in place, gently mark the dough through the paper into 2 in squares with the back of a knife, without breaking the paper. Carefully peel back the top piece of baking paper.

5  Transfer the bottom layer, with the scored cracker dough, directly onto the oven shelf, rack, or dehydrator. (If using the dehydrator, dehydrate at 115°F for 8 hours until crisp.)

6  Bake in the oven for 12 minutes, then check the crackers. The ones on the outside will be nicely toasted and golden, so snap these off and put to one side (they will crisp up as they cool). Return the rest of the crackers to the oven for a few more minutes, until also crisp and toasted.

7  Leave the crackers to cool on a wire rack for 20 minutes, then finish snapping them and enjoy alone or serve with dips. These will keep for 1 week in a sealed container in the fridge.

# TOASTED COCONUT CHIPS

An easy snack to whip up for any last-minute visitors or if you need a handful of crunch to satisfy a craving or boost your energy. Toasting the coconut flakes brings out their rich, nutty flavor, which you can enjoy with all your favorite spices. Sprinkle them onto soups and curries or simple salads for added flair and a sizzle when the hot chips hit the dressing. Keep a close eye on them as they can burn quickly – even after you take them off the heat, the hot pan will continue to cook them. When they're done, transfer to a bowl immediately and serve.

SERVES 2

3 ½ oz unsweetened coconut flakes or chips

**FOR THE INDIAN SPICED MIX**

1 tsp ground cumin

1 tsp ground coriander

½ tsp ground turmeric

a tiny pinch of cayenne pepper

a pinch of sea salt

**FOR THE SMOKED PAPRIKA MIX**

1 tsp sweet smoked paprika and a tiny pinch of cayenne pepper (or just use 1 tsp hot smoked paprika)

a pinch of sea salt

**FOR THE SWEET SPICED MIX**

1 tsp ground cinnamon

1 tsp ground ginger

**1** Add the coconut flakes to a hot dry frying pan, then turn down the heat to medium.

**2** Keep your eye on them and keep moving them with a wooden spatula. They should be golden and toasted after a minute.

**3** Take the pan off the heat, then add your chosen spices, stirring them through and tossing around a few times so they don't stick.

**4** Serve them warm or cool, then transfer to a glass airtight jar. They will keep for up to a week, just refresh in the oven to serve.

# CHICKPEA CRUNCHIES

Good for party snacks and food on the go. When you get a "crunch craving," these chickpea snacks deliver and make a more interesting bar snack than deep-fried habas fritas or tortilla chips. Experiment with flavors – we like salt and vinegar, garam masala, or wasabi powder. We've also included a sweet variation using maple syrup, so you can tailor this snack to fit sweet and savory needs!

SERVES 2

2 tsp coconut oil

1 tin of chickpeas
(9 oz drained weight)

### FOR THE SPICED CHICKPEAS

1 tsp sea salt

1 tsp black pepper

½ tsp ground cumin

¼ tsp cayenne pepper
(or less if you like –
these are pretty spicy)

### FOR THE SWEET CHICKPEAS

1 tsp ground cinnamon

1½ tsp maple syrup

a tiny pinch sea salt

**1**  Preheat the oven to fan 390°F.

**2**  Carefully warm the coconut oil in a pan over a gentle heat.

**3**  Meanwhile, drain the chickpeas, rinse, pat dry, and remove any of the loose chickpea skins that easily pop off as these can burn.

**4**  Mix the heated coconut oil and all the other ingredients for either the spiced or sweet chickpea crunchies in a bowl and ensure the chickpeas are evenly coated.

**5**  Spread onto a baking tray and bake in the oven for 30–35 minutes, giving the tray a shake every now and then until the chickpeas are golden and crunchy.

✚ **MAKE A DOUBLE BATCH** and store in a glass jar for a couple of days. After that, you can rebake them for 5–10 minutes to get the crunch back.

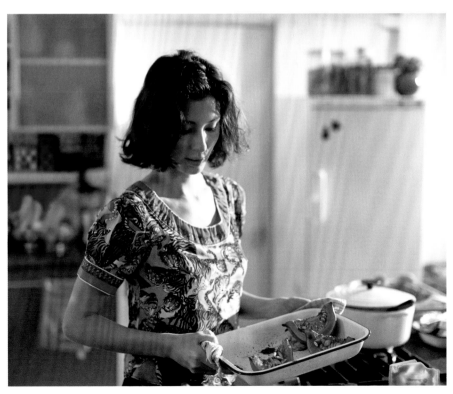

# TAHINI BLISS BALLS

Bliss Balls are nutrient-dense snacks, typically made from dried fruits and nuts, and have been around since the raw-food trend began in the seventies. They're currently enjoying a resurgence, thanks to a renewed interest in gluten-free whole foods.

Our Bliss Balls are easy to make at home so you can tailor them to your taste buds and avoid the overly sweet, shop-bought varieties that use a high ratio of dried fruit to bind them. They are a brilliant snack to have on the go and a great pre- and post-workout snack.

Our recipe is a hunger-busting mixture of fats and protein thanks to a combination of light tahini and creamed coconut balanced with raw honey. Add a little more honey and cacao and you've got a dessert.

No need for a food processor, just stir everything together and roll into balls. Make batches of Bliss Balls and, if you store them in a well-sealed glass container, they'll last for ages in the fridge or freezer.

MAKES ABOUT
16 BLISS BALLS

**FOR THE COCONUT BLISS BALLS**

7 oz bar of creamed coconut or coconut butter

3 tbsp light tahini

1 tbsp raw honey

a pinch of sea salt

a handful of cacao nibs

**FOR THE CHOCOLATE BLISS BALLS**

7 oz bar of creamed coconut or coconut butter

3 tbsp light tahini

1½–2½ tbsp raw honey

2 tbsp cacao powder

¼ tsp sea salt

a handful of cacao nibs

**1** In cold weather, place the unopened packet of creamed coconut in a bowl of warm water to melt it through (you can massage the packet to help it along). In warm weather, the creamed coconut will already be fluid enough.

**2** When it's soft all the way through, pour the coconut into a bowl and mix in the rest of the ingredients for either flavor ball, except the cacao nibs (avoid the tahini oil on the surface of the jar, just pour this off and use in salad dressings).

**3** Depending on the temperature of the day, you can either roll these straight into balls or cool the mix a little in the fridge to make it easier to work with.

**4** Take a spoonful of the mixture and gently roll into a ball between your palms. If the balls are very soft and delicate, refrigerate a little before the next stage.

**5** Roughly chop the cacao nibs if they are large or break them up a little with a rolling pin.

**6** Lightly roll each ball in the cacao nibs and then gently roll them again between your palms to push the nibs in for a smooth surface and so that they don't get knocked off easily.

**7** Store in the fridge or freezer and bring them to room temperature to enjoy, unless you're after a cold treat or need them to last for longer in your bag.

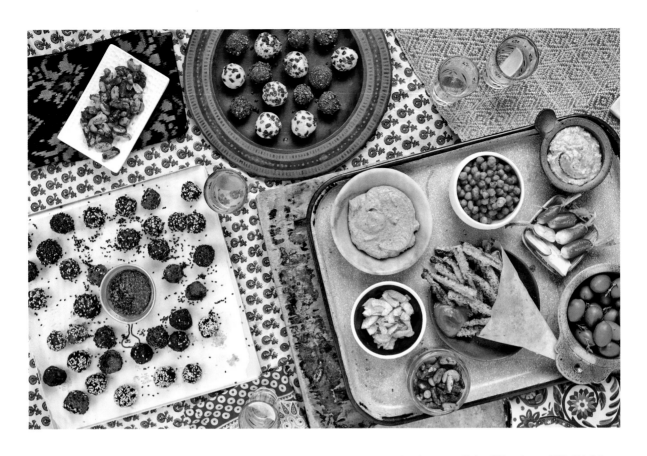

**LEFT TO RIGHT:** Southwestern Spiced Nuts (page 119), Falafel and Italian Veg Balls (page 118), Tahini Bliss Balls (opposite), Lemon Parsley Cashew Dip (page 233), Toasted Coconut Chips (page 122), Baked Zucchini Fries (page 110) with Probiotic Ketchup (page 306), Chickpea Crunchies (page 123), Mung Bean Hummus (page 232), radishes, and green olives.

# BAKED BROCCOLI FRITTERS AND SPICY AVOCADO DIP

MAKES 30 SMALL
FRITTERS

If there was ever a way to make broccoli palatable and delectable, it has to be the fritter. Broccoli is one of the most popular vegetable health heroes and whether these little florets are steamed, stir-fried, oven-roasted, munched raw or even juiced to extract their goodness, it's all good. But not everyone thinks so, and that's where these little caramelized, kid-friendly patties come into their own. Serve the fritters with a big salad of baby spinach, watercress, arugula, chopped radishes, cucumbers and red peppers and some toasted walnuts. This recipe makes up a big batch, and is an ideal snack to keep in the freezer.

## FOR THE FRITTERS

2 large broccoli, stalks and heads, about 2 lb total

2 large scallions, finely sliced or 1 small onion, finely diced

3 garlic cloves, diced

1 tsp lemon zest

3 ½ oz or more of ground almonds

2 ¾ oz parmesan, grated

a large handful of chopped fresh cilantro, parsley, dill, or basil (we used cilantro)

¼ tsp sea salt, plus more to taste

black pepper

1 tsp ground cumin, chili, or smoked paprika (optional)

1–2 eggs

coconut oil or ghee, to fry

## FOR THE SPICY AVOCADO DIP

2 large avocados

4 tbsp lime or lemon juice

4 tbsp extra virgin olive oil

4 tbsp full-fat probiotic natural yogurt

2 scallions, handful of fresh chives or 1 small onion, finely diced

2 garlic cloves, diced

¼ tsp or more of cayenne pepper, minced red chili, or jalapeño peppers, to taste (for children/ non-chili lovers, just split the avocado dip into two portions and add chili to one portion)

sea salt and black pepper

## TO GARNISH

fresh herbs, such as cilantro, to garnish

**1** Preheat the oven to fan 325°F.

**2** Grate the whole broccoli on the coarse teeth of your grater (the fine teeth will make it too watery) or using a food processor. We find a hand grater produces a less wet mixture, but it's a bit more effort.

**3** Combine the fritter ingredients (except the egg) in a large bowl with your hands. Mix in one of the beaten eggs with your hands or a wooden spoon, making sure not to overmix as the mixture can become too wet. If the mixture is too wet, add more ground almonds. If too dry, crack the other egg, whisk it, and add a little to the mixture, adding more if needed.

**4** Take a spoonful to make a tester fritter and fry in a little ghee or coconut oil for a few minutes on each side. Try this one for flavor, then adjust the seasoning if you need to for the rest of the mixture.

**5** Once you're happy with the flavor, shape the mixture, making about 30 patties 1 ½ in in diameter and spread over 2 baking trays. Bake for 20–25 minutes until firm and brown.

**6** To make the spicy avocado dip, blend all the ingredients together with 2 tablespoons water and slowly add cayenne pepper or chili to your taste. Garnish with some fresh herbs and serve with the fritters and a salad.

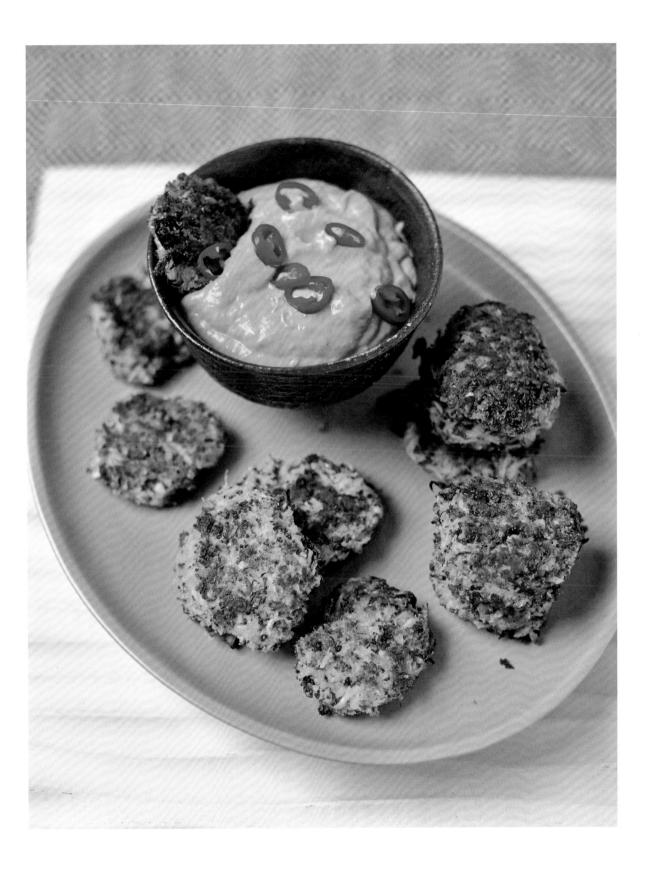

# APPLE RINGS FIVE WAYS

MAKES SNACKS FOR 4,
WITH LEFTOVER DIPS
FOR ANOTHER DAY

Say hello to the new vehicle for tasty toppings: the apple ring! A fresh apple, sliced into discs, replaces crackers and bread. This will totally transform your 4pm snack attacks. Apples are one of the few fresh, unprocessed foods in our urban lives that can be found all year round and easily picked up on the go. Take an apple, wash it and slice through cross sections at any width you desire. Top with your favorite spread!

**FOR THE CINNAMON-SPICED ALMOND BUTTER**

1 jar of almond butter, about 6 oz

1 tbsp ground cinnamon

1 tsp ground nutmeg

1 tsp vanilla extract

1 tbsp raw honey

✚ **IF YOU'VE GOT A SPARE MOMENT AND A FOOD PROCESSOR**, then make your own Nut Butter (pages 303)

**1**  Open the jar of almond butter and pour out some of the almond oil (save this for a salad dressing), then add the rest of the ingredients to the jar and mix well. This will keep for up to 2 weeks in the fridge.

---

**FOR THE FETA AND TAHINI DIP**

2 ½ oz feta

1½ tbsp tahini

¼ tsp lemon zest

1 tbsp lemon juice

1½ tsp extra virgin olive oil

1 tbsp fresh parsley, cilantro, or mint, chopped

black pepper

✚ **THIS IS ALSO NICE SPOONED INTO CELERY STICKS** or stuffed into apples and baked.

**1**  Mash the ingredients together with a fork or throw into your food processor. Add a touch more olive oil if you like to loosen the spread, but for easier transport keep it dry. Store in a jar in the fridge and use within a week.

---

**FOR THE CHOCOLATE HEMP SPREAD**

¾ oz cacao powder

¼ cup coconut oil

1 oz hemp hearts (shelled hemp seeds)

a tiny pinch of sea salt

1 tbsp raw honey

✚ **ROLL THIS MIX INTO BLISS BALL TRUFFLES**, instead of topping the apple, it works really well.

**1**  Blend the ingredients together or melt the coconut oil and mix into the other ingredients. This will keep for up to 2 weeks in the fridge.

---

**FOR THE CHEDDAR AND CHUTNEY**

✚ **NO CHUTNEY?** Try our Goji Marmalade page 48.

**1**  Top the apple slices with your favorite cheddar and chutney.

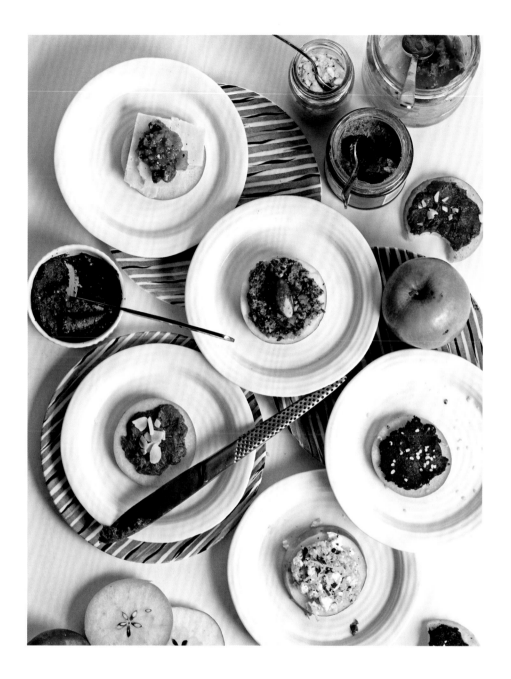

**FOR THE BRAZIL PESTO TOPPING**

just under an ounce fresh
  basil

1 tbsp extra virgin olive oil

½ tbsp lemon juice

1 garlic clove

12 Brazil nuts (about 1 ¾ oz)

sea salt and black pepper

**1**  Make up this chunky version of our easy Brazil Nut Pesto (page 198). This time we reduce the liquid content to create a savory, chunky nut topping. Keep in the fridge and use within a week.

# MEAT AND FISH

ATING MEAT HAS POLARIZED OPINION IN THE WORLD OF NUTRITION. It's either promoted as essential to our well-being or it's argued that eating meat is not necessary at all. Naturally, different bodies have different needs and different preferences for food and so everyone needs to find their own balance.

For us, eating from both the plant and animal kingdom makes sense nutritionally and makes us feel our best, so we regularly eat meat and fish as well as butter, eggs, fat, and liver.

Every now and then we'll enjoy a whole baked fish or a juicy steak but generally we eat smaller portions of meat and fish and prefer foods like beef, lamb, and pork earlier in the day for better digestion before bed.

The quality of the meat is very important. We aim to be ethical omnivores and choose meat from animals that have not been intensively reared (factory farmed) but that have roamed freely and eaten a diet that is natural to them (no GM feeds). Look for organic, pasture-raised (grass fed) meat and dairy, poultry and eggs, and wild or organic, sustainable (environmentally friendly) fish and seafood, including both fresh and tinned options. These quality animal products are richer in micronutrients than their conventional counterparts, which in turn will benefit you.

We realize that these products can sometimes be expensive but eating quality meat doesn't have to mean spending more money. Look for the cheaper, less popular cuts of meat (try our Beef Shin Stew on page 160 or Chicken Liver Mousse page 168), and explore the fish counter for some of the less fashionable fish that are just as tasty and nutritious as more familiar varieties. The money you save on this can be invested in better quality food.

Like meat, fish reared naturally will be better for you nutritionally. Farmed fish are often given pesticides and antibiotics and though fattier (with more flesh to eat), they provide less usable omega-3 fatty acids than wild fish. They also tend to be fed pellets that can contain GM crops like soy and corn, whereas wild caught fish eat a natural diet of other fish, algae, and sea vegetables.

Overfishing and the pollution of the oceans are very real issues, so we need to find a healthy and sustainable way of eating fish and seafood. Look for a supplier of wild fish, caught in a traditional, environmentally friendly way e.g. short lines and pole-caught fish rather than trawled varieties; and look for shellfish that are handpicked rather than dredged. Also find a source of farmed fish, preferably from local fisheries, that is both organically reared and sustainable. It is important that the fundamentals of organic farming practices (health, ecology, fairness, and care) are applied to fish and shellfish too.

Thankfully, most supermarkets are now aware of the issue of sustainability and acknowledge the source of their fish. The good news is fish in good supply usually costs less too.

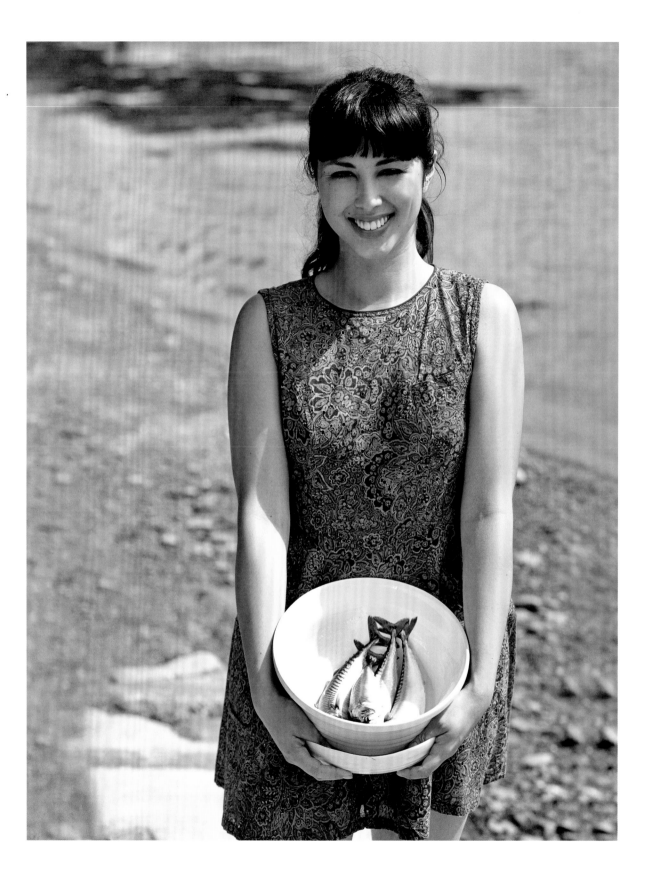

# FISH AND CELERY ROOT CHIPS WITH TARTAR SAUCE

Our take on this quintessential British dish. Instead of refined oil and glutenous batter, we use a mix of chickpea and arrowroot flour and shallow fry the fish in ghee, coconut oil, or beef fat. Use any sustainable white fish.

Our oven-baked chips are made from celery root, which has a subtle celery flavor and makes a great chip. Dip the chips into homemade tartar sauce, below, and Probiotic Ketchup (page 306). Serve with salty and nutritious sea beans, sautéed in butter (don't add salt), or try our Watercress Salad (page 92).

**SERVES 2**

### FOR THE FISH AND CHIPS

1 celery root

3 tbsp ghee, coconut oil, duck, or beef fat, plus extra for greasing

2 tbsp arrowroot flour

4 tbsp chickpea flour

1 egg, beaten

2 x 5 oz firm white fish fillets

sea salt and black pepper

### FOR THE TARTAR SAUCE

1 egg yolk

½ tsp Dijon mustard

¾ cup avocado oil, macadamia oil, or extra virgin olive oil (though delicious, the avocado oil will give a green hue to your sauce!)

2 tbsp lemon juice

½ tbsp capers, roughly chopped

1 tbsp cornichons or gherkins, roughly chopped

½ garlic clove, diced

a large pinch of roughly chopped fresh tarragon or dill (optional)

**1**   Preheat the oven to fan 375°F. Wash and peel the celery root (you might need to use a knife as the skin is thick). Slice off the top and bottom and cut the celery root into thumb-thick slices, and then into fat chip shapes.

**2**   Spread the chips out on a large baking tray, dot with ghee, oil, or fat and season with sea salt.

**3**   Bake for 15 minutes, remove the tray and use two spatulas to toss the chips and coat them in the melted ghee. Return the tray to the oven and bake for another 25–30 minutes or until golden brown.

**4**   To make the tartar sauce start by making a mayonnaise. Use a blender or hand-held whisk to beat together the egg yolk, Dijon mustard, and some sea salt and black pepper.

**5**   Slowly blend or whisk in the oil, a drop at a time, making sure that the oil is thoroughly incorporated before adding the next drop. Once you start to see the yolk thickening, you can add the oil at a slightly faster rate.

**6**   Pour the mayonnaise into a bowl, stir in the other ingredients, then leave to chill.

**7**   Mix the flours together with a tiny pinch of sea salt and pepper and then divide between 2 plates. Set out a bowl of beaten egg.

**8**   Rinse each fish fillet and pat dry with kitchen paper before seasoning both sides of the fish with sea salt. It is important that the fish is dry for the coating to stick.

**9**   Press each fillet firmly into the first plate of flour to coat on all sides, then into the bowl of beaten egg, and then into the last plate of flour to coat, patting an even layer on each side.

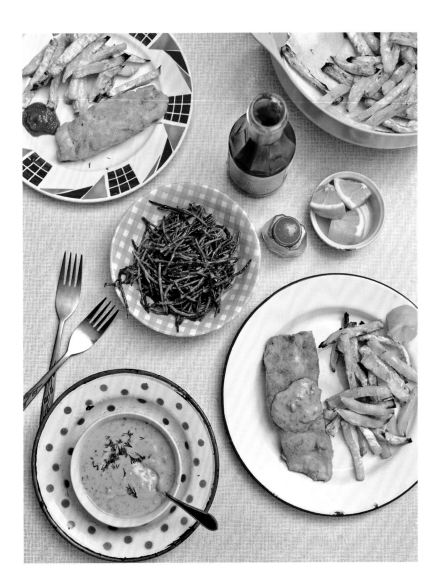

**10** Heat up a frying pan with 1 tablespoon of the ghee until a pinch of leftover flour sizzles when dropped in.

**11** Fry the fish for 3 minutes (you might need to cook them in 2 batches) until crisp and crunchy on the underside, using the remaining tablespoon of ghee if you need it.

**12** Carefully turn the fish to fry the other side for about 2–3 minutes or until golden brown and cooked through. If your fish is particularly thick, you may want to finish it off in the oven preheated to fan 390°F until cooked through.

**13** Serve the fish with the celery root chips, tartar sauce, and some sea beans. Eat any extra tartar sauce within about 2 days and keep refrigerated at all times until serving.

# MACKEREL WITH MISO CARROT DRESSING

Tasty, sweet, and succulent, mackerel is prized for its abundance of omega-3 fatty acids, making it quite possibly our favorite fish. Mackerel partners well with many flavors, but especially horseradish. For a smoky tang, try roasting with cumin, lemon, and garlic or grill with ginger and soy sauce. Here we lightly sear some fillets, and serve with Summer Lime Coleslaw (page 80) topped with miso carrot dressing. The carrot gives texture, color, and bulk to our dressing, and the unpasteurised miso adds a rich flavor, as well as probiotics, to your meal.

SERVES 4

**FOR THE MACKEREL**

8 small mackerel fillets or 4 large ones

1 tsp ghee or coconut oil

sea salt and black pepper

1 tbsp sesame seeds

1 tbsp chives

**FOR THE COLESLAW**

1 x quantity of Summer Lime Coleslaw (without the dressing page 80)

2 tbsp sesame seeds (replace the peanuts in the coleslaw with these)

**FOR THE MISO CARROT DRESSING**

1 large carrot, grated or roughly chopped

2–4 tbsp unpasteurised miso paste (depends on strength of the paste)

a thumb-sized piece of fresh root ginger (about 1 ½ oz) – unpeeled if organic – grated or roughly chopped

1 tsp raw runny honey

juice of 1 lemon or lime

a pinch of sea salt and black pepper (depends how salty the miso paste is)

5 tbsp extra virgin olive oil

**1**   Combine all the dressing ingredients, except for the olive oil, in a blender. Pulse a few times then add 4 tablespoons of water and blend until nearly smooth. Slowly add the oil and continue to blend until smooth. If you need to, add another tablespoon or more of water until the dressing has reached your desired consistency. Leave the dressing to chill a little if you have the time (this is easy to make in advance and will keep well in a sterilized jar).

**2**   Gently toast the sesame seeds for the mackerel and the coleslaw in a dry pan – they will be ready when they start to pop and jump out of the pan. Set to one side.

**3**   Make the Summer Lime Coleslaw following the method on page 80 but swap the peanuts for 2 tablespoons of the toasted sesame seeds. Spoon some of the miso carrot dressing over the coleslaw.

**4**   Season the mackerel. Using the same pan, heat the ghee or coconut oil over a high heat and fry the mackerel fillets skin-side-down to get a crispy, golden skin. After about 45 seconds, flip the mackerel over and cook the flesh side for a further 30 seconds – when the flesh goes from transparent to opaque it is ready. You can also cook the mackerel in the broiler, if preferred.

**5**   Arrange the mackerel on a plate and garnish with the remaining sesame seeds and chives. Serve with the bowl of coleslaw and another bowl of dressing ready to spoon over as needed.

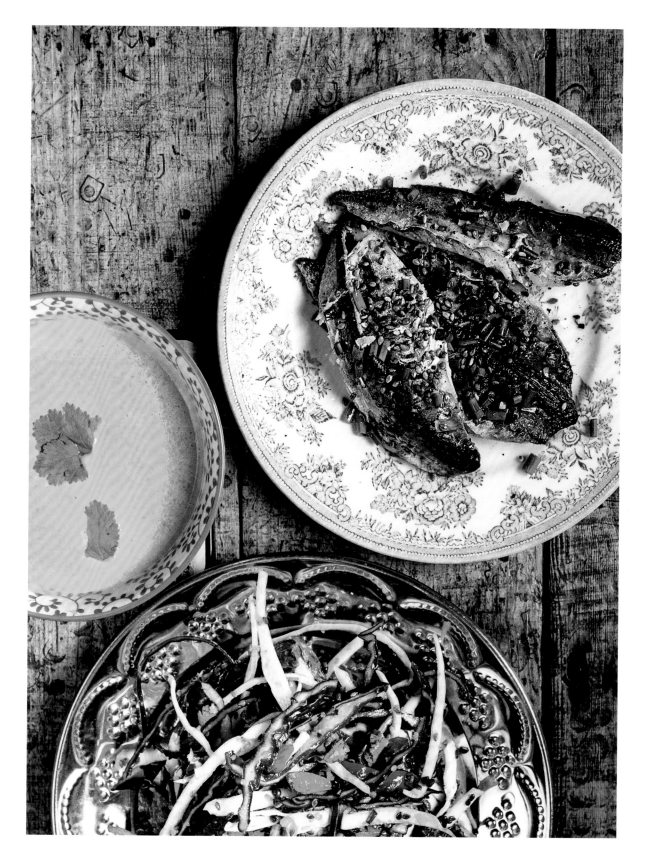

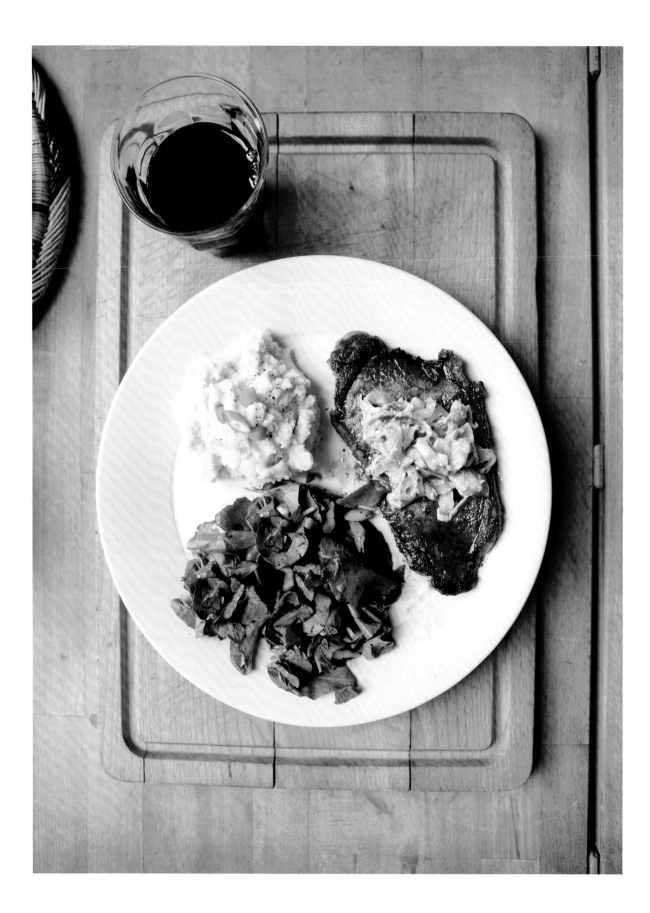

## STEAK WITH MUSTARD LEEK SAUCE AND WATERCRESS SALAD

The perfect weekend lunch – a juicy, caramelized steak. We used grass-fed sirloin here, but ribeye is delicious too – ask the butcher to keep the fat on for the best taste. There is a lot of goodness in grass-fed beef fat. Fat is necessary for nutrient absorption, as well as healthy brain and cell function. We top the steaks with an easy mustard and leek sauce and serve with a couple of vegetable sides. Our favorites are Leek and Kale Salad (but leave out the mint, page 146), Cauliflower Mash (page 104), or a simple watercress salad. The mustard leek sauce is also good with a salmon steak – with some chopped dill stirred in too.

SERVES 2

**FOR THE STEAK**

1 tsp ghee or beef or duck fat

2 good-quality aged steaks, like sirloin or ribeye, fat on

sea salt and black pepper

**FOR THE MUSTARD LEEK SAUCE**

1 large leek, sliced (or 1 onion, halved and then sliced)

1 tbsp good-quality Dijon mustard

a splash of wine, bone broth or water (optional)

**FOR THE WATERCRESS SALAD**

a bunch of watercress or other leaves, such as arugula or baby spinach

1 scallion, sliced

3 tbsp extra virgin olive oil

1 tbsp lemon juice

**1**  Heat the ghee or fat in a frying pan over a high heat until very hot (smoking).

**2**  Season the steaks on each side. Fry the steaks in the hot pan until cooked to your liking, bearing in mind that they'll continue to cook after you take them off the heat. We like medium rare, so just under a couple of minutes on each side based on a ¾ in thick sirloin in a very hot pan. Rare is 1½ minutes, medium is just over a couple of minutes on each side. Once you start frying the steaks, don't touch them, leave to caramelise until you flip them over. Only cook 2 steaks in one pan and space them apart from each other. In order to really caramalise the fat, we use tongs to hold and cook the steak on its edges.

**3**  Transfer the steaks to a plate, cover with another plate or shallow bowl and rest for 5 minutes to allow the juices that have been drawn to the surface to relax back into the meat.

**4**  Using the same frying pan, sweat the leek or onion in the meat juices and fat over a low heat for 3 minutes or until soft. Stir in the mustard and season. Add a splash of wine, bone broth, or water if you want to make the sauce thinner.

**5**  Put the watercress and scallion in a mixing bowl. Drizzle with the extra virgin olive oil and lemon juice and season to taste. Divide the salad between 2 serving plates. Add the steak and spoon the mustard leek sauce over the top.

# BEEF RAGU AND COURGETTI

The new way to spaghetti bolognese! Rather than heavy, glutenous pasta, we use "courgetti" – long strands of raw zucchini ("zoodles" might be more apt for you as our courgette is your zucchini!) cut using a spiralizer or julienne peeler. If you don't have one of these, try a vegetable peeler for very wide ribbons, pappardelle-style. For our beef ragu, we like to squeeze in as many vegetables as possible to make the meaty sauce go further, even using zucchinis again and carrots for added sweetness. It's also a good place to hide a nutritious chicken liver – finely dice and cook the liver with the sauce for a rich flavor.

SERVES 4

2 tbsp ghee or butter

2 onions, finely chopped

4 garlic cloves, diced

2 dried bay leaves

¼ tsp mixed spice (or try a tiny pinch of nutmeg)

2 tsp dried oregano

14 oz minced beef (chuck or braising steak and don't go for lean meat)

a large glass of red wine, about 9 oz

14 large tomatoes, roughly chopped, or 2 tins of chopped tomatoes or 24 oz passata

2 tsp tomato purée

¾ cup bone broth (page 300) or water (you won't need as much if using chopped tomatoes)

2 large carrots, finely grated

1 large handful of fresh parsley, finely chopped

4 large zucchinis

sea salt and black pepper

**TO SERVE**

extra virgin olive oil

2 handfuls of grated parmesan

**1** Heat the ghee or butter in a large saucepan and gently fry the onion over a low heat until softened, but not browned (about 10 minutes). Add the garlic, bay leaves, mixed spice, oregano (and any other herbs that you choose) and fry for a further 2 minutes.

**2** Increase the heat and add the beef to the pan, using a wooden spatula to break it up as you cook.

**3** After 5 minutes, pour in the red wine and stir to deglaze the pan, then add the tomatoes, tomato purée, and bone broth or water.

**4** Bring to the boil, cover with a lid, leaving the lid just slightly off, then reduce to a gentle simmer, stirring occasionally, for 2½ hours until rich and thickened. It is even better after 3–4 hours – keep an eye on it and add more liquid if needed.

**5** Add the grated carrots 15 minutes before the end of cooking. Turn up the heat to a medium simmer and season with sea salt, a good grind of pepper, and the fresh parsley.

**6** Meanwhile, use a spiralizer or julienne peeler to make the courgetti. Or use a regular vegetable peeler to slice the zucchinis lengthways into very wide ribbons, which you can then slice in half. You might want to cut the long strands in half to make them easier to eat.

**7** Soften the courgetti in a pan with a little butter, stirring over a low heat for 3 minutes. Alternatively, save washing up another pan by just running some of the hot sauce through your spirals – the heat and salt in the sauce will soften them.

**8** Drizzle each bowl of ragu and courgetti with extra virgin olive oil and serve with parmesan for everyone to help themselves.

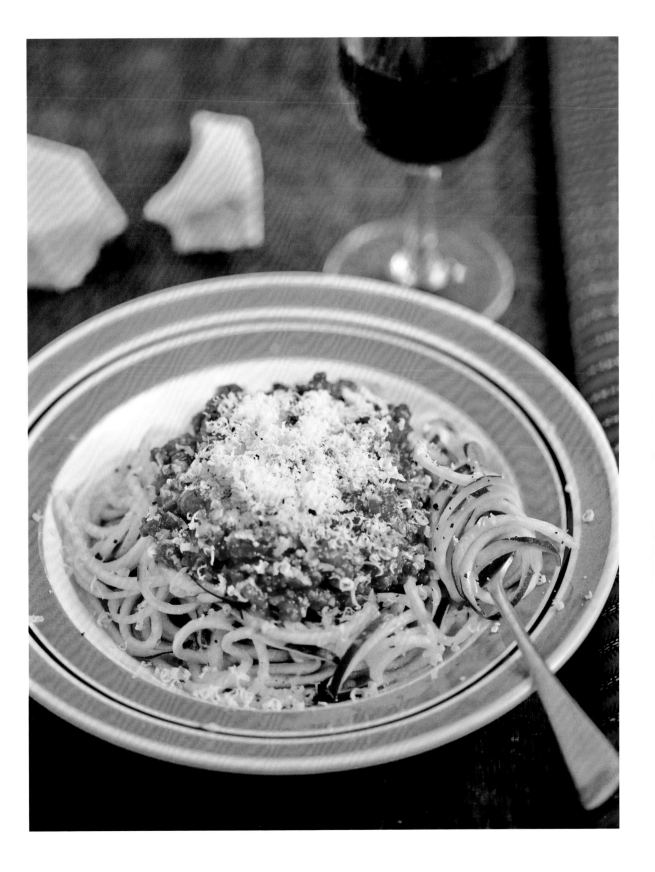

# SARDINE BUTTER

Tinned sardines are a wonderfully cheap and nourishing food that you can keep in your cupboard at all times – a handy emergency snack. This is our favorite way to eat them and an appealing one for people who are squeamish about the look of them. Once mashed together with quality butter, sea salt, and plenty of black pepper and lemon juice, these humble sardines turn into something utterly delicious. Add some chopped chives, red onion or capers and we are in our food heaven.

We use sardine butter like a pate and enjoy with crudité. It makes a delicious topping for steamed green beans or a crunchy salad. But we really like to eat it squashed into Flax Sandwich Bread (page 272) with lots of watercress to offset its richness.

MAKES 6 OZ BUTTER

3 oz butter at room temperature, cut into small cubes

3 ½ oz tin of sardines (3 oz drained weight)

grated zest and juice of ½ an unwaxed lemon

1 tbsp chopped fresh chives

sea salt and black pepper

**OPTIONAL**

capers, finely sliced shallot, or red onion

**1**  Place the room temperature butter in a medium bowl. Drain the sardines and add them to the bowl. Use a fork to mash the butter and sardines together.

**2**  Add the lemon zest and juice, chives, and plenty of sea salt and black pepper to taste, and mix in with the same mashing technique to incorporate. Add capers or finely sliced shallot or red onion, if desired.

**3**  Serve in a ramekin or pile onto a piece of baking parchment, roll into a log, and chill to make it easier to slice.

**4**  Use the butter to top hot vegetables, a salad, or serve with Flax Sandwich Bread (page 272) fresh from the oven.

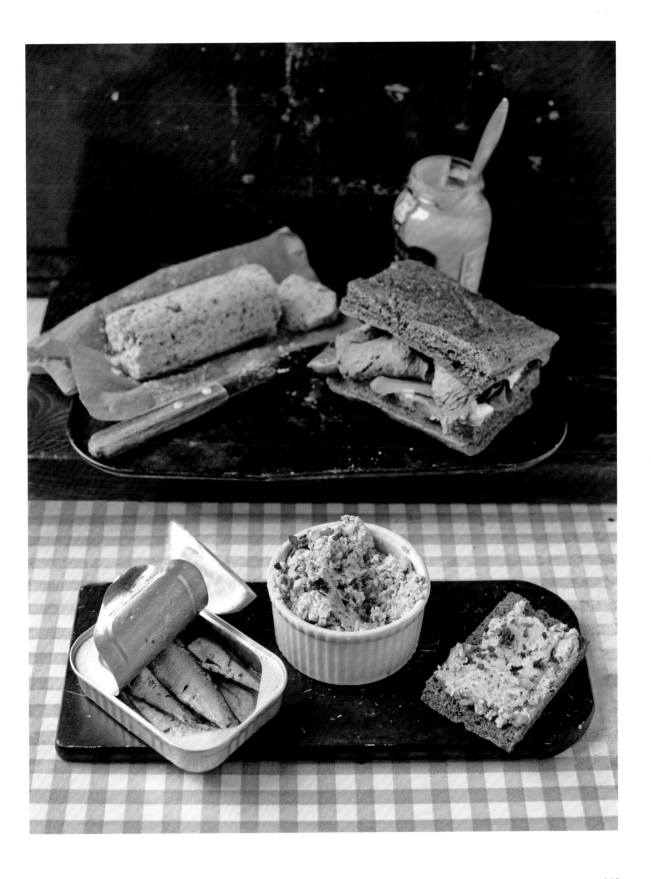

# LAMB MEATBALLS AND CAULIFLOWER TABBOULEH

We've turned a classic Middle Eastern tabbouleh into a gluten-free delight. The rich flavors of lamb work well with the zesty salad, but beef is good too. To make your meat go further, you can add finely grated carrot, shredded celery, and even the carrot pulp from your juicer. For a change, pair your cauliflower tabbouleh with grilled halloumi instead of the meatballs (look for the traditionally made goats' or sheep's milk halloumi).

SERVES 4

### FOR THE MEATBALLS

18 oz minced lamb or beef (don't go for lean mince)

1 egg

1 small onion, finely chopped

3 garlic cloves, diced

1 tsp sea salt

½ tsp black pepper

a large pinch of ground cumin

a large pinch of ground cinnamon

1 tbsp ghee, for frying

a pinch of ground chili or a little fresh chili (optional)

### FOR THE TABBOULEH

2 cauliflowers

1 tbsp ghee or butter

2 red onions or 2 bunches of scallions, finely chopped

4 large tomatoes, diced

3 large handfuls of fresh parsley, finely chopped

a large handful of fresh mint leaves, finely chopped

juice of 1 lemon

6 tbsp extra virgin olive oil

sea salt and black pepper

### TOPPINGS

chopped radishes, nuts, or seeds (such as almonds, pistachios, or sunflower seeds and preferably "crispy" activated, page 300), to garnish

**1** First make the tabbouleh. Remove the cauliflower leaves and the tough end of the stalk. Grate the cauliflower into rice-sized pieces using the slicing attachment of a food processor or the coarse side of a hand-held grater.

**2** Steam the grated cauliflower in a saucepan, lid on, with a couple of tablespoons of water and the ghee or butter. Over a medium heat, it should take roughly 4–6 minutes for the cauliflower to cook (not too soft!). Check there is enough water at the bottom of the pan so that the cauliflower doesn't burn. Drain any excess water and tip the steamed cauliflower into a large serving bowl.

**3** While the cauliflower cools, chop up the rest of the tabbouleh ingredients, then combine everything together. Taste for seasoning.

**4** In a large bowl, combine all the meatball ingredients, except the ghee, and mix well.

**5** In a wide saucepan over a medium heat, add a little ghee and fry a small piece of the meatball mixture and taste to check for seasoning. Adjust the remaining mixture as necessary.

**6** Wet your hands and shape the mince mixture into balls. We use roughly 1½ teaspoons of the mixture per meatball to make about 20 balls, but make them any size you like. Just remember, the larger they are, the longer they'll take to cook.

**7** Heat up a little more ghee and, over a medium-high heat, fry the meatballs in a few batches until lightly browned on all sides and cooked through – this should take about 6–7 minutes. You can always brown the meatballs in advance and finish them off in the oven later if you're having people round.

**8** Serve the meatballs with the tabbouleh and your choice of toppings scattered over the top. If there are any leftovers, eat cold the next day with some homemade Lemon Parsley Cashew Dip (page 233).

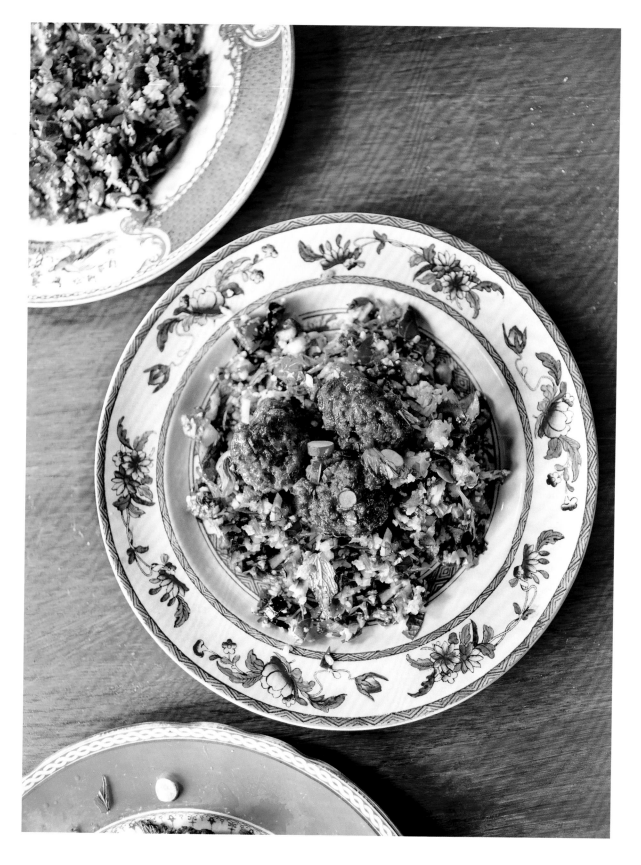

# SLOW-ROASTED LAMB WITH ANCHOVIES

SERVES 6

We use shoulder of lamb here, which is a cheap cut that's more widely available and easy-to-prepare. Since it doesn't carve well, thanks to the bone, we slow-roast the shoulder until the meat falls apart, remembering to save the bone to make a broth.

We serve this with a minty leek and kale salad and some Cauliflower Mash (page 104). Make Shepherd's Pie (page 164) with any leftover meat.

## FOR THE LAMB

a shoulder of lamb on the bone, about 5 ½ lb, at room temperature

2 tbsp ghee or beef or duck fat

8 garlic cloves, peeled and halved

a small jar of anchovies (about 10 anchovies)

2 tbsp fresh thyme leaves or use 1 tbsp dried thyme (but fresh thyme would be ideal)

a large glass (8 ½ oz) of red or white wine

2 dried bay leaves

sea salt and black pepper

## FOR THE LEEK AND KALE SALAD

1 ⅓ lb (stalks removed), leaves finely chopped

1 leek, finely sliced

3 tbsp fresh mint, finely sliced

6 tbsp extra virgin olive oil

3 tbsp lemon juice

**1**  Preheat the oven to its maximum temperature.

**2**  Place the lamb in a large ovenproof dish or stainless steel roasting pan and rub with the ghee or fat. Season with a little sea salt (not too much as the anchovies are salty) and black pepper.

**3**  Make 10 incisions into the fat of the lamb, about 1 ½ in deep, and fill with the garlic, anchovies and thyme.

**4**  Pour over the wine, add the bay leaves, cover with a tight-fitting lid and place in the oven.

**5**  Turn the oven heat down immediately to fan 325°F and cook for 3–3 ½ hours until the meat is tender enough to fall apart easily.

**6**  Start the kale salad while the lamb is slow cooking. Put the kale leaves in a large bowl with the leek and mint leaves. Using your hands. massage the leaves with the extra virgin olive oil, lemon juice, and some salt and pepper for a minute, then set aside to marinate. The kale will start to relax and soften almost straight away, but this salad will be really tender after 1–2 hours.

**7**  When the lamb is cooked, drain the gravy from the bottom of the pan into a small saucepan, reduce if necessary, and check for seasoning.

**8**  Keep the lamb covered and allow to rest in the pan for at least 15 minutes before serving with the hot gravy and leek and kale salad.

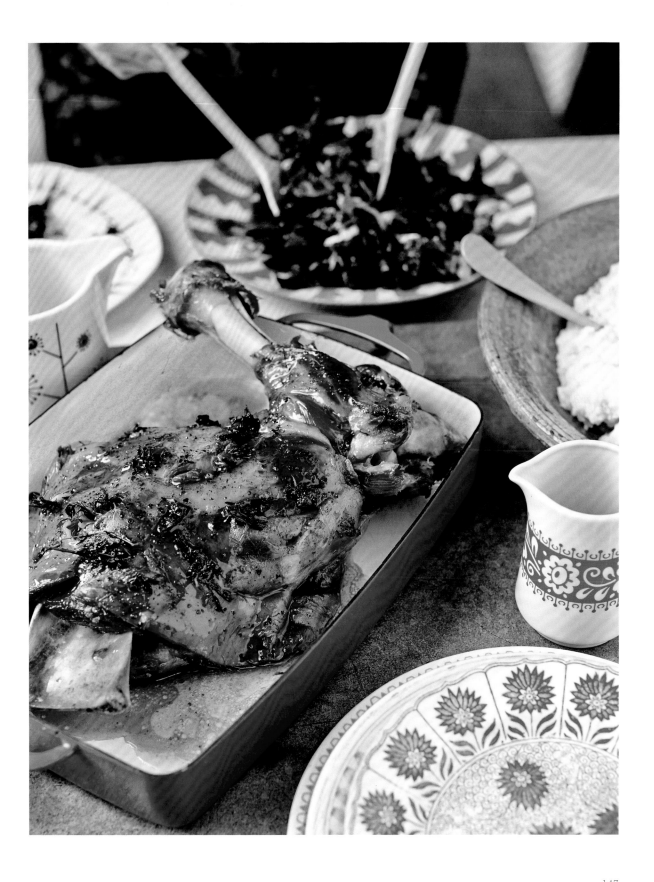

# SAUSAGE AND CIDER STEW

A one-pot meal is the way to go when entertaining – sausage and cider stew, perfect for autumn evenings, has become our Bonfire Night special. Protein-rich sausages are best combined with less starchy vegetables for better digestion. The best for this dish has to be the good old savoy cabbage because the gravy from the stew clings to its textured leaves, but any cabbage will do, and rutabaga makes an excellent alternative to potato.

Delicious with Cauliflower Mash (page 104), Garlic Lemon Green Beans (page 113), and some homemade Sauerkraut (pages 306–307) for a fresh tang and a helping of probiotics.

SERVES 6

2 tbsp ghee

10 large gluten-free sausages

2 medium onions, diced

2 medium leeks, sliced

4 garlic cloves, diced

3 celery sticks, diced

2 cups strong cider

2 tbsp tomato purée

2 tbsp mustard (depending on strength)

3 large pinches of dried mixed herbs (a combination of thyme, rosemary and sage) or double the amount if using fresh

2 dried bay leaves

2 large handfuls of chopped fresh parsley leaves and finely chopped stalks

2 cups bone broth (page 300) or vegetable stock

2 rutabagas, peeled and diced

4 large carrots, roughly chopped

sea salt and black pepper

**1**  Heat 1 tablespoon of the ghee in a large pan or casserole dish over a medium heat. Brown the sausages, then set aside. Do this in two batches to avoid overcrowding, otherwise they will start to steam rather than brown.

**2**  In the same pan, heat the remaining ghee over a medium heat and add the onions, leeks, garlic, and celery. Sauté for 5 minutes or more until soft.

**3**  Pour in the cider to deglaze the pan, turn up the heat, and let it bubble away until it reduces. Use a wooden spatula to scrape the bottom of the pan and release any caramelized, browned bits.

**4**  Add the tomato purée, mustard, and herbs, including the parsley stalk ends but not the fresh parsley leaves, and stir.

**5**  Add the broth or stock and bring to boil. Throw in the rest of the vegetables, cover the pan, reduce the heat to a medium simmer, and cook for 30 minutes or more until the vegetables are tender.

**6**  Meanwhile, slice each sausage into thirds at an angle and add to the pan for the last 15 minutes of cooking. Season to taste with sea salt and pepper.

**7**  Add more liquid for a soupier stew or cook without a lid for a thicker, richer sauce if preferred. Alternatively, remove some of the sauce and vegetables and blend to make a thick, creamy sauce before stirring it back into the pan. Stir in the parsley leaves to serve.

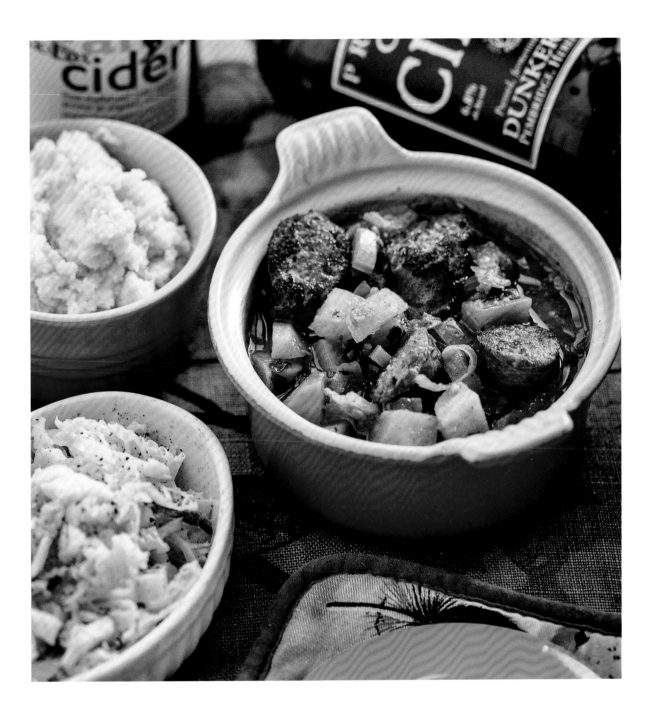

# CHICKEN CURRY AND CAULIFLOWER RICE

Curry that's so good for you, we say eat it for breakfast! We love this chicken curry for lunch, leaving us more than enough time to digest the meat before bed. Cumin and coriander are full of antioxidants and help with digestion. Turmeric, the "superstar spice," is known to have anti-inflammatory properties. By skipping the starchy rice and serving this curry with cauliflower and crunchy raw cabbage, you're treating yourself to two portions of vegetables.

SERVES 4

## FOR THE CHICKEN CURRY

2 tbsp ghee or coconut oil

4 large chicken thighs or drumsticks, skin on

3 tsp ground cumin

2 tsp ground coriander

3 tsp ground turmeric

2 tsp garam masala

2 tsp fennel seeds (we like these whole, but you could grind them first)

a pinch of dried or fresh chili, to taste, or ½–1 tsp cayenne pepper (add a little at the start, then adjust), optional

2 large onions, sliced or chopped

6 garlic cloves, diced

2 tbsp tomato purée

4 large tomatoes, chopped

2 cups bone broth (page 300) or vegetable stock

10 ½ oz green beans or any other green vegetables, such as zucchini, broccoli or sugar snap peas

2 large handfuls of spinach or other greens

juice of ½ a lime or lemon

sea salt and black pepper

## TO SERVE

Pilaf-style Cauliflower Rice (page 102)

a small handful of flaked almonds, toasted

1 tbsp raisins

## FOR THE RED CABBAGE SALAD

1 red cabbage

1 tbsp sesame oil (not toasted) or extra virgin olive oil

a small handful of chopped fresh cilantro or mint

grated zest and juice of 1 unwaxed lime or lemon

**1** Gently toast the flaked almonds (for the rice) for a minute in a wide, dry pan with a lid over a low heat, then set aside.

**2** Heat 1 tablespoon of the ghee or coconut oil over a medium heat in the same pan. Season the chicken thighs or drumsticks with a little sea salt and pepper, then brown for a few minutes on each side until golden. Remove the chicken and set aside.

**3** Lower the heat in the pan and add all the spices, including the chili or cayenne pepper, if using. Keep the spices moving so that they don't burn and let them fry gently for 1 minute.

**4** Add the rest of the ghee or coconut oil and the onions and fry for 5 minutes before adding the garlic, a large pinch of sea salt, and pepper, followed by the tomato purée and turn up the heat.

**5** Add the chicken back in, the chopped tomatoes, and the hot broth or stock.

**6** Simmer over a medium heat, covered, for 35 minutes. The slower it cooks, the better – add a little water if needs be. It also tastes even better the next day.

**7** Meanwhile, prepare the salad by finely shredding the red cabbage with a knife or in a food processor and heaping onto a serving dish. Add the oil, cilantro or mint, zest and juice of the lime or lemon to a jam jar, shaking with the lid on to make the dressing, then taste for seasoning and mix with the cabbage.

**8** After the 35 minutes of chicken cooking, add the green beans and leave to simmer for a further 4 minutes. Turn off the heat and check the chicken is tender and cooked through using a knife. Add the lemon or lime juice and check the seasoning.

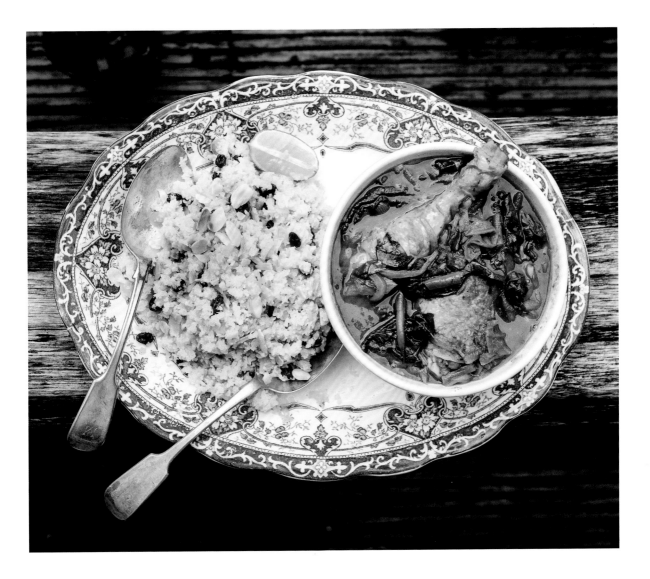

**9** Place the spinach on top, cover with a lid and let the residual heat wilt the spinach for 5 minutes while you prepare the cauliflower rice.

**10** Serve with the Pilaf-style Cauliflower Rice, chicken curry, and the red cabbage salad.

# ROAST DUCK WITH CRANBERRY AND ORANGE JAM

This is a favorite recipe of ours to serve at a family gathering, such as Christmas. Duck meat is so juicy that it can be cooked in advance, left to rest, then served at room temperature with some piping hot gravy.

Orange is a classic partner to duck and cranberries are "of the holiday season," so a cranberry and orange jam fits the bill. The recipe makes enough for about 15 portions, so the leftovers will see you through your festive season (it's great as a chutney with cheese).

Carve the duck at the table and serve with a platter of low-starch roasted veg, such as turnip, red cabbage, carrots, onions, and that Christmas-dinner-must-have, sprouts, or Roasted Vegetables (page 192), Kohlrabi Dauphinoise (page 211), and Red Cabbage, Bacon, and Apple Salad (page 96).

DUCK SERVES 4 AND THE JAM MAKES 15 PORTIONS

## FOR THE ROAST DUCK

1 duck, about 3 ¾ lb (ask your butcher for advice – some breeds of ducks have lighter frames than others, which will affect the cooking time even if the weight is the same)

2 tsp ghee

sea salt and black pepper

## FOR THE CRANBERRY AND ORANGE JAM

1 ⅓ lb dried cranberries

1 juniper berry, crushed

3 star anise

¾ cup port

grated zest and juice of 1 unwaxed orange

grated zest and juice of 1 unwaxed lemon

2 large pinches of sea salt

2 pinches of black pepper

1 tbsp maple syrup

2 small pinches of ground nutmeg

**1** Remove the duck from fridge at least 2 hours before cooking to bring it up to room temperature. Preheat the oven to fan 425°F.

**2** Wash the duck inside and out and pat dry. Remove the giblets if there are any (keep to make a gravy or add to a stew). Use a skewer or very sharp knife to prick the duck (not too deep) about 10 times all over its body, especially in the fatty bits at the breast.

**3** Rub the duck all over with the ghee and some salt and pepper (throw a pinch of salt and pepper inside the duck too), then place on a wire rack with a deep roasting tray underneath to catch all the fat.

**4** Roast for 40 minutes, keeping an eye out to check the skin does not burn and turning down the heat if the skin darkens too much – it should be golden rather than brown.

**5** Roast for another 20 mins at fan 350°F. Use a skewer to poke between the thighs to check if the duck is cooked – the juices should run clear. Otherwise, keep cooking for another 15 minutes and then check again.

**6** Turn up the oven again to fan 425°F for a final 8 minutes to make crispy skin.

**7** Remove the duck from the oven, cover, and leave to rest for 15 minutes. With caution, pour the duck fat into a sterilized jar and leave to cool before adding the lid. Keep in the fridge and use for roasts and stir-fries etc.

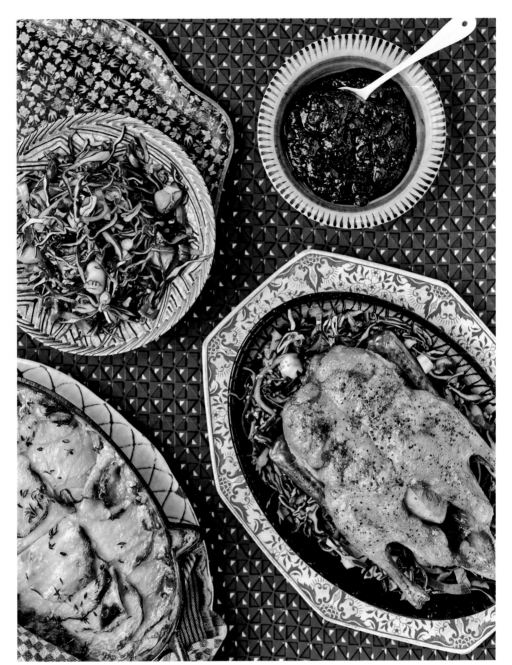

**LEFT TO RIGHT**:
Kohlrabi Dauphinoise
(page 211), Red
Cabbage, Bacon, and
Apple Salad (page 96),
and Roast Duck with
Cranberry and Orange
Jam (opposite)

**8**  To make the jam, simmer all the ingredients
together with 3 ⅓ cup water in a pan for 15 minutes.
Blitz with a hand-held blender or mash with a potato
masher to make a thick sauce but leave a few lumps
for texture.

**9**  If the jam is too thin, simmer in the pan for
5 minutes to allow it to reduce. If you want more of a
pouring sauce, just add some bone broth or water and
blend until smooth.

# MUM'S BAKED TROUT

This was an almost impossible recipe to get off our mum. Many emails back and forth and endless variations and suggestions. She says she changes it every time, but we've worked out that this is the basic version – lots of lemon, onion, and tomatoes. As they cook with the fish, their juices create a delicious sauce. If she fancies it, she makes it "more Filipino" and adds a dash of tamari and grated ginger or some of her roasted red chilies that we love. Serve hot from the oven with a simple, crisp salad and some buttered green beans.

SERVES 2-3 PEOPLE

1 large whole trout, about 1 ⅓ lb, or 2 small trout (ask your fishmonger to prepare the fish so you can stuff it)

1 large onion, preferably red for color and sweetness, halved

1 large tomato, finely chopped or 6 cherry tomatoes, finely chopped

1 lemon

10 cherry tomatoes on the vine, kept whole

4 scallions, kept whole

sea salt and black pepper

**1** Preheat the oven to fan 390°F.

**2** Make 5 shallow slices on an angle into the top side of the fish. Season the fish inside and out and place on parchment paper on a baking tray.

**3** Slice half of the onion into thin slices and finely dice the other half.

**4** Mix together the finely chopped tomato, the diced onion, juice of half the lemon, and some salt and pepper, then fill the fish cavity with the mixture.

**5** Arrange the cherry tomatoes, scallions, and the sliced onion around the fish on the tray, then season and squeeze the rest of the lemon all over, leaving the lemon halves on the tray.

**6** Bake for 20 minutes or until cooked through.

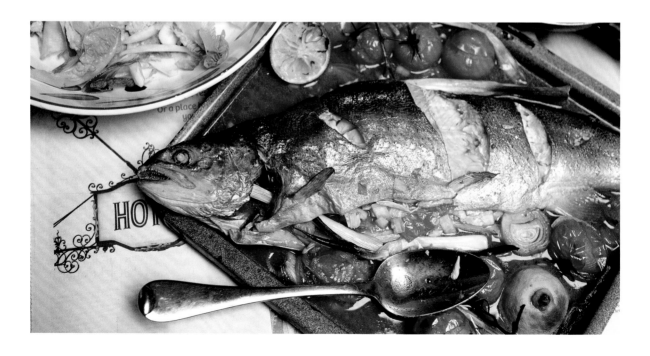

## SEA BREAM TERIYAKI

If you don't have time to marinate the fish, don't worry, because this sauce is rich in flavor and can be reduced on the stove and poured over instead. Make up the sauce while the oven is heating up, then bake the fish until it's just cooked through. Any leftover sauce is great with a chicken salad or added to a stir fry. Serve this dish with Broccoli Slaw (page 88), Carrot, Radish, and Seaweed Salad (page 86), Cauliflower Rice (page 102), or Spring Greens with Blood Orange Dressing (page 221).

SERVES 2

**FOR THE SEA BREAM**

2 large sea bream fillets (about 10 ½ oz, ask your fishmonger to descale)

1 tbsp ghee or coconut oil

2 scallions, sliced on the angle

**FOR THE TERIYAKI SAUCE**

¼ cup tamari

2 tbsp apple cider vinegar

1½ tbsp maple syrup

1 garlic clove, finely grated

1 tsp fresh root ginger (unpeeled if organic), finely grated or chopped (optional)

a pinch of white or black pepper or some fresh red chili or chili flakes (optional)

**1**  First make the sauce. Whisk together the tamari, apple cider vinegar, maple syrup, garlic, ginger, pepper, and chili, if using, to make the teriyaki marinade.

**2**  Make six shallow cuts in the fish's skin, lay the fish in a shallow dish and pour over the teriyaki sauce. Cover with a plate and put in the fridge for 1 hour. If you use a more robust fish like salmon, you can marinate it for much longer, but sea bream is quite delicate.

**3**  Preheat the oven to fan 350°F. Rub the ghee or coconut oil into the bottom of an ovenproof dish. Drain the fish, reserving the marinade, then place the fish into the dish, skin side up, and bake for 5–7 minutes until just cooked through.

**4**  Meanwhile, heat the reserved marinade at a simmer for a few minutes.

**5**  Serve immediately, spooning the hot teriyaki sauce over the fish and scatter over the spring onion.

# FISH PIE WITH CELERY ROOT MASH

If you're having people over, then try this fish pie — you can make it up in advance, ready to pop in the oven. Use a large serving dish or try individual pots, which look great for presentation and are good for freezing in portions. Celery root is not the prettiest of vegetables, but once you've peeled off the knobbly outer layer and cooked it up, you'll find the creamy mash makes a satisfying topping to the veg-packed fish filling and you won't miss potatoes at all. For an extra twist, stir through a little tamarind paste with the wine to give it a Worcestershire sauce-type kick. Serve with a Watercress Salad (page 139) or Garlic Lemon Green Beans (page 113).

SERVES 4

### FOR THE FISH FILLING

1 large onion (or 2 onions if no leeks), finely chopped

1 large leek (or 2 leeks if no onions), finely chopped

1 carrot, finely diced

1 celery stick, finely diced

½ fennel bulb, finely diced (you could add the fennel fronds to the sauce in place of dried dill)

1 tsp dried dill

1 bay leaf

1 tbsp ghee

½ cup white wine

1 ⅓ lb fish (we used 10 ½ oz wild salmon and 10 ½ oz undyed smoked haddock)

2 tbsp arrowroot, to thicken the sauce

a handful of fresh parsley, chopped

sea salt and black pepper

### FOR THE CELERY ROOT MASH

2 medium celery root, about 2 ¼ lb in total, peeled and cut into ¾ in cubes

1 ¾ oz butter

just under an ounce parmesan, grated

**1** First make the celery root mash. Steam the celery root cubes in a pan with a little water, lid on, for about 15 minutes until tender. Drain well and then roughly mash with the butter and some seasoning using a vegetable masher or pulse a few times with a hand-held blender.

**2** Preheat the oven to fan 350°F.

**3** Fry the onion and/or leek, carrot, celery, fennel, dried dill, and bay leaf in the ghee in a large pan over a medium heat for about 10 minutes until almost tender.

**4** Add the wine to the softened veg mix, stir, and simmer until the wine has evaporated.

**5** Add 2 cups hot water to the pan and bring to a simmer over a medium heat. Add the fish, cover, and poach for about 5 minutes until cooked through. Remove the fish and set aside.

**6** Mix the arrowroot in a cup with a little cold water until smooth then add it to the pan. Stir constantly for a few minutes as the sauce thickens up, then take off the heat and stir through the chopped parsley and season.

**7** Flake the fish into a round 10 in diameter oven dish that is 2 in deep. Sit the dish on a baking tray in case the sauce runs over during cooking, then pour the veg sauce over the fish.

**8** Cover with the roughly mashed celery root and bake for 30 minutes to heat through.

**9** Preheat the broiler. Cover the mash with the grated parmesan and cook on high for 5 minutes until the top is golden.

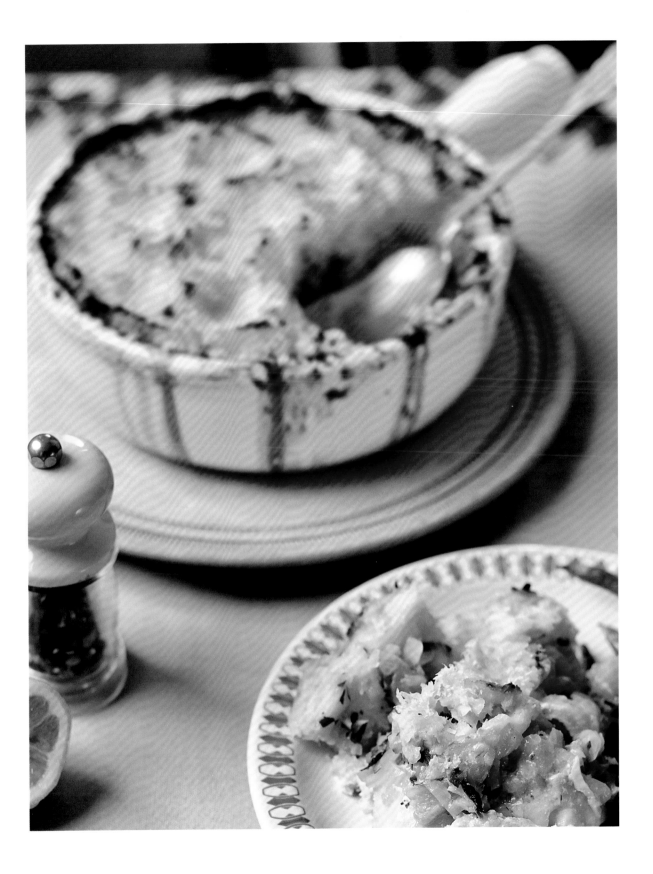

## SALMON WITH ARGENTINIAN CHIMICHURRI SAUCE

Chimichurri sauce is traditionally served with a good rare steak, but we also love how the apple cider vinegar and the bitter, antioxidant-rich fresh herbs cut through the richness of a beautifully grilled piece of salmon. Serve with Braised Fennel with Lemon and Rosemary (page 109). Chimichurri works with plenty of other dishes too, especially robust ones, and livens up a simple meal. Also try mackerel and other oily fish, adding a dash more vinegar to cut through the fattiness.

Try the Columbian version of a chimichurri sauce with half parsley and half cilantro or blend it smooth and add another 4 tablespoons extra virgin olive oil and 1 tablespoon more apple cider vinegar to make a tangy green dressing for any salad.

SERVES 2 WITH EXTRA
CHIMICHURRI SAUCE

**FOR THE SALMON**

2 salmon fillets, skin on

1 tsp ghee or coconut oil, for crispy skin

sea salt and black pepper

lime wedges, to serve

**FOR THE CHIMICHURRI SAUCE**

3 large handfuls of fresh parsley (stalks included if you're blending it smooth or save the stalks for juicing or soups)

1 small onion or shallot or 3 scallions

4 garlic cloves

1 tsp dried oregano or thyme

a fresh green chili or a pinch of chili powder, to taste

6 tbsp extra virgin olive oil

1½ tbsp apple cider vinegar

**1**  Preheat the oven to fan 350°F.

**2**  To make the chimichurri sauce, use a knife or food processor to finely chop all the ingredients together, then stir through the extra virgin olive oil and apple cider vinegar at the last minute. Season to taste. The sauce can be blended quite chunky (traditional) or smooth, depending on your preference.

**3**  Pat the salmon fillets dry, then season on both sides, rubbing the skin side with a little ghee or oil. Place in a frying pan (preferably one that can go in the oven), skin side down, and cook for a few minutes to get a crispy skin.

**4**  Transfer to the oven and bake for 5 minutes or until cooked through.

**5**  Serve the salmon hot with braised fennel, lime wedges, and a big spoonful of chimichurri sauce. Alternatively, for a packed lunch, let the salmon cool, then flake and serve in a big salad with the chimichurri sauce as a dressing.

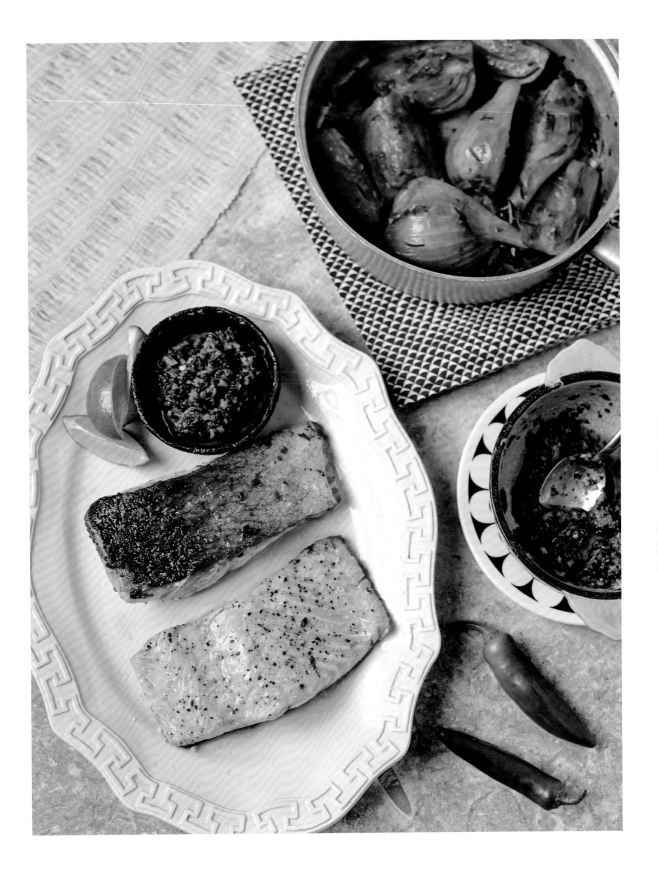

## OSSO BUCCO BEEF SHIN WITH OAK-SMOKED TOMATOES

A slow-cooked, one pot, melt-in-the-mouth stew with a sweet and smoky gravy. Our friends Lizzie and Richard from Wild Beef gave us the tip for adding oak-smoked, sun-dried tomatoes. If you have trouble finding these, then use fresh or tinned tomatoes instead, reducing the amount of water and upping the tomato purée to keep it rich. A few pinches of smoked sweet paprika will provide the subtle smoky flavor. The stew freezes beautifully and tastes even better the next day, and even the day after that, so don't be put off by the number of people the recipe serves. This dish really is easy peasy – quick prep, slow cook, and maximum appreciation from everyone who is lucky enough to eat it. Serve with a Watercress Salad (page 139) in summer or Cauliflower Mash (page 104) in winter.

SERVES 8

4 ½ lb beef shin, cut into rounds with marrow bones included

1 tbsp ghee or butter

3 large onions, roughly diced

2 celery sticks, diced

6 carrots, chopped into large batons (you don't want them to disintegrate during the cooking)

2 tbsp tomato purée

2 dried bay leaves

2 x 6 ½ oz containers of oak-smoked tomatoes, drained

1 large white or savoy cabbage, halved and shredded

2 handfuls of chopped fresh parsley, to garnish

sea salt and black pepper

**1** If using the oven, preheat to fan 275°F.

**2** If the butcher has not already done it, start by removing the tough outer skin from the beef shins, but leave the fat on. Season the meat with sea salt and black pepper.

**3** Heat the ghee or butter in a casserole dish over a low heat and gently fry the onion, celery, and carrot for 5 minutes before adding the beef shins, tomato purée, bay leaves, and drained smoked tomatoes.

**4** Add enough hot water to just cover everything and bring up to a gentle simmer.

**5** Pop the lid on and bake in the oven for 3–4 hours, checking and stirring occasionally. If you are cooking on the stove top, simmer away gently for 3–4 hours. You can start cooking this up to 8 hours in advance and keep it on the lowest simmer.

**6** Check your stew for seasoning 10 minutes before serving, then pile up the shredded cabbage on top, put the lid on and let the cabbage wilt over a gentle heat before serving, garnished with parsley.

✚ **WE OFTEN USE OUR SLOW COOKER** and keep it bubbling all day. If you are using a slow cooker from scratch, add all the ingredients to your pot on low and let it cook for 6–8 hours. Use less water, filling just two-thirds of the way up.

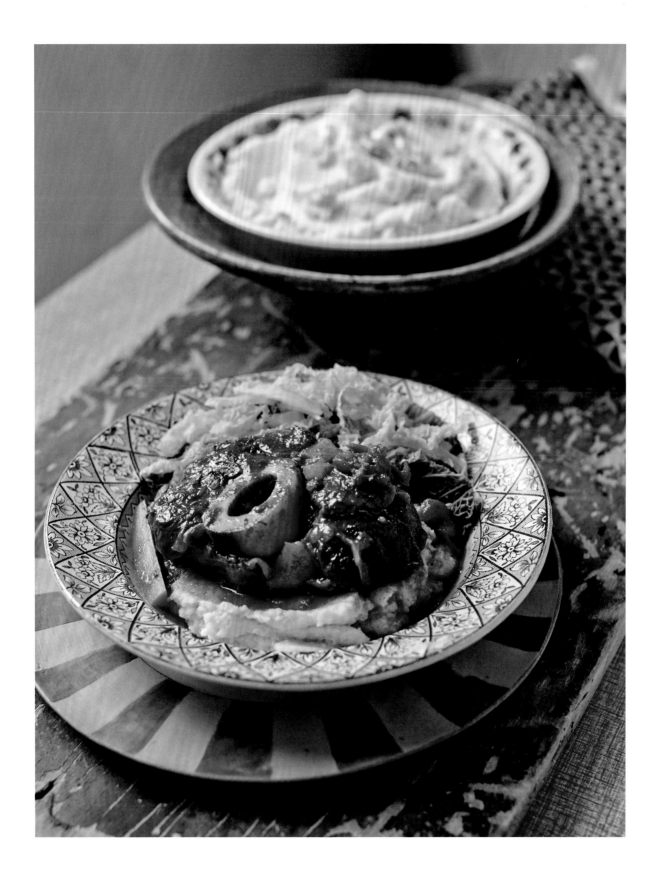

## SRI LANKAN LAMB CURRY

**SERVES 4**

Sweet coconut, earthy spices, and juicy lamb. Making your own spice mix from fresh makes all the difference and is easy, it's just a bit of measuring!

Enjoy this curry with Cauliflower Rice (page 102), Broccoli Rice (page 170), or Summer Lime Coleslaw (page 80) and greens like chard or spinach added towards the end of the cooking time. We cook this on the stove for a few hours or for 6–8 hours on low in a slow cooker. Leftover sauce will go nicely with some roasted squash wedges the next day or pour over coleslaw to warm it up.

**FOR THE LAMB CURRY**

1 tbsp ghee or coconut oil

2 onions, halved and finely sliced

3 garlic cloves, grated

a thumb-sized piece of fresh root ginger (about 1 ½ oz) – unpeeled if organic – grated

18 oz stewing lamb (from lamb shoulder is delicious), cubed

1 tin of full-fat coconut milk

2 cups bone broth (page 300) or water

2 large carrots, diced

2 zucchinis, diced

1 red pepper, roughly diced

juice of 1 lemon or lime

2 large handfuls fresh cilantro, chopped

sea salt and black pepper

**FOR THE SRI LANKAN SPICE MIX**

1 tbsp ground cumin

1 tbsp ground coriander

1 tsp fennel seeds

¼ tsp chili powder or fresh chili, to taste

½ tsp ground turmeric

¼ tsp ground cinnamon

¼ tsp ground cloves

¼ tsp ground cardamom

**1** Heat the ghee or coconut oil in a large casserole dish over a low heat and gently fry the onion, garlic, ginger, and all the spices for the Sri Lankan spice mix for 10 minutes until soft.

**2** Add the lamb, coconut milk, and broth, then turn the heat up and leave to simmer for 2–3 hours until the lamb is tender.

**3** Add the carrot and turn up the heat to a medium simmer. After 8 minutes, add the zucchini and red pepper.

**4** After another 8 minutes, check all the veg is tender and season, if needed. Squeeze in some lemon or lime juice to taste and add half of the fresh cilantro.

**5** Serve each bowl with more fresh cilantro on top.

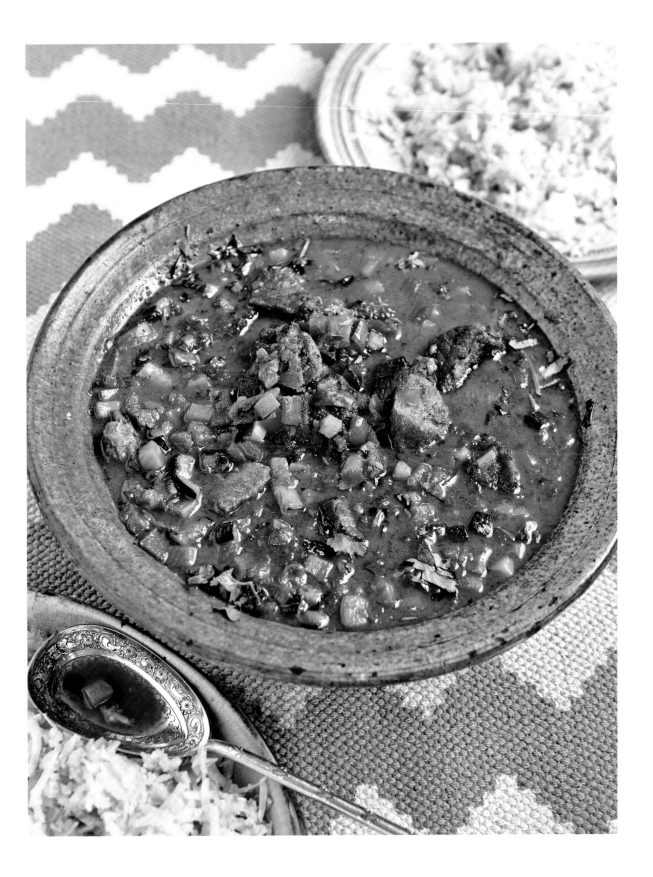

# SHEPHERD'S PIE

The beauty of shepherd's pie is that it's a fantastically frugal way of using less tender and less popular cuts of lamb. By using this trick you can afford to step up the quality of the meat that you buy – after all every part of a naturally reared animal is nutritious, not just the "premium" cuts.

While the traditional pie is topped with potato, we've used our popular Cauliflower Mash (page 104) here instead. When you mash it, give it a kick with some of the following: mustard, snipped fresh chives, finely sliced spring onion, horseradish, garlic, nutmeg, some caramelized onions and leeks, or crumble in any cheese.

Serve your Shepherd's Pie with some seasonal buttered veg like spring greens, purple sprouted broccoli, and Garlic Lemon Green Beans (page 113) or keep it light with a Watercress Salad (page 139).

SERVES 4

## FOR THE SHEPHERD'S PIE FILLING

1 tbsp ghee or duck fat

18 oz minced lamb (ask your butcher to mince the lamb and don't go for lean meat)

1 large onion or leek, finely chopped

1 celery stick, finely diced

2 carrots, finely diced

2 dried bay leaves

1 tsp dried rosemary or 2 tsp fresh rosemary, roughly chopped

1 tsp dried thyme or 2 tsp fresh thyme (save some to garnish)

1 garlic clove, diced

1 zucchini, finely diced

1 tbsp tomato purée

8 $\frac{1}{2}$ oz red wine

2 cups bone broth (page 300)

a small handful of fresh parsley, roughly chopped

sea salt and black pepper

## FOR THE TOPPING

Cauliflower Mash (page 104)

a sprinkle of fresh chives or fresh thyme leaves, to garnish

a little butter

**1** Heat half the ghee in a large pan over a medium heat and brown the mince for a few minutes. Set aside.

**2** In the same pan, add the remaining ghee and sauté the onion, celery, carrot, bay leaves, rosemary, and thyme for 5 minutes. Add the garlic and zucchini and gently fry for a further minute.

**3** Return the mince to the pan and stir in the tomato purée and red wine. Cook over a medium heat for a few minutes until the liquid has reduced.

**4** Add the broth and simmer with the lid on for at least 30 minutes. We like to slow cook the sauce for up to an hour, adding more broth or water if it starts to get dry.

**5** Stir through the fresh parsley and taste for seasoning.

**6** Meanwhile, preheat the oven to fan 390°F.

**7** You can either use individual 5 x 6 in ramekins or pie dishes (great for freezing portions) or a 7 $\frac{1}{2}$ in square baking dish, that is 2 in deep (or the rough equivalent of an oval dish). Fill your dish two-thirds full with the lamb mixture and top with the Cauliflower Mash, using a fork to crisscross over the top. Dot with some butter.

**8** Bake for 25–30 minutes until golden. Finish with a sprinkle of chives or some fresh thyme leaves.

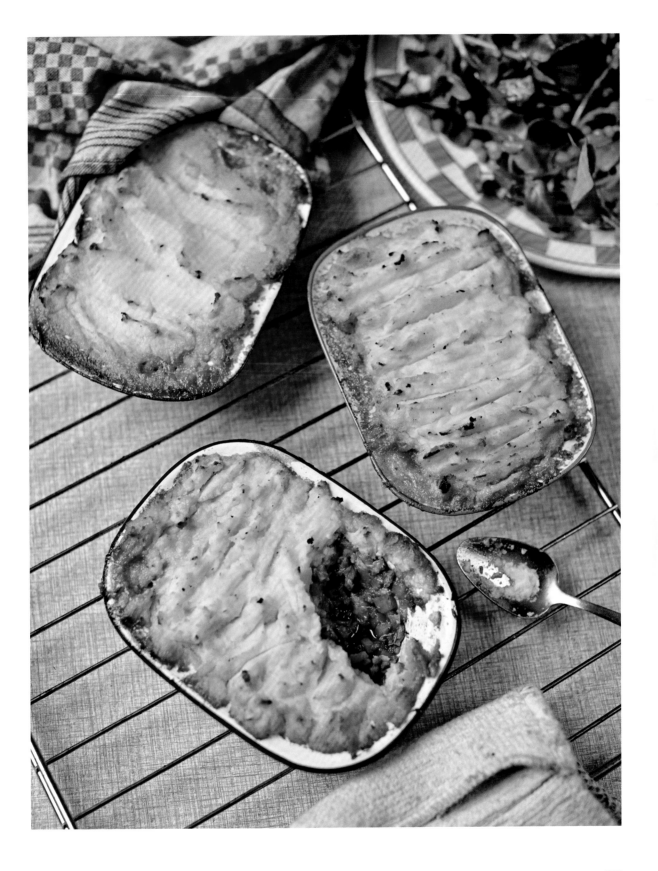

# PABLO'S CHICKEN

We named this dish after Pablo, our cousin's husband, because he's a fried chicken fiend who challenged us to make him a healthy version that would keep him happy. Here it is – no breadcrumbs, no vegetable oil, no need to deep fry! Succulent chicken baked in a homemade spice mix with a crisp nutty crust, perfect hot or cold. Serve with some Probiotic Ketchup (page 306), Thai Sweet Chili Sauce (page 228), or just a squeeze of lemon and either Summer Lime Coleslaw, Quicker-than-toast Zucchini Salad, or Fennel, Cucumber, and Dill Salad (pages 80, 84, and 97).

SERVES 4

**FOR THE CHICKEN**

6 ½ oz ground almonds or use Sun Flour (page 302)

2 eggs

6 pieces of chicken (use a mix of drumsticks and thighs), skin on

1 tbsp ghee

sea salt and black pepper

**FOR THE SPICE MIX**

3 tsp hot smoked paprika or 2 ½ tsp smoked sweet paprika with ½ tsp cayenne pepper

1½ tsp ground cumin

1½ tsp sea salt

1 tsp dried thyme

1 tsp dried oregano

¾ tsp onion powder (optional)

¾ tsp garlic powder (optional)

**1** Preheat the oven to fan 350°F and line a baking tray with baking parchment.

**2** Mix the ground almonds and ingredients for the spice mix in a bowl. In a second bowl, beat the eggs.

**3** Dip the chicken pieces, one at a time, in the egg, then coat in the mix of ground almonds and spices and lay on the baking tray.

**4** Gently heat the ghee and use a spoon to drizzle it over the pieces.

**5** Bake for 45 minutes until golden and sprinkle with some sea salt and pepper.

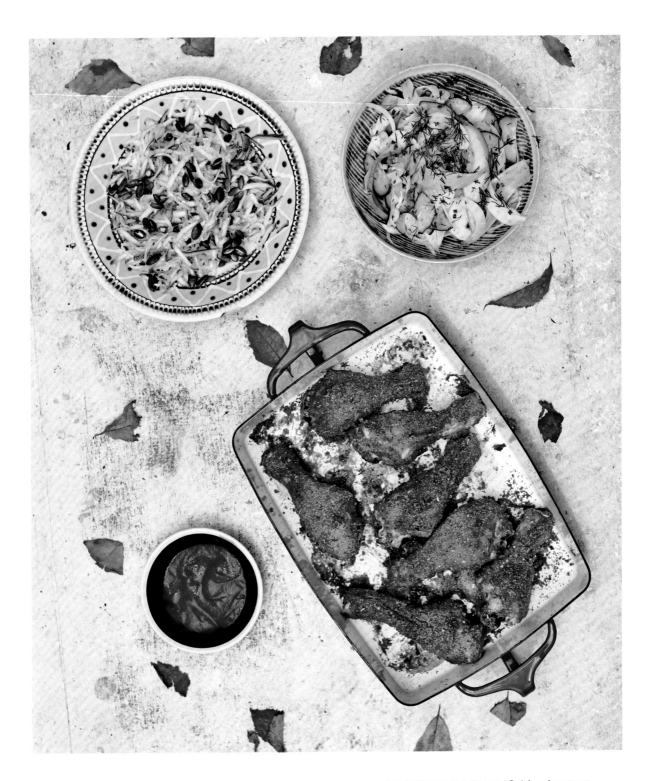

**ANTI-CLOCKWISE FROM TOP LEFT:** Quicker-than-toast Zucchini Salad (page 84), Probiotic Ketchup (page 306), Pablo's Chicken (opposite), Fennel, Cucumber, and Dill Salad (page 97).

# BAKED CHICKEN LIVER MOUSSE

This is our easy chicken liver mousse. Smoother and finer than pâté (which we love too) and so easy because we just blitz everything then pour it straight into a dish and bake. We've also given the option of a water bath below because the slow cooking results in a smoother mousse, but we must confess we sometimes don't bother.

Organic chicken livers are incredibly nutritious and, luckily, one of the cheapest meats you can buy. Enjoy the mousse smoothed onto our Flax Sandwich Bread (page 272) or Carrot and Flax Crackers (page 121). Serve with Fennel, Cucumber, and Dill Salad (page 97) or our favorite way to eat this is sliced and served on top of any stir-fried veg.

**SERVES 6-8**

½ apple, cored and peeled (no need to peel if you have a strong blender)

½ small onion

3 ½ oz butter at room temperature

7 oz fresh (not frozen) chicken livers (any leftover liver can be thrown into a ragu for a richer sauce)

1 tsp sea salt

½ tsp allspice

½ tsp ground white pepper

2 eggs

**OPTIONAL**

1–2 tbsp Cognac if you want to jazz it up

**1** Preheat the oven to fan 250°F. Butter and line a 5 ½ x 2 ¾ in loaf tin, if you are using this instead of individual ramekins.

**2** If you have a strong blender and room temperature butter, then throw all the ingredients in, pulse a few times, and blend until smooth. Otherwise, finely chop the apple and onion. Melt the butter in a pan and cook the apple and onion until softened, then add to a blender or food processor.

**3** Add the chicken livers, sea salt, allspice, white pepper, and eggs and blend until completely smooth. Add the Cognac, if using.

**4** Pour the liver mixture into four or five 3 in ramekins, filling almost to the top, or a 5 ½ x 2 ¾ in buttered or lined loaf tin. Tap the bottom lightly on the work surface to get rid of air bubbles.

**5** Place the ramekins or tin inside a deep baking tray, fill with freshly boiled water until the water is halfway up the sides, and pop in the oven.

**6** If using ramekins, cook for 20–25 minutes or about 30–35 if using a loaf tin. You know the liver mousse is done when it is set around the edges and the center is only very slightly wobbly.

**7** Let the dish cool a little and serve hot or cold straight from the ramekins or loaf tin. Alternatively, if you used a lined tin, cover with a plate and turn upside down to remove the mousse. Slice and serve or refrigerate the mousse until needed.

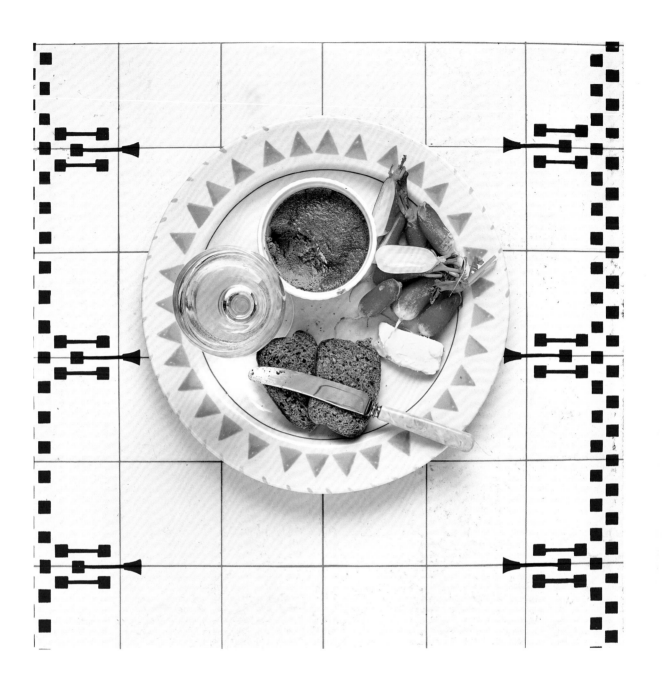

# CHICKEN ADOBO WITH BROCCOLI RICE

Chicken Adobo is one of the national dishes of the Philippines and was one of our favorite meals growing up. You can see the Spanish and Chinese influences on Filipino cuisine in this dish. The chicken is simmered in soy, or in our version tamari, and vinegar; adobo means marinade in Spanish.

Our mum grew up eating adobo with white rice but surprised herself by enjoying cauliflower and broccoli rice instead – both give the perfect texture for soaking up the rich gravy.

SERVES 4

### FOR THE CHICKEN

1 tbsp coconut oil

4 large chicken thighs, skin on

5 garlic cloves, diced

3 ⅓ cup bone broth (page 300) or vegetable stock

3 dried bay leaves

1 tsp freshly ground white or black pepper

1 tsp whole black peppercorns

3½ tbsp apple cider vinegar

2 tbsp tamari (no extra salt needed as tamari is salty)

### FOR THE BROCCOLI RICE

1 head of broccoli including stalk, about 12 oz

2 scallions, finely sliced or 1 tbsp snipped fresh chives

sea salt and black pepper

**1** Heat the coconut oil over a medium-high heat in a wide pan with a lid. Once the oil is hot, place the chicken thighs into the oil and brown lightly, lid off, for about 3 minutes on each side. Remove the browned chicken from the pan and set aside.

**2** Lower the heat and add the garlic. Sauté for another 30 seconds until starting to color before adding the broth, bay leaves, pepper, peppercorns, and apple cider vinegar. Stir and bring the sauce to a simmer.

**3** Add the chicken back to the sauce in the pan, turn the heat down to low, and cover. Simmer the chicken in the sauce for 10 minutes, then turn the chicken over, cover and cook for another 5–8 minutes until the chicken is cooked through. Add the tamari to the sauce and stir through.

**4** We like lots of sauce to go with our broccoli rice, but if you'd like it thicker, remove the chicken and keep it warm (you can remove the skin at this point too, put it on a baking tray and bake it until crispy – it'll be super tasty with all the adobo flavors), then reduce the sauce, uncovered, for a few minutes over a medium simmer.

**5** To make the broccoli rice, use a food processor or the coarse teeth on a grater to grate the whole broccoli including the stalk into rice-sized pieces. Steam the broccoli in a pan with a few tablespoons of water, lid on, for 3–4 minutes until tender with a little bite, stirring halfway through. Season to taste and stir through the spring onion or chives, then serve immediately with the chicken.

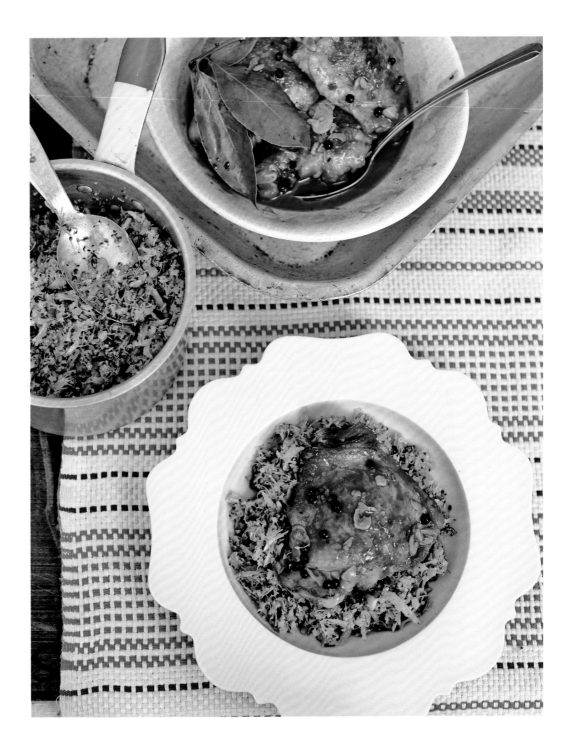

+ **TRY STEAMING THE BROCCOLI RICE** with some finely grated ginger or garlic, use coconut milk instead of water, season with ½ tsp tamari instead of salt or a few drops of toasted sesame oil to taste.

+ **FOR A REALLY QUICK TAKE ON EGG FRIED RICE**, scramble an egg and stir it through Broccoli Rice with a splash of tamari and toasted sesame oil.

171

# SESAME CHICKEN SALAD WITH CUCUMBER NOODLES

A refreshing summer salad with cucumber noodles and Asian flavors. This is the perfect way to use up leftover chicken or serve instead with a little fish or sliced seared beef. We love raw chopped bok choy, but you can substitute with Chinese-style cabbage or finely shredded English cabbage. Eat this within a few hours as the cucumber will start to get watery or make everything else up in advance and prepare the cucumber noodles just before serving. If you're taking this for lunch, pack the chicken first, then arrange all the veg on top so they don't get squashed, and take your dressing in a separate jar.

SERVES 2

## FOR THE SALAD

2 tbsp black or white sesame seeds

2 cucumbers

1 small head of romaine or cos lettuce, shredded into ribbons

1 small head of bok choy or 5 oz Chinese cabbage, shredded into ribbons

3 scallions, thinly sliced

a handful of fresh cilantro, roughly chopped

9 oz cooked shredded chicken

## FOR THE SESAME DRESSING

5 tbsp sesame oil (not toasted) or extra virgin olive oil

2 tbsp toasted sesame oil

juice of 1 lime or 3 tbsp lemon juice

2 tsp raw runny honey

1 tsp tamari or sea salt

## OPTIONAL

1 finely chopped red chili, to garnish

**1** Gently toast the sesame seeds in a dry pan until fragrant.

**2** Use a spiralizer or julienne peeler to make the cucumber noodles. Or use a regular vegetable peeler to slice the cucumbers lengthways into wide pappardelle-style ribbons. You might want to cut the long, spiralized strands in half to make them easier to eat.

**3** Prepare the dressing by whisking together all the ingredients in a bowl or shaking them together in a jam jar.

**4** Add the lettuce, bok choy, scallion, and cilantro to a bowl.

**5** Pour over the dressing and mix everything together (hands are best).

**6** Plate up with some shredded chicken and top with toasted sesame seeds. Serve immediately.

## ✛ NO LEFTOVER CHICKEN?

Roast 2 large chicken thighs at fan 390°F/ Gas mark 7 for 25–30 minutes until cooked, then shred quickly with 2 forks to cool the meat quickly.

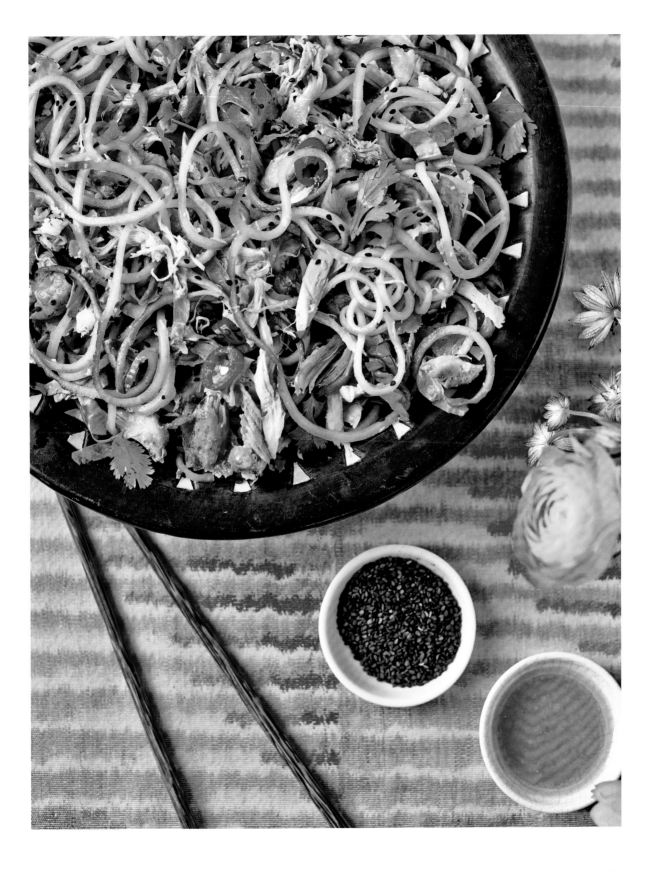

# DUCK TAMARIND LETTUCE WRAPS

We're big on Asian flavors, so the ingredients for this easy sauce are in our cupboard at all times. You'll probably know the tangy tamarind flavor from Thai and Southeast Asian cooking – our Mum cooks with the super-sour tamarind fruit all the time. Look for tamarind paste, which is just the fruit mixed with water, as it's easier to use than the blocks of tamarind, which contain some seeds. The sauce can be made in advance and you'll have leftovers to use in stir fries and salads – it will transform a buckwheat noodle stir-fry or leftover roast veg. Collect the duck fat in a jar for frying or roasting meats or veg in the week. Serve the wraps with Broccoli Slaw (page 88) or Carrot, Radish, and Seaweed Salad (page 86).

SERVES 2

**FOR THE DUCK**

2 duck legs, about 14 oz

½ cucumber

4 scallions

1 red chili

2 Little Gem lettuces, leaves separated

a small handful of fresh cilantro, roughly chopped

1 lime, cut into wedges

sea salt and black pepper

**FOR THE TAMARIND SAUCE**

3 tbsp almond or peanut butter (chunky or smooth)

4 tbsp tamarind paste

1½ tbsp maple syrup

2 large garlic cloves, grated

1 teaspoon tamari

some fresh or dried chili, to taste (optional)

**1** Preheat the oven to fan 350°F.

**2** Pat the duck legs dry with kitchen towel, prick the skin all over, and rub sea salt and pepper into the duck. Roast in the oven for 60–75 minutes on a wire rack. Then remove the duck, drain the fat, and leave the duck to sit for 10 minutes under foil or somewhere warm while you prepare the sauce.

**3** Mix all the tamarind sauce ingredients together with ½ cup water, then simmer with the lid on for 8 minutes. If it's not thick enough, take the lid off and leave it to reduce until thick enough to cling to a piece of cucumber or spring onion.

**4** Thinly julienne the cucumber and scallion and slice the red chili.

**5** Shred the duck using two forks – don't forget to include the crispy skin.

**6** Let everyone help themselves or assemble them on a platter to serve. Pile up each lettuce leaf with duck, cucumber, scallion, chili, and cilantro, squeeze over the lime juice and add a dollop of tamarind sauce.

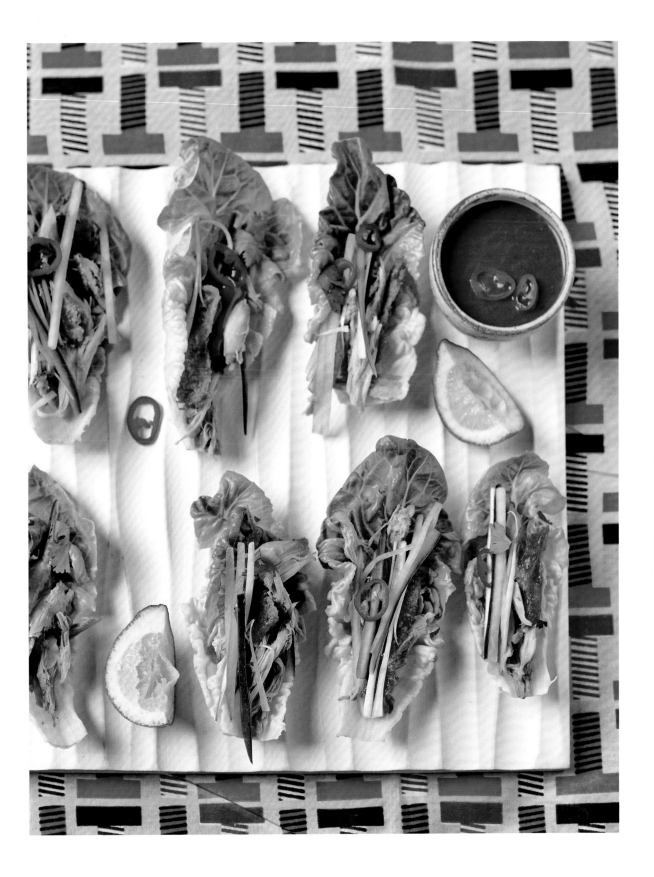

# MOROCCAN CHICKEN STEW

One of our favorite one-pot dishes. Once you prep everything and put the lid on, you can leave this simmering on the stove for 40 minutes while it cooks slowly, then add a handful of leaves to serve. We sometimes make this with fish fillets instead, which are quicker to cook – just add them in to poach once you're happy with the flavor and thickness of the sauce. This is also good with Cauliflower Rice (page 102) or Fennel, Cucumber, and Dill Salad (page 97). Any leftover sauce from the stew can be enjoyed the next day with some steamed quinoa and fresh veggies. Save the bones and add to the stock pot.

SERVES 4

a large handful of flaked almonds

1 tbsp ghee

2 red onions, finely sliced

4 garlic cloves, diced

a thumb-sized piece of fresh root ginger (about 1 ½ oz) – unpeeled if organic – finely grated or 2 tsp ground ginger

1 tsp ground cumin

1 tsp ground cinnamon

½ tsp smoked sweet paprika

4 chicken thighs, skin on

2 red peppers, deseeded and sliced into thin strips

1 large lemon, cut into 6 thick slices

a handful of green olives, stones removed

8 ½ oz bone broth (page 300) or vegetable stock

4 pitted dates or dried apricots, chopped

5 oz green beans, halved

a handful each of fresh cilantro and parsley

sea salt and black pepper

**OPTIONAL**

a small pinch of chili powder or 1 fresh chili, chopped

**1**  In a large, dry pan, gently toast the flaked almonds for a minute – don't take your eyes off them as they burn easily. Set the almonds aside.

**2**  In the same pan, heat the ghee, then gently cook the onion for 8 minutes until softened. Add the garlic, ginger, and spices and fry for another minute.

**3**  Add the chicken thighs and cook until colored lightly on both sides.

**4**  Add the red pepper slices, lemon slices, olives, the broth, and dates or apricots. Simmer with the lid on for about 40 minutes until the chicken is cooked through.

**5**  If you find the sauce is too watery, take the lid off and leave it to reduce a little. If the sauce is too thick, add a few more tablespoons of water.

**6**  Add the halved green beans for the last 4 minutes cooking time.

**7**  Season to taste and top with the cilantro and parsley and the toasted flaked almonds to serve.

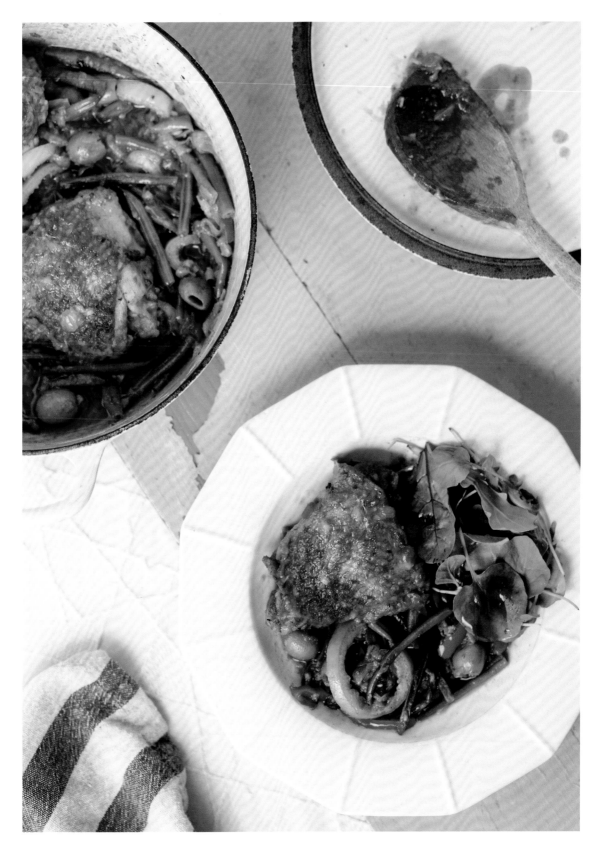

# PRAWN LAKSA

A curry rich with Malaysian spices and coconut that comes together in just 20 minutes. We use small or regular-sized prawns, but for guests we serve with a couple of big prawns, shell on, for effect. Choose cold water prawns rather than tropical and look for the sustainable logo. Lemongrass is worth seeking out with its citrus flavor and slightly gingery taste, otherwise use lime or lemon zest.

Kelp noodles are a great alternative to glass noodles so we always have them in our storecupboards ready to add to Asian-inspired salads and soups. If you can't get kelp noodles, substitute with Zucchini Noodles (page 66) or Cucumber Noodles (page 172) or serve with Cauliflower Rice made with ½ tsp turmeric (page 102).

SERVES 2

2 ¾ oz kelp noodles

1 tbsp peanuts (preferably "crispy" activated page 302)

1 large onion, halved

a thumb-sized piece of fresh root ginger (about 1 ½ oz) – unpeeled if organic

1 red chili

3 garlic cloves

1 tsp coriander seeds

1 tbsp coconut oil

2 lemongrass, each chopped into 4 pieces and roughly bashed or zest of 1 unwaxed lime or ½ unwaxed lemon

2 tsp ground turmeric

½ cup bone broth (page 300), fish/shellfish stock, or vegetable stock

1 tin of full-fat coconut milk

4 ¼ oz snow peas

5 oz fresh raw unpeeled prawns (use peeled if easier for you, but we like to keep them whole)

3 ½ oz rainbow chard or other greens, finely chop the stems on the angle and slice the leaves into 3 pieces

1 tbsp tamari

juice of 1 lime or ½ lemon

a handful of fresh cilantro, plus more to serve

**1**  Follow the kelp noodle packet instructions (they normally say to soak them for 10 minutes in warm water, then rinse them).

**2**  In a large, dry pan, toast the peanuts over a gentle heat for a minute until golden – giving the pan a shake to make sure they are golden all over. Set the nuts aside.

**3**  Blend the onion, ginger, chili, garlic, and coriander seeds in a blender or food processor to make a paste or finely chop with a knife and bash the coriander seeds.

**4**  Using the same pan, heat up the coconut oil and add the paste, the chopped and roughly bashed lemongrass or lime zest, and the turmeric and fry for a few minutes.

**5**  Add the broth and coconut milk and turn up the heat to a medium simmer.

**6**  Add the snow peas and prawns to the pan and cook for 2–3 minutes, depending on their size and whether they have the shell on, until pink and tender. Take off the heat and stir through the kelp noodles.

**7**  Meanwhile, in a separate pan, steam the chopped chard stems and leaves with a little water, covered, for 2 minutes until tender. Season to taste.

**8**  Stir the tamari, lime juice, and fresh cilantro through the laksa and check for seasoning – you might want to add a little more tamari or lime juice, to taste. You can fish out the lemongrass, if you like, or just leave it in and eat around it.

**9**  To serve, divide the prawns between two bowls and ladle over the soup, top with chard, more cilantro, and the toasted peanuts.

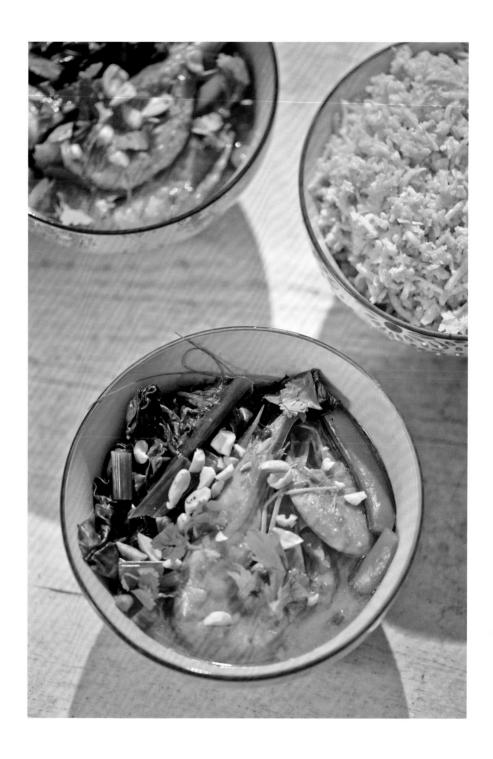

✚ **EXPERIMENT** — we also enjoy this with beef or some poached fish… For a vegetarian version, add some squash and juicy chunks of eggplant.

# CUCUMBER MAKI CRAB ROLLS

Rice-free sushi? We love sashimi (that's just the raw fish), but you need to be able to access high-quality and super-fresh fish – something that most of us can't really do. So, our Cucumber Maki Crab Rolls are a great faux option. They are perfect for entertaining and there's no rolling technique needed either – it's actually a pretty easy dish despite its creativity!

This is a good way of using up leftover poached or smoked salmon. It's also a nice way of eating the expensive treat of some crab as a little goes a long way once you've mixed it with the other ingredients. Avocado is a must and so is a mayonnaise. An old-school melon baller will give you an easier job and a neater finish.

MAKES 10–12 PIECES

### FOR THE CRAB ROLLS

3 ½ oz crabmeat, mixed or just white

½ avocado, diced

2 scallions, sliced

1 tbsp Ginger Poppy Seed Mayonnaise (page 88) or full-fat probiotic yogurt

2 tsp lime juice

½ red chili, finely chopped or a sprinkle of chili flakes, to taste

1 large cucumber

black or white sesame seeds, to garnish

sea salt

### TO SERVE

tamari

wasabi paste (or 1 tbsp tamari mixed into the paste with ½ tbsp water)

a few slices of pickled ginger

**1** Drain any liquid from the crab and put it in a bowl with the avocado, spring onion, mayonnaise, lime juice, and a pinch of salt. Mix very carefully to avoid crushing the ingredients and then stir in the chili, to taste.

**2** Wash the cucumber and remove one end. Cut the cucumber into even 1 in thick slices.

**3** Use a small knife to carefully cut out the flesh from the center of the cucumber, leaving just a few millimetres of flesh all the way around. We found the neatest way was to use a melon baller to scoop the seeds out, leaving the bottom of the cucumber intact.

**4** Distribute the crabmeat mixture between each cucumber roll. Finish with a sprinkle of sesame seeds and serve with the tamari, wasabi, or pickled ginger.

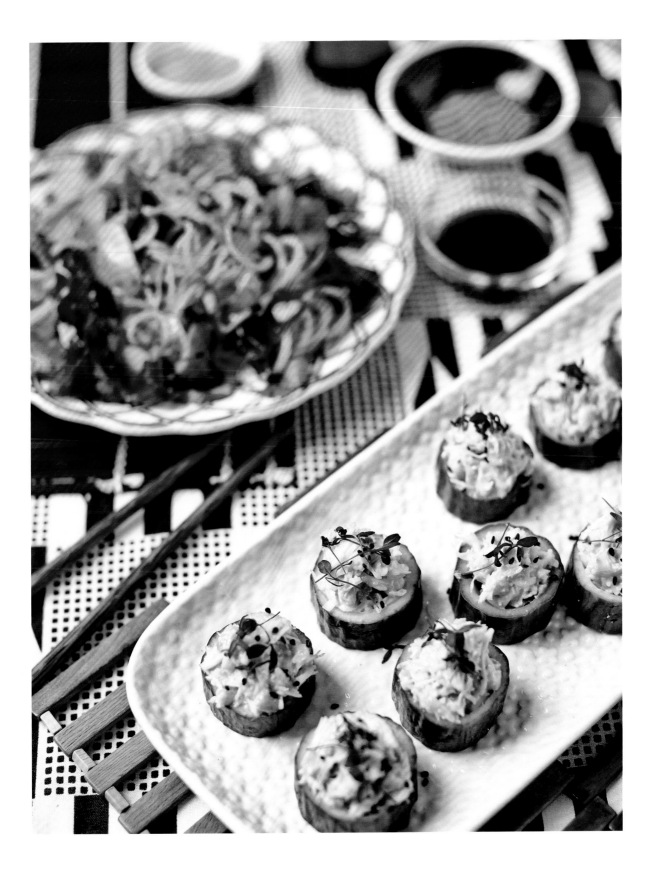

# VEGETABLE MAINS

**T**HIS CHAPTER CELEBRATES PLANT-BASED MAINS, perfect for breakfast, lunch, and supper and, again, demonstrates our simple food combining principles (see page 14 for more information). Without meat, high-starch vegetables are comfortably digested along with pseudocereals, legumes, and nuts, as well as low-starch veg. By substituting these nutrient-rich whole foods for conventional carbs, you will have more sustained energy throughout the day.

We love getting creative with our cooking and have reinvented some classic dishes, using quinoa to make risotto, ground almonds to make pastry, and kohlrabi in a dauphinoise. We make pizza bases from cauliflower, burritos from buckwheat, and turn zucchinis into spaghetti and cucumbers into noodles.

We include nourishing bone broth wherever possible and plenty of extra-virgin olive oil, coconut cream, egg yolks, and other animal fats, such as cheese and butter, to help absorb the fat-soluble vitamins in the vegetables. You can also add a little meat and fish to give a deeper flavor, such as cured meat on our Flower Power Pizzas (page 194) and anchovies in our Courgetti Puttanesca (page 210), while still eating a dish that's rich in plant foods. For vegetarians, the recipes can be adapted to suit your tastes by using a homemade vegetable stock, or water.

We always recommend buying organic food when you can. Finding a great local producer and sticking to seasonal eating will keep costs down. However, if you cannot buy all of your fruit and veg organic, prioritize the ones where you eat the skin over those that you peel (for more info see pages 12 and 308).

Organic dried legumes are cheap and organic pseudocereals are so nutrient-rich compared to grains like pasta or rice that any extra cost is money well spent on your health. These dry goods also keep for a long time so you can make savings by buying in bulk.

Before you tuck into dried legumes and pseudocereals, they need a little preparation to make them easier to digest, especially if you base your diet around them. Turn to page 14 for an explanation of why soaking and "activating" is important and turn to page 300 for instructions on how to do these crucial but simple jobs.

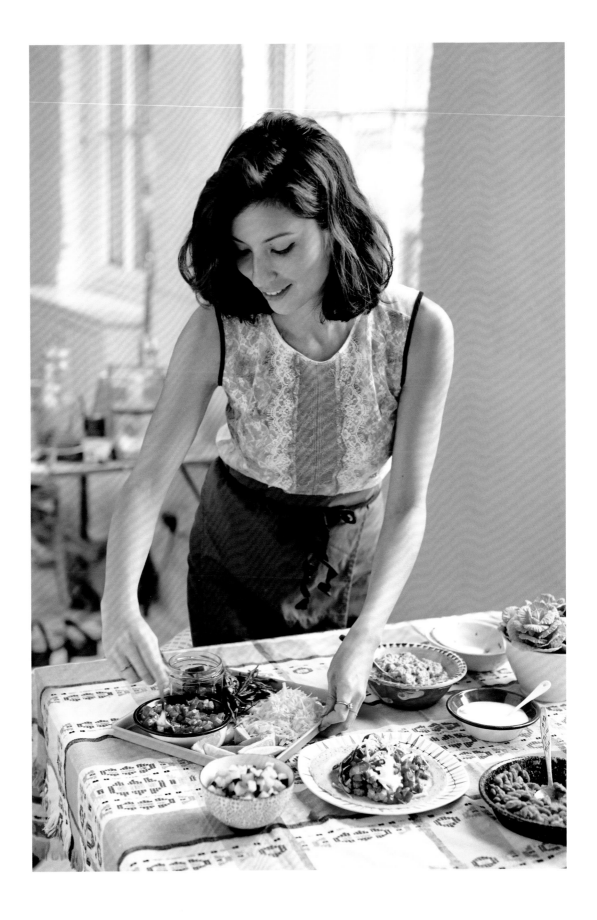

# MUNG DAHL

Mung dahl/dhal/dal/daal – so many ways to spell it – we chose dahl! This is our secret weapon for counteracting indulgences, or indeed any time we are feeling a little less than our best. It is a great dish to stockpile in your freezer and it's a favorite amongst clients. Soothing and easy to eat, you'll thank yourself that you've got some ready and waiting after a long day. The medicinal spices used to flavor this simple dish can be chosen and combined according to your constitution. A good dose of garlic, onions, and ginger make this an immune-boosting dish.

SERVES 6

6 cups bone broth (page 300) or water (you might want to add less or more depending on how soupy you like your dahl)

18 oz green mung beans (or soak and boil your own, page 300)

1 tbsp ground cumin

1 tbsp ground turmeric

2 tsp ground coriander

6 cardamom pods, crushed

dried or fresh chili, to taste (optional)

1 tbsp ghee or coconut oil

4 large onions, sliced

6 garlic cloves, grated

2 thumb-sized pieces of fresh root ginger (about 2 ¾ oz) – unpeeled if organic – grated or finely diced

4 large carrots, finely diced

2 celery sticks, finely diced

2 large pinches of sea salt or 1 tbsp tamari, to taste

2 large pinches of black pepper

3 large handfuls of fresh cilantro, finely chop the stems and roughly chop the leaves

8 large handfuls of greens, such as baby spinach, spinach, winter greens or kale (stalks removed)

juice of 1 lime or lemon

1 lime or lemon, cut into wedges to serve

**1**  Bring the broth or water to boil in a large saucepan with a lid, add the mung beans, and simmer over a medium heat, with the lid on, for 20 minutes.

**2**  Meanwhile, dry fry the spices in a large deep frying pan for 1 minute over a medium heat or until fragrant – keep stirring to prevent burning. Add the chili now if you want this dahl to have a little kick.

**3**  Add the ghee or coconut oil to the pan and fry the onion and spices for 10 minutes until the onion is soft, stirring occasionally. Add the garlic and ginger and fry for a further 5 minutes over a gentle heat, until softened and starting to caramelize.

**4**  After the mung beans have had their 20 minutes of cooking time, add the diced carrot and celery and the fried onion, garlic, and ginger mix, keeping back 6 tablespoons of this mix to garnish the bowls at the end.

**5**  Add the salt or tamari, pepper, and the finely chopped cilantro stalks and continue to cook, with the lid on, for a further 15 minutes over a medium heat until tender. Add more liquid if needed and stir at the bottom of the pan to prevent burning.

**6**  Finely slice the kale leaves and winter greens, if using, or roughly chop the spinach (baby spinach doesn't need to be chopped).

**7**  If you're using kale or a "tougher" green veg, then add it now. If using spinach, then stir in just before serving to wilt the leaves and finish with the lime or lemon juice.

**8**  To serve, top each bowl of dahl with a spoonful of the spiced fried onions, the chopped cilantro leaves, and a wedge of lime or lemon.

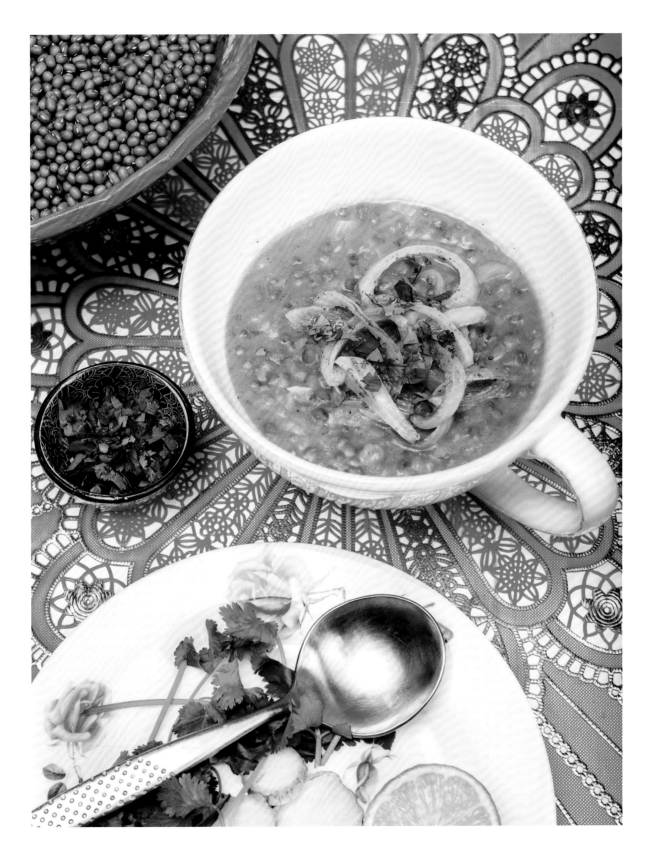

# LENTIL AND DINOSAUR KALE STEW WITH CHERMOULA DRIZZLE

Chermoula is a Moroccan blend of spices that is earthy, smoky, and slightly sweet thanks to smoked paprika and cinnamon. A drizzle of chermoula spices transforms roast chicken, roast cauliflower (see page 108), and this hearty lentil stew.

You could use any lentils here, but nutty brown lentils are delicious in this stew and hold their shape and texture. Dinosaur kale, or black leaf kale, is a leafy cabbage that is traditionally used in Tuscan cooking and we love adding it to lots of our dishes. You can also use spinach, kale, beet greens or Swiss chard.

SERVES 6

## FOR THE LENTIL AND DINOSAUR KALE STEW

1 tbsp ghee

2 large onions, diced

2 tsp ground cumin

2 tsp dried thyme

3 carrots, diced

3 celery sticks, diced

3 garlic cloves, diced

18 oz brown lentils (activated overnight page 300)

6 cups bone broth (page 300) or water

2 zucchinis (when in season), diced or ½ small squash (when in season), diced

14 oz dinosaur kale, finely shredded, or kale (stalks removed)

juice of 1 lemon

a large handful of roughly chopped fresh cilantro

a large handful of roughly chopped fresh parsley

sea salt and black pepper

## FOR THE CHERMOULA DRIZZLE

3 tbsp ghee

1 tbsp ground cumin

1 tbsp smoked sweet paprika

1 tsp ground coriander

½ tsp ground cinnamon

3 garlic cloves, grated

1 tsp chili flakes (optional)

**1** Heat the ghee in a frying pan over a low heat and gently fry the onion, cumin, and thyme for about 10 minutes until soft.

**2** Add the carrot, celery, and garlic and cook for a further 5 minutes.

**3** Add the lentils and the bone broth and simmer for 45 minutes, adding the squash after 20 minutes, if using, or the zucchinis after 30 minutes.

**4** In the meantime, make the chermoula drizzle by heating the ghee in a small pan and frying the cumin, paprika, coriander, and cinnamon for 30 seconds until fragrant, stirring frequently to prevent sticking. Add the garlic, and the chili if using, and stir for another 20 seconds. Add a little splash of water to stop the spices burning.

**5** When the lentils are tender, stir through the dinosaur kale or kale and cook for a final 5 minutes. Turn off the heat and stir through the lemon juice and fresh herbs to serve. Season to taste.

**6** Top each serving with some of the chermoula drizzle.

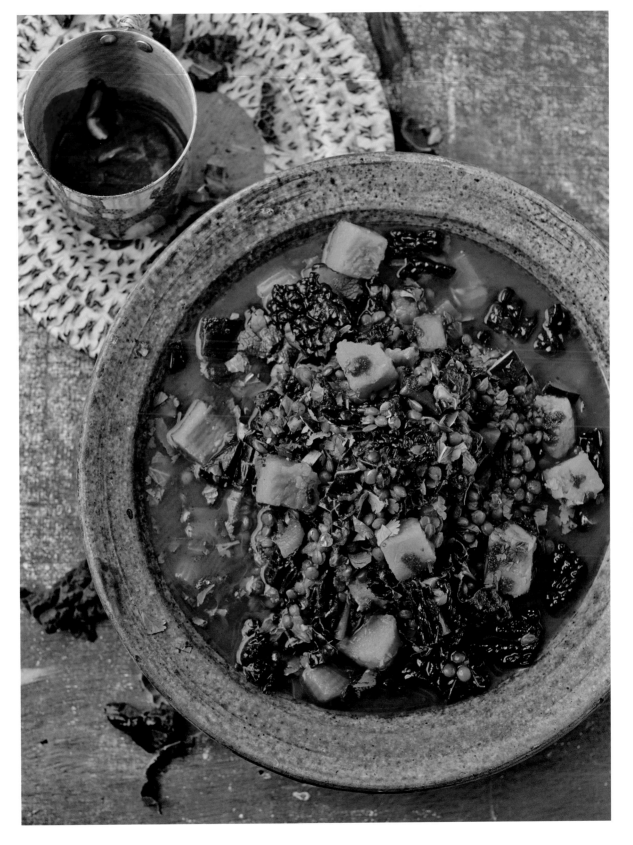

## MUSHROOM QUINOA NUT ROAST WITH A CHESTNUT APRICOT TOPPING

SERVES 10–12

Nut roasts have a reputation for being bland and heavy on the tummy because, although nuts are highly nutritious, more than a handful can be hard to digest. We use protein-rich quinoa to bulk out the loaf instead, flavored with a mushroom duxelle. Black quinoa is nice for presentation, but any color of quinoa will do.

We also created a delicious topping, which doubles up as a stuffing. It adds another stage to the recipe, but is well worth it. The topping has a sweet, caramelized flavor and the duxelles quinoa base is deep and rich. When entertaining, make up the nut roast and any stuffing balls in advance so that they're ready to pop in the oven, helping to minimize your time in the kitchen. This makes plenty and extras will freeze well.

**FOR THE CHESTNUT APRICOT TOPPING (MAKE DOUBLE IF YOU WANT STUFFING BALLS AS WELL)**

1 ¾ oz butter

2 medium onions, chopped

4 oz organic unsulphured dried apricots (brown/dark), roughly chopped into ½ in pieces

7 oz cooked chestnuts, roughly chopped into ½ in pieces

8 large fresh sage leaves, finely chopped

3 ½ oz ground almonds

sea salt and black pepper

**FOR THE NUT ROAST BASE**

3 tbsp chia seeds

6 tbsp lemon juice

1 tsp butter or ghee

4 medium onions, finely chopped

4 tsp fresh thyme leaves or 2 tsp dried thyme

roughly 1 ½ lb (26 oz) mushrooms, grated (we use a food processor)

6 ½ oz quinoa (activated overnight page 300)

1 ¾ oz Madeira or white wine

3 ½ oz pine nuts

3 ½ oz pistachios

4 oz ground almonds

a small handful of fresh parsley, finely chopped

tamari or sea salt, to taste

**1**  Preheat the oven to fan 325°F. Grease a 14 x 5 ½ x 4 in loaf tin with some softened butter and line with baking parchment, taking 2 rectangular pieces and crossing them in the middle to cover both sides.

**2**  To make the topping, heat the butter in a frying pan over a medium heat and fry the onion lightly for a few minutes so that it still has bite. Add the apricots, chestnuts, and sage and cook for a further 5 minutes. Add salt and pepper, to taste.

**3**  Remove from the heat and fold in the ground almonds. If making these into stuffing balls, roll into 2 in balls and bake for 20 minutes until golden brown. Otherwise, follow the instructions below to use it in the nut roast.

**4**  Press the stuffing mixture firmly into the bottom of the prepared loaf tin and set to one side.

**5**  To make the nut roast, make a chia gel by mixing the chia seeds with the lemon juice in a bowl and leave to one side.

**6**  Heat the butter or ghee in a pan over a medium heat and fry the onion with a pinch of salt for about 8 minutes until soft and translucent.

**7**  Add the thyme and grated mushrooms, drained quinoa, and Madeira and stir to mix everything together. Cover with a lid and cook for 25 minutes, stirring regularly.

**8**  Remove the lid and cook for a further 20 minutes, continuing to stir regularly. (You want the excess liquid to evaporate and for the mixture to become sticky.)

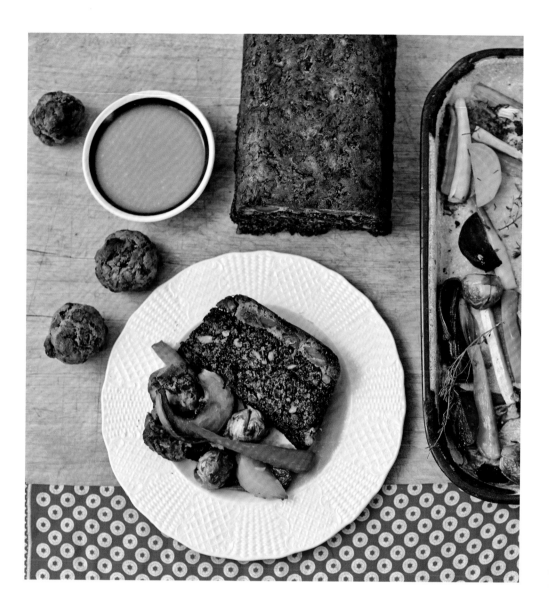

**9** Meanwhile, toast the pine nuts and pistachios on a baking tray in the preheated oven for about 2–3 minutes until lightly browned. They are easily burnt, so watch them!

**10** Add the toasted pine nuts and the pistachios to the nut roast mixture. Stir in the ground almonds, chopped parsley, and chia lemon gel. Add some tamari or sea salt to taste.

**11** Pour the nut roast mix into the loaf tin covering the topping and press down firmly. Bake in the preheated oven, on the middle shelf, for 1½ hours or until firm to touch.

**12** Leave to cool for 5–10 minutes, then cover with a large serving plate or wooden board and flip the pan over to turn it out. Rest for another 5 minutes before slicing to serve.

# ROASTED VEGETABLES WITH WHITE WINE MISO GRAVY

This is a fantastic dish for when you have those carb cravings – which is always inevitable as the weather turns cold. As well as the vegetables used here you could try fennel, cauliflower, squash, rutabaga, turnip, celery root, beets, and whole bulbs of garlic. Far better to snack on than multicolored sweets and cookies!

The dry heat of roasting caramelizes the natural sugars in your food to intensify the flavor, plus basting vegetables with coconut oil reduces their moisture loss so that you can enjoy them crispy on the outside and tender on the inside. This is also great made with beef dripping, as well as ghee, and duck fat (for more on good fats see page 11).

Delicious, smooth, and light on the tummy, we love miso. It's an Asian flavor but we wanted to keep this dish as "British" in taste as possible so we use whole onions to thicken this tangy gravy.

SERVES 4 AS A MAIN COURSE OR 10 AS A SIDE DISH (GREAT FOR CHRISTMAS DAY)

## FOR THE VEGETABLES

4 large handfuls of Brussels sprouts

4 large carrots

2 red onions or leeks

4 large parsnips (leave out the starchy parsnips if serving with meat and use cauliflower or more Brussels instead)

1 large broccoli

3–4 heaped tbsp coconut oil

fresh herbs such as rosemary or thyme

sea salt and black pepper

## FOR THE WHITE WINE MISO GRAVY

2 white onions, about 3 ½ oz

8 ½ oz white wine

1 tbsp tamari

1–2 tbsp unpasteurized miso paste, depending on strength

any fresh or dried herbs (optional)

**1** Preheat the oven to fan 350°F.

**2** Slice off the Brussels sprouts ends and halve any large sprouts so they are all the same size. Top and tail the carrots and cut the carrots and all the other vegetables into equal-sized chunks.

**3** Arrange the vegetables in a ceramic or glass ovenproof dish and distribute the oil equally around them.

**4** Season with salt and pepper, scatter over the herbs, then roast in the oven for 20 minutes.

**5** Remove the dish and stir to coat the vegetables. Roast for another 25–35 minutes or so until the vegetables are just tender.

**6** Meanwhile, to make the gravy, quarter the onions and simmer in a small saucepan, lid off, with the white wine and 8 ½ oz water for about 25 minutes until the onion has softened.

**7** Add the tamari, 1 tablespoon of the miso, and the herbs, if using, and blend until smooth, adding more water to reach your desired gravy consistency.

**8** Add black pepper or any seasoning you like, including more miso and tamari for a stronger flavor.

**9** Serve the miso gravy in a jug alongside the dish of roasted veg.

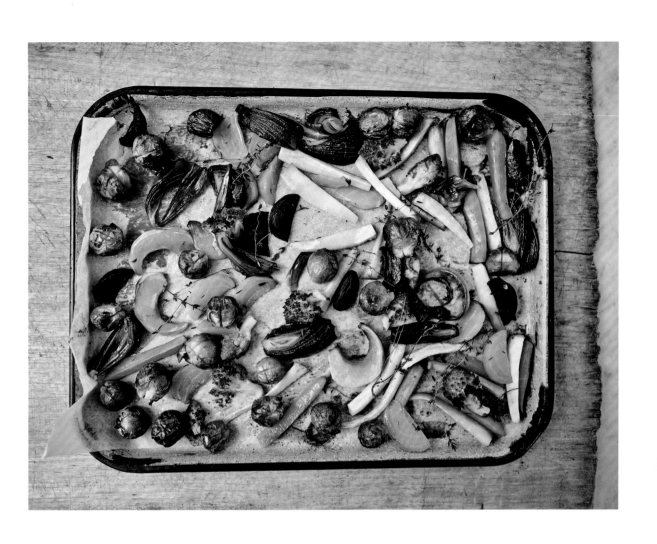

# FLOWER POWER PIZZA

This is not quite as simple as the Socca Pizza on pages 218–220, but no pancake skills are required for this. We sneak some cauliflower (the flower!) into the pizza base and then use protein-rich ingredients like almonds, egg white, and buckwheat – that's the power part.

If you plan to cover your pizza with lots of protein in the form of meat, we recommend using more ground almonds rather than buckwheat flour for better food combining. Try the toppings from our Socca Pizzas or our tangy Puttanesca sauce (page 210), as well as the tomato sauce below.

Double the recipe to make two pizzas, then you can freeze one of the pizza bases or freeze a constructed pizza ready to pop in the oven later that week. Stick the leftover egg yolk in a smoothie, bake it on top of your pizza, or make a mayo or tartar sauce (page 134).

**MAKES 1 PIZZA**

**FOR THE TOMATO SAUCE (MAKE THIS UP IN ADVANCE OR USE PASSATA IF YOU'RE IN A RUSH)**

3 garlic cloves, or diced

1 tbsp ghee

12 large tomatoes, roughly chopped

2 tsp dried oregano or 1 tbsp fresh oregano leaves

sea salt and black pepper

1 fresh or dried chili, finely sliced or chopped (optional)

**FOR THE PIZZA BASE**

5 oz cauliflower (about ¼ of a head without the stalk)

1 egg white, beaten

1 ¾ oz ground almonds

1 ½ oz buckwheat flour

½ tsp sea salt

½ tsp black pepper

¼ tsp baking soda

Choose your favorite toppings from the options opposite or try the toppings on page 220.

**1** Preheat the oven to fan 350°F. Line a baking tray with parchment paper and lightly grease with butter, ghee, or coconut oil.

**2** Make the tomato sauce: gently heat the ghee in a pan over a medium heat and fry the garlic for 1 minute, then add the chopped tomatoes, oregano, salt and pepper, and a little chili, if you like.

**3** Cook the tomatoes down to a thick sauce over a medium heat, lid off, which will take about 15 minutes, then mash the tomatoes with your spatula or blend to a paste if you like things less rustic.

**4** While the sauce is cooking, grate the cauliflower into rice-sized pieces using a hand grater or food processor.

**5** Put all of the pizza base ingredients into a bowl and mix well with a spoon, or add to the food processor and blend, to form a sticky dough.

**6** Spread the dough out with the back of the spoon on the prepared tray, shaping it into a 12 in-diameter.

**7** Bake in the oven for about 20 minutes, flipping it over after 15 minutes to cook the underside.

**8** Choose your pizza topping from the options opposite and cook as instructed.

**9** Serve the pizza with a big green salad and drizzle over some Brazil Nut Pesto (page 198), if you like.

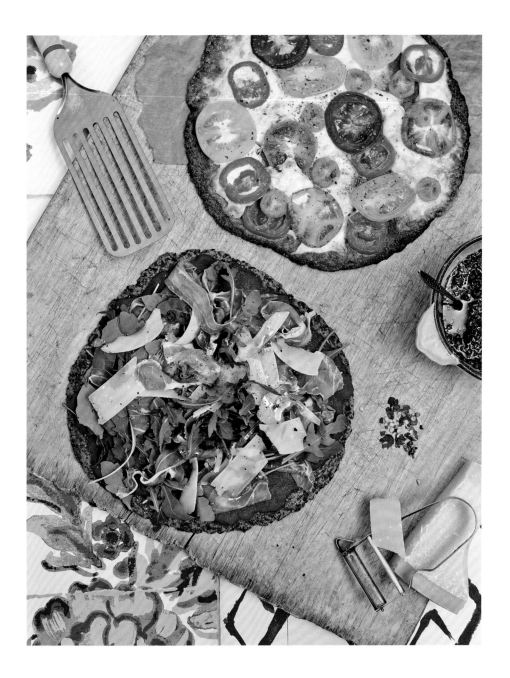

**+ FOR A PARMA HAM AND ARUGULA TOPPING:** spread the tomato sauce over the base of the pizza with the back of a spoon. If you've made the sauce in advance and it's cold, rebake the tomato-topped pizza for 5 minutes before adding your toppings. Top with 4 slices of Parma ham torn into small pieces, 2 handfuls of arugula, and some parmesan shavings. Add chili flakes, if you like.

**+ FOR A TOMATO AND MOZZARELLA TOPPING:** pull apart 1 medium mozzarella ball into small pieces and arrange over the base of the pizza. Slice 2 handfuls of fresh tomatoes into ½ in-thick slices (a mixture of colors looks good) and arrange over the pizza. Add chili flakes, if desired. Bake for 10–15 minutes until the mozzarella is melted and bubbling.

# ZUCCHINI AND EGGPLANT CURRY

A simple one-pot supper that is warming for the soul. Red split lentils provide a quick-and-easy creamy base without the need to soak them. The coconut and ginger have incredible immune-boosting properties and, as usual, we like to sneak nourishing homemade broth into all our cooking. With this fragrant curry, the bone broth is purely for the nutritional value, so you can afford to skip it if you don't have any on hand (but please don't be tempted to use stock cubes).

Try this curry with Toasted Coconut Green Beans (page 112), Cauliflower Rice (page 102), or Broccoli Rice (page 170), or serve with a pile of watercress on top, or add in lots of finely shredded cabbage towards the end of the cooking time.

SERVES 4 AS A ONE-POT MEAL OR 6 IF SERVED WITH A SIDE DISH

a handful of peanuts or cashew nuts (preferably "crispy" activated, page 300)

7 oz bar of creamed coconut (use the oil for frying) or 2 tins of full-fat coconut milk plus 2 tbsp coconut oil or ghee, for frying

2 large onions, diced

2 thumb-sized pieces of fresh root ginger (about 2 ¾ oz) – unpeeled if organic – grated

6 large garlic cloves, diced

7 oz red split lentils, rinsed (no need to soak these)

2 cups - 1 quart bone broth (page 300) or water (use a little less if you are using coconut milk and depending on how thick or saucy you want your curry to be)

1 large eggplant, chopped into ⅔ in pieces

4 large tomatoes, quartered

2 large zucchinis, diced

grated zest and juice of 1 unwaxed lime or lemon (avoid the bitter white pith)

2½–3 tsp tamari or 2 large pinches of sea salt

1 tsp maple syrup

a handful of roughly chopped fresh herbs, such as cilantro, mint, or basil (Thai basil if you can get it)

**1** In a large wide pan, dry fry the peanuts or cashews for a few minutes to toast them, roughly chop, and then set aside.

**2** In the same pan, heat the coconut oil over a medium heat and fry the onion, ginger, and garlic for 10 minutes until soft (don't let the onion and garlic go brown).

**3** Add the lentils, the roughly chopped coconut solids or coconut milk, and then most of the bone broth or water (a bit less if you're using the coconut milk), and stir well. This should be enough liquid for the coconut solids to dissolve, but keep an eye on the liquid levels so that the lentils don't stick and burn at the bottom.

**4** After 6 minutes of cooking over a medium-high heat, add the eggplant and stir.

**5** After a further 10 minutes, add the tomato, zucchini, lime or lemon zest, and the tamari or salt. Add more bone broth or water if you think your curry needs it.

**6** After 6 minutes, turn off the heat and add the lime or lemon juice, the maple syrup and fresh herbs, then stir and taste. You might need a little more tamari or salt or lime or lemon juice to add sourness.

**7** Top with the nuts and serve with watercress or your chosen side dish. If we're having guests round, we like to serve our curry with some little bowls of extras (nuts, herbs, lemon or lime wedges, and a bowl of tamari or sea salt) so everyone can help themselves to extra toppings.

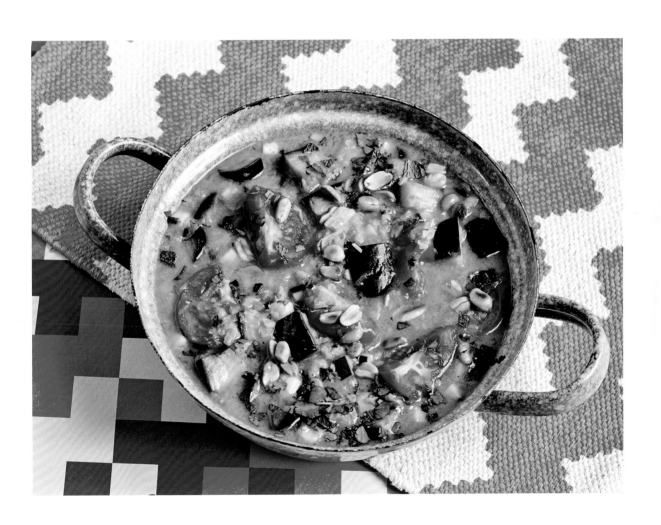

# QUINOA AND ROASTED VEGETABLE SALAD WITH BRAZIL NUT PESTO

This simple recipe is delicious eaten hot or cold and makes an excellent packed lunch. Roasting vegetables is an easy way to cook up lots of veg at the same time and use up any older ones, while pesto is a fast and fancy way to jazz up anything – always make extra and keep it in the fridge.

Instead of pine nuts and parmesan, we've used selenium-rich Brazil nuts here to add that creamy texture. Brazil nuts are also one of the few nuts and seeds that don't require soaking, so we always rely on them for last minute food and they taste delicious alongside the traditional basil in this pesto. Feel free to add in any fresh herbs you have – parsley, mint, and dill work and you can even try a little arugula or watercress. This would also be delicious with buckwheat groats instead of quinoa.

SERVES 4

### FOR THE ROASTED VEGETABLE SALAD

roughly chop any vegetables you like, the more colors, the better, we suggest:

4 large carrots, roughly chopped

1 large red pepper, roughly chopped

2 handfuls of cherry tomatoes or 4 large tomatoes, halved

1 large onion (we used red for color), roughly chopped

3 large beets, well scrubbed and chopped into small chunks or little wedges as they take the longest to cook

1 tbsp ghee or coconut oil

a handful of fresh herbs, such as thyme, rosemary, or 2 tbsp mixed dried herbs

fresh leaves, such as arugula, corn salad, and watercress, to serve

sea salt and black pepper

### FOR THE QUINOA

8 ½ oz bone broth (page 300) or water

9 oz quinoa (activated overnight page 300)

### FOR THE BRAZIL NUT PESTO

12 Brazil nuts

2 garlic cloves

3 large handfuls of fresh basil (stalks and all if you're using a strong blender)

1 ⅓ cup extra virgin olive oil

4 tbsp lemon juice or 2 tbsp apple cider vinegar

**1**  Preheat the oven to fan 390°F.

**2**  Lay the roughly chopped vegetables in a single layer on a large roasting tray, sprinkle with salt and pepper, and add your dollops of ghee or coconut oil. Scatter over the herbs.

**3**  Roast for 30–40 minutes or until the veg is tender (pierce with a knife to check). Halfway through the roasting time, use a wooden spatula to turn the veg.

**4**  Meanwhile, make the pesto. Blitz everything together in a food processor or with a hand blender (the more nuts you add, the thicker and creamier your pesto will be, but if you want it thinner, add more oil and lemon juice). Alternatively, grab a sharp knife and finely chop the garlic, basil, and nuts, then whisk with the olive oil and lemon juice. Season to taste.

**5**  Bring the broth to boil in a pan, add your drained quinoa, and cook for 12 minutes (see page 301 for how to cook perfect quinoa).

**6**  Combine the quinoa and roasted veg in a big serving bowl, toss in your pesto, and then the fresh salad leaves. Or, if preferred, serve your fresh salad leaves on the side with a little lemon juice and olive oil.

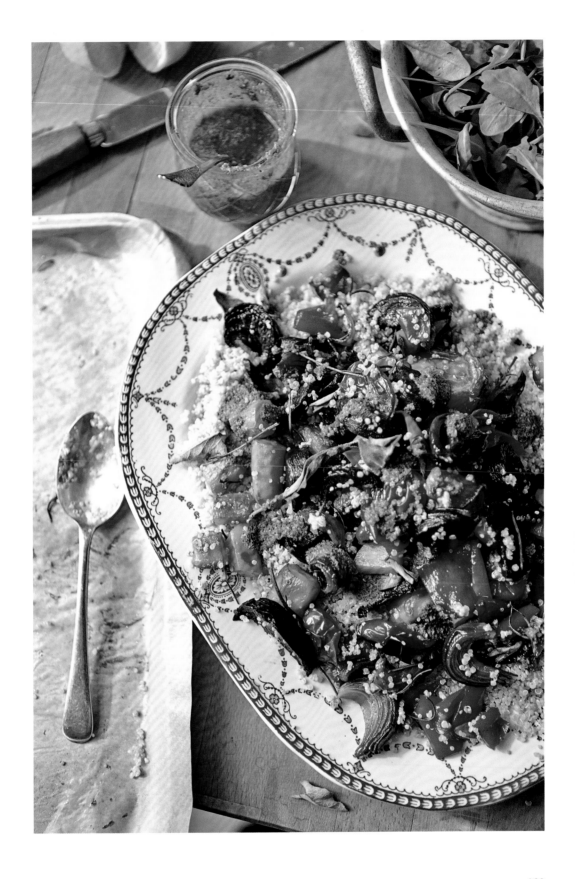

# HOT BUCKWHEAT NOODLE SALAD

This is our 15-minute "please everyone" meal – a colorful dish that looks impressive and always goes down well with guests. Eat it for supper and catch up on your veg intake, enjoying the leftovers cold for a packed lunch the next day.

We always use a high ratio of vegetables in a meal to help pack in as much nutrient-dense food as possible. Here we use 100 percent buckwheat noodles, also known as soba noodles. Their high nutritional value, along with plenty of veg, means that you don't need to eat a mountain to feel satisfied.

**SERVES 2 WITH A THIRD PORTION FOR A PACKED LUNCH THE NEXT DAY**

### FOR THE NOODLE SALAD

6 oz buckwheat noodles (soba)

extra virgin olive oil

2 tbsp coconut oil

1 small red onion or 3 scallions, finely sliced

a large handful of finely chopped carrots

a large handful of shredded cabbage (we like red for color, but white/savoy are good)

a large handful of any other crunchy veg, such as broccoli florets, sliced fennel, or radishes

2 handfuls of leaves, such as watercress, baby spinach, or sliced lettuce

### FOR THE DRESSING

juice and zest of 1 unwaxed lime or lemon (avoid the bitter white pith)

1 tbsp toasted sesame oil

2 tbsp extra virgin olive oil

1 garlic clove, grated

sea salt and pepper (white pepper is especially good in Asian dishes)

a splash of tamari

### FOR THE TOPPING

a small handful of any nuts or seeds, such as cashew nuts, peanuts, almonds, sesame seeds, sunflower seeds, or poppy seeds (preferably "crispy" activated, page 300)

a handful of fresh herbs, such as cilantro, mint, chives, basil, or Thai basil

**1** Make the dressing by adding everything to a jam jar and shaking well.

**2** Cook the buckwheat noodles according to the packet, using plenty of water. During the first minute of cooking use two forks to stir and separate the noodles.

**3** When tender, drain and rinse with cold water for about 15 seconds to stop them cooking further. Set aside to drain then toss a little extra virgin olive oil through to stop the noodles sticking.

**4** Over a medium heat, dry toast your nuts or seeds in a frying pan until golden brown then set aside. This only takes a minute so keep your eye on that pan.

**5** Turn the heat up and add in the coconut oil and onion. After 30 seconds or so, add the "hardest" vegetables, like the carrots, and stir-fry over a high heat for 2 minutes. Add the rest of the vegetables and stir-fry for a further minute – you want to lightly cook the vegetables to retain their crunch and bright colors. Cook the vegetables a little more if you prefer, adding a few tablespoons of water helps to steam them if they catch on the bottom of the pan.

**6** Turn off the heat, add the cooked noodles, and toss.

**7** Add any raw leaves now. Spoon over the dressing and toss everything together. Top with the toasted nuts or seeds and herbs and let everyone help themselves from the hot frying pan.

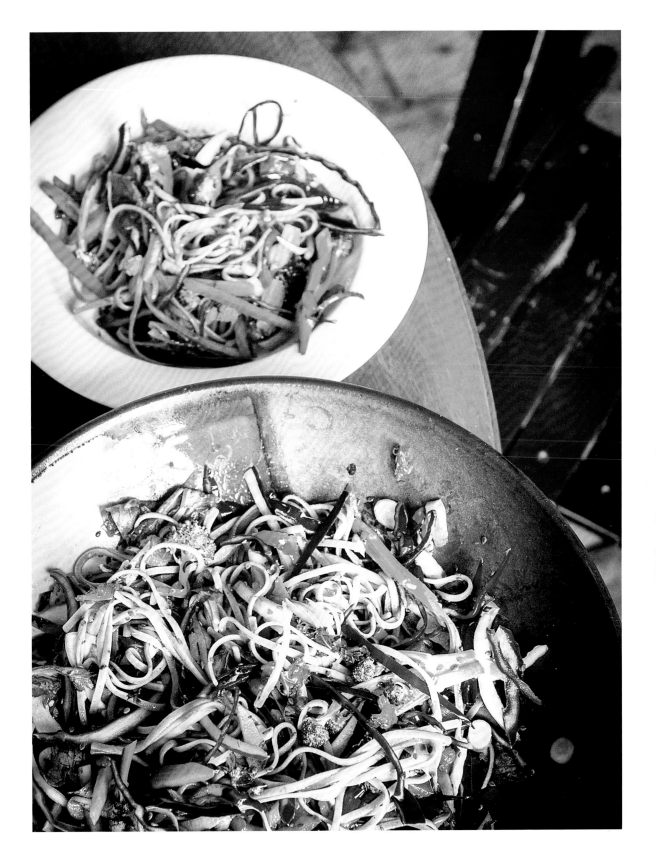

# CARAMELIZED GARLIC TART WITH ALMOND CRUST

Sweet caramelized garlic and butternut squash combine with creamy goats' cheese and the aniseed flavors of tarragon to make a delicious, uniquely flavored tart with a twist: we use ground almonds to make a nutritious and gluten-free crust. Serve the tart hot from the oven with a green salad for lunch or take a thick slice for food on the go – and it's always a winner at picnics.

SERVES 4–5

**FOR THE FILLING**

9 oz butternut squash, skin on, deseeded

3 bulbs of garlic, cloves peeled

1 oz butter

1 tbsp maple syrup

1 tbsp apple cider vinegar

2 eggs

7 tbsp full-fat probiotic natural yogurt

2 oz mature cheddar, grated

2 ½ oz goats' cheese

3 tsp chopped fresh tarragon, parsley or sage

sea salt and black pepper

**FOR THE PASTRY**

13 ¼ oz ground almonds

1 tsp sea salt

½ tsp baking soda

1 oz butter at room temperature

2 eggs

**1**  Preheat the oven to fan 350°F. Halve and roast the butternut squash in the oven for about 40–50 minutes, cut-side up, until cooked through and tender.

**2**  Mix the pastry ingredients together to form a dough and roll into a ⅛ in-thick disc between two pieces of parchment paper. Line a 9 ½ in ceramic tart dish with the almond pastry, trimming away the excess. Line with greaseproof paper, fill with baking beans and put into the fridge for 20 minutes.

**3**  Bake for 10 minutes, remove the beans and bake for a further 10 minutes. Set aside.

**4**  Meanwhile, put the garlic in a small pan with a few tablespoons of water. Simmer for a few minutes until almost tender. Add the butter, increase the heat, and cook until the water has evaporated and the garlic is starting to brown.

**5**  Add the maple syrup, cider vinegar, and a pinch of sea salt and simmer for 10 minutes, until most of the liquid has evaporated and the cloves are coated in dark syrup.

**6**  Peel the skin from the roasted squash, chop into ¾ in pieces and arrange in the tart base. Whisk the eggs, yogurt, and grated cheddar together with a pinch of salt and a few good grinds of black pepper and pour over the squash in the tart.

**7**  Scatter pieces of goats' cheese and caramelized garlic over the tart, drizzle over the syrup, and sprinkle with the tarragon.

**8**  Reduce the oven heat to fan 325°F and bake the tart for 30 minutes, until it is set and the top goes golden brown. Eat warm or at room temperature with a crisp seasonal salad.

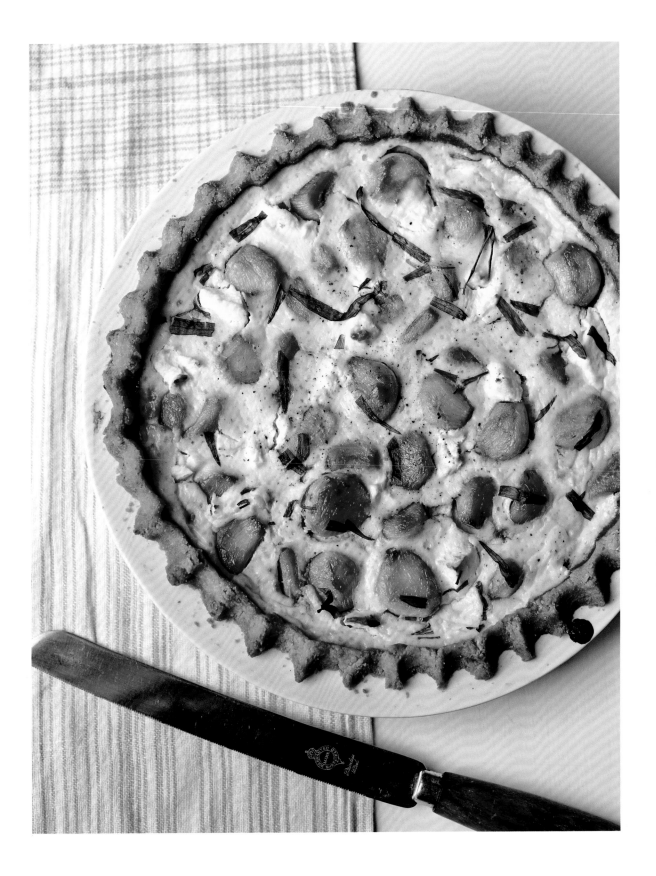

# ASPARAGUS AND PEA RISOTTO WITH MINT AND PARSLEY OIL

In this asparagus risotto, we use the lighter and more nourishing quinoa instead of risotto rice, which can leave you feeling bloated and heavy (Italians, please don't be too annoyed, we know risotto means rice!). You don't have to watch the pan while making this risotto because quinoa is more forgiving than rice and soaking quinoa speeds the whole process up.

We think of May as "asparagus month" and eat our way through plenty of it in order to get our yearly fix. Out of the short asparagus season, choose another seasonal green veg – green beans, broad beans, purple sprouting broccoli, zucchinis, and spinach are all good.

The mint and parsley oil can be made in advance. The mint goes perfectly with the peas and the lemon zest balances the richness of the risotto. This oil is delicious with so many things and is particularly good with fish, dolloped onto the Mung Bean Hummus (page 232) or added to stews.

**SERVES 4 OR 2 WITH LEFTOVERS TO MAKE 10 RISOTTO BALLS**

## FOR THE RISOTTO

2 tbsp ghee

2 medium leeks or onions, diced

2 garlic cloves, diced

½ tsp dried oregano or thyme or 1 tsp fresh oregano or thyme leaves

9 oz white quinoa (activated overnight page 300)

3 ½ cup bone broth (page 300) or veg stock

a large bunch of asparagus, about 1 ½ lb

2 small handfuls of frozen or freshly shelled peas

1 tbsp lemon juice

1 ¾ oz parmesan, grated

sea salt and black pepper

## FOR THE MINT AND PARSLEY OIL

¾ cup extra virgin olive oil

1 garlic clove, grated

grated zest of 1 unwaxed lemon (avoid the bitter white pith)

1 oz fresh parsley, finely chopped

⅓ oz fresh mint leaves, finely chopped

sea salt and black pepper

**1** Heat the ghee in a pan over a medium heat and soften the leek or onion for 8 minutes, stirring occasionally.

**2** Meanwhile, prepare the mint and parsley oil by mixing everything together in a bowl.

**3** Add the garlic, oregano, and thyme to the pan and fry for another 30 seconds. Add the drained quinoa and stir to mix.

**4** Pour in most of the broth, turn up the heat to bring to boil, then turn down to a medium simmer and leave to cook for 13 minutes.

**5** Meanwhile, prepare the asparagus by snapping off the woody ends and discarding them. Chop the remaining asparagus spears into 3 pieces on the angle.

**6** After the quinoa has cooked for 13 minutes it should be tender. Try a little and if not, leave it to cook longer. When the quinoa is cooked, stir through the asparagus and peas and leave to simmer for just a few minutes until the asparagus is tender, then turn off the heat. You might want to add another ladle or so of bone broth if the risotto is getting dry as the quinoa will continue to suck up any liquid for the next few minutes.

**7** Gently fold through the lemon juice, grated parmesan, and check for seasoning. Serve each bowl of risotto with a drizzle of mint and parsley oil.

✚ **THERE ARE LOTS OF POSSIBLE VARIATIONS FOR THIS RISOTTO.** Swap the peas for broad beans or swap the white quinoa for red or black quinoa, which both take about 5 minutes longer to cook.

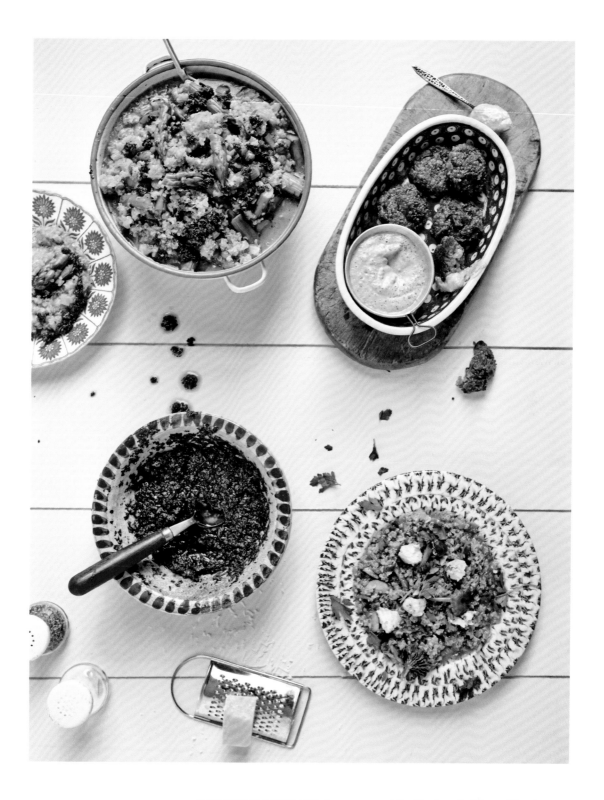

**CLOCKWISE FROM TOP LEFT**: Asparagus and Pea Risotto with Mint and Parsley Oil (opposite), Quinoa Risotto Balls (page 207), Mushroom and Stilton Quinoa Risotto (page 206), and Mint and Parsley Oil (opposite).

# MUSHROOM AND STILTON QUINOA RISOTTO

SERVES 4 OR 2 WITH
LEFTOVERS TO MAKE
10 RISOTTO BALLS

We cook this quinoa just like a risotto with the bonus that it's actually quicker and easier to make and, of course, packs more of a protein punch than the traditional dish. Plus you can turn any leftovers into risotto balls/arancini (opposite).

We use white quinoa, but look out for red and black quinoa, which are nuttier and keep more of an al dente bite no matter how long you cook them. Serve this with a simple watercress salad (try our recipe on page 139).

**FOR THE RISOTTO**

⅔ cup hot water

3 tbsp dried porcini mushrooms

1 tbsp ghee

2 medium onions, diced

3 celery sticks, diced

4 garlic cloves, diced

1½ tsp dried thyme or 3 tsp fresh thyme leaves

14 oz mushrooms, sliced and stalks chopped (we use a mix of chestnut mushrooms and chanterelles)

9 oz white quinoa (activated overnight page 300)

¾ cup white wine or 1 tbsp apple cider vinegar

3 cup bone broth (page 300) or vegetable stock

4 oz stilton or any blue cheese (gorgonzola or taleggio would be delicious)

a handful of fresh parsley

grated zest of 1 unwaxed lemon (avoid the bitter white pith)

1 tbsp lemon juice

sea salt and black pepper

**1** Add the hot water to a bowl with the porcini mushrooms and leave to soak for 20 minutes.

**2** Meanwhile, heat up the ghee in a pan over a medium heat and gently fry the onion and celery for about 8 minutes, until softened.

**3** Add the garlic, thyme, and the fresh mushrooms (not the porcini), stir and leave to cook for a few minutes.

**4** Add the drained quinoa to the pan over a medium heat, stir, and leave for a minute until the quinoa is almost sticking.

**5** Add the white wine or vinegar and stir to deglaze the pan of all the juicy sticky bits.

**6** Pour in most of the broth, turn up the heat to bring to boil, then turn down to a medium simmer.

**7** After 8 minutes of cooking, the quinoa should be on its way to being tender, so roughly chop the porcini mushrooms before throwing them in with the soaking liquid, turning up the heat because the soaking liquid will cool the heat in the pan.

**8** After 5 more minutes, taste the quinoa. It should be cooked and tender with a nutty texture. Turn off the heat and add another ladle of broth if you want a more saucy risotto. Bear in mind the risotto will continue "sucking up" the liquid for the next few minutes.

**9** Stir through the stilton, parsley, lemon zest, lemon juice, and salt and pepper, to taste. At this point, taste, taste, taste! Add more lemon for freshness if you like it or stir through a last half ladleful of hot bone broth if you think it could do with a little more sauce.

**10** Serve each person with a few ladlefuls of risotto and the watercress salad, if using. We like to serve with a small bowl of crumbled stilton for everyone to help themselves to a little more.

# QUINOA RISOTTO BALLS

Any leftover quinoa risotto is delicious the next day, but we just love making these balls with the leftover risotto and they make an excellent packed lunch or starter.

This recipe assumes you've eaten two portions of the risotto and so now have two portions left to make about 10 balls. The mint and parsley oil is delicious as a dipping sauce for these balls (page 204). We throw in a little arrowroot to hold the structure together, but if you don't have any, roll them small and they'll be a great texture once baked.

MAKES 10 RISOTTO BALLS

1 ½ – 2 oz arrowroot (or try chickpea flour)

2 portions of cold risotto (see pages 204 and 206)

mint and parsley oil (page 204)

sea salt and black pepper

**1** Preheat the oven to fan 350°F.

**2** Mix the arrowroot or chickpea flour into the leftover quinoa risotto and combine well.

**3** Take about 1 tablespoon of risotto and roll into balls. Place on a baking tray.

**4** Bake for 20–30 minutes until golden. Serve with the mint and parsley oil for dipping.

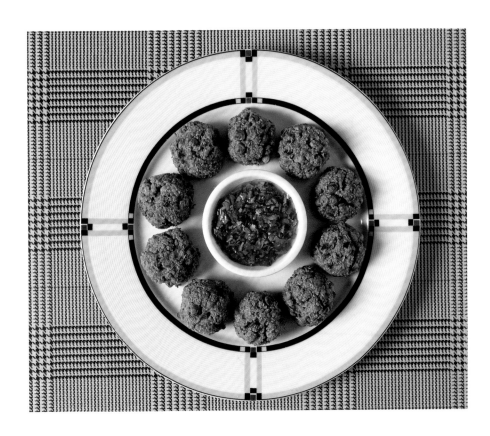

## SMOKY BAKED BEANS

Our beans aren't really "baked" as in the traditional recipes – we cook them on top of the stove but you could pop the pot in the oven and cook them until sticky. Cooking up your own dried beans is easy and much cheaper than buying ready made. Always soak them first or you can use tinned beans for faster results – follow steps 2 and 3, add the beans at step 4 and then simmer for 20 minutes.

SERVES 6 (WE LIKE TO MAKE A BIG BATCH OF THIS AND FREEZE ANY LEFT OVER)

This is a delicious and filling main. We like a bowl of these with some Summer Lime Coleslaw (page 80) and serve them without meat for better food combining (page 14).

18 oz dried cannellini or haricot beans (activated overnight, see page 300) or 6 tins of cooked beans (drained weight 3 ⅓ lb)

2 dried bay leaves

1 tbsp ghee

2 large onions, diced

2 celery sticks, finely chopped

4 garlic cloves, finely grated

2 tsp ground cumin

1 tsp smoked hot paprika or ½ tsp smoked sweet paprika and ½ tsp cayenne pepper (or a little more if you like it spicier)

1½ tsp dried oregano or 3 tsp fresh oregano

1½ tsp dried thyme or 3 tsp fresh thyme

2 tbsp tomato purée

2 tins of tomatoes or 1 ¾ lb passata

2 tbsp good-quality molasses or 1–2 tbsp maple syrup (but molasses is best)

1 quart bone broth (page 300) or vegetable stock

½–1 tbsp tamari

3 tbsp butter

sea salt and black pepper

**1**  If using dried activated beans, heat a large pan with plenty of hot water (about half a gallon) and cook the beans and the bay leaves with the lid on at a medium simmer for about 80–90 minutes until tender. Try a few beans – sometimes you get a tender one and the others are still hard.

**2**  In a separate large pan, heat the ghee over a medium heat and fry the diced onion for 10 minutes, until soft.

**3**  Add the celery, garlic, spices, and herbs, stir, and leave to cook for 5 minutes over a gentle heat.

**4**  Turn the heat up, add the tomato purée, tomatoes or passata, molasses, some sea salt and pepper, and the bone broth, and cook at a medium simmer for 30 minutes.

**5**  Add the cooked beans or the drained and rinsed tinned beans, if using, and simmer for a further 30 minutes (or longer if you've got the time). Remove the lid towards the end of the cooking time if needed to create a thick and sticky sauce coating the beans.

**6**  Add ½ tablespoon tamari, then taste before you add more as tamari is very salty. Season to taste, stir through the butter, and serve.

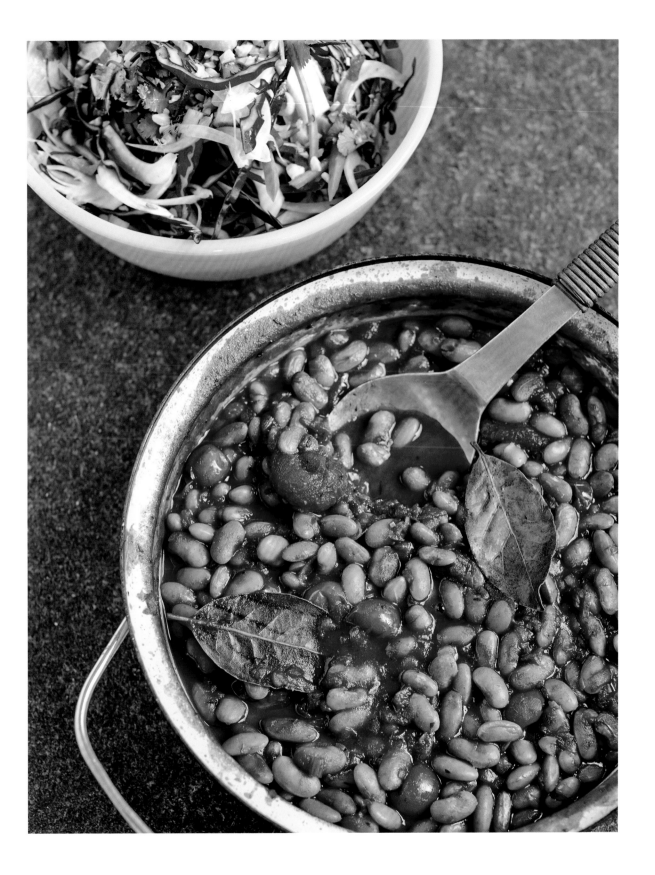

# COURGETTI PUTTANESCA

We enjoy "courgetti" (zucchini vegetable noodles, see page 140) with all the classic Italian sauces, but find it particularly delectable when you team its delicate refreshing flavor with deep, rich, and salty flavors like the much-loved puttanesca. This recipe is a great quick standby for supper as you can keep most of these ingredients in the cupboard. The anchovies add a delicious depth, but it's still tasty without them if you're not an anchovy fan – just add more olives or capers or even some bacon.

SERVES 4

2 tsp ghee

3 garlic cloves, diced

½ tsp chili flakes or a little fresh chili, to taste

8 anchovies, drained and chopped

just over 3 oz pitted olives (drained weight), chopped a bit if you like (we like them whole)

1½ tbsp small capers, rinsed and drained

2 tins of chopped tomatoes

a large handful of fresh parsley, finely chopped, saving a little for the garnish

6 large zucchinis

1 tbsp butter

extra virgin olive oil, to serve

sea salt and black pepper

**1**  Heat the ghee in a pan over a low heat and very gently fry the garlic and chili flakes for 1 minute – don't let them brown or burn.

**2**  Add the anchovies and stir and cook for 30 seconds, using your wooden spoon to bash them up a little as they fry.

**3**  Add the olives, capers, and tomatoes, turn up the heat and simmer for 10 minutes until you have a very thick and rich sauce. Add the parsley and season to taste, you won't need much salt as the anchovies are naturally very salty.

**4**  While the sauce is simmering, use a spiralizer or julienne peeler to make the courgetti. Or use a regular vegetable peeler to slice the zucchinis lengthways into very wide ribbons, which you can then slice in half. You might want to cut the long strands in half to make them easier to eat.

**5**  Soften the courgetti in a pan with a little butter, stirring over a low heat for 3 minutes. Alternatively, save washing up another pan by just running some of the hot sauce through your courgetti – the heat and salt in the sauce will soften them.

**6**  Serve the courgetti with the sauce. Add a generous sprinkling of parsley and a drizzle of extra virgin olive oil to each bowl before serving.

# KOHLRABI DAUPHINOISE

A dauphinoise is the perfect comfort food on a cold, autumn day. As always, we like to make a classic dish much healthier, so we've used homemade bone broth to replace half the cream and swapped the high-starch potato for kohlrabi.

Thanks to the fat from the cream and the bone broth, this is a very satisfying meal when served with a salad, like our Red Cabbage, Bacon, and Apple Salad on page 96. If you haven't any bone broth, but you can get hold of quality probiotic cream, then use this for all the liquid content – both options are delicious.

**SERVES 4**

1 tbsp butter or ghee, plus extra for greasing

2 medium onions, sliced

2 tsp fresh thyme leaves

½ cup bone broth (page 300) or water

½ cup unpasteurized double cream, sour cream, or crème fraîche or use more bone broth

2 garlic cloves, finely diced

1 ¾ lb kohlrabi, about, 2–4 kohlrabi

sea salt and black pepper

**OPTIONAL**

¼ tsp ground nutmeg or 1 tsp lemon zest (avoid the bitter white pith)

**1**  Preheat the oven to fan 350°F and grease a 8 x 10 ½ in baking dish with butter or ghee.

**2**  Heat the butter or ghee in a pan over a medium heat and gently fry the onion and thyme leaves for 5 minutes.

**3**  Add the bone broth and bring to boil, reduce the heat, add the cream, garlic, and some salt and pepper, and simmer for a few minutes.

**4**  Peel and slice the kohlrabi into thin $^{1}/_{16}$ - $^{1}/_{8}$ in rounds, using a mandolin if you have one.

**5**  Lay the kohlrabi slices in the prepared baking dish, overlapping the slices slightly. Top the kohlrabi with the cream sauce and/or bone broth, cover with baking parchment and bake for 1 hour.

**6**  After an hour, remove the baking parchment and return to the oven for a further 30–40 minutes until the top is golden brown and the kohlrabi is tender.

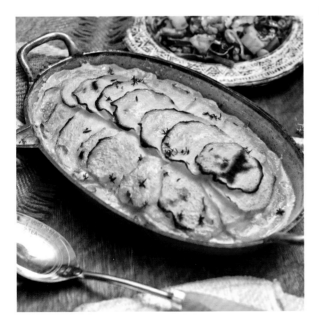

# MALAYSIAN LENTIL AND SQUASH CURRY

Malaysian food is rich in coconut and full of flavor. This Malaysian spice mix is one of our favorites. There are nine different elements to the mix, but you've probably got quite a few already and we use all of them in other recipes, so they are well worth getting. Red lentils are the go-to lentil when you've forgotten to soak some or want a quick supper because they don't need soaking and cook in 20 minutes. This is delicious on its own, eaten like a stew, or served with some Cauliflower Rice (page 102), Quicker-than-toast Zucchini Salad (page 84), Toasted Coconut Green Beans (page 112), or our Summer Lime Coleslaw (page 80) on the side. We swap the squash for 4 large zucchinis in the summer. This freezes really well and is so hearty and delicious that you'll forget that it's health food.

**SERVES 6**

## FOR THE LENTIL AND SQUASH CURRY

1 tbsp coconut oil

2 tins of full-fat coconut milk

3 medium onions, chopped

3 garlic cloves, diced

3 thumb-sized pieces of fresh root ginger (about 4 1/4 oz) – unpeeled if organic – grated or finely chopped

1 squash, about 2 1/4 lb, peeled and diced into 1 in chunks

3 cup bone broth (page 300) or vegetable stock

18 oz red split lentils (no need to soak)

14 oz spinach or use cabbage or seasonal greens, sliced

juice of 1 small lime or 1/2 large lemon

2 2/3 oz fresh cilantro, roughly chopped

sea salt and black pepper

## FOR THE MALAYSIAN SPICE MIX

2 green cardamom pods or 1/4 tsp ground green cardamom

1/2 tsp yellow mustard seeds

2 tbsp ground cumin

2 tsp ground turmeric

2 tsp fennel seeds

2 tbsp ground coriander

1/2 tsp ground cinnamon

1/2 tsp chili flakes, or more or less to your taste

1/4 tsp ground clove

**1**  First, make the Malaysian spice mix. If using whole cardamoms, remove the shells and crush along with the mustard seeds with the back of your knife or in a pestle and mortar. Add all the spices to a large saucepan and gently toast for a minute or so until fragrant, stirring to prevent the spices burning.

**2**  Add the coconut oil and fry the onion for 10 minutes, until softened. Add the garlic and ginger and fry for a few more minutes.

**3**  Add the coconut milk, squash, and the broth. If using zucchinis instead of squash, add them 10 minutes before the end of the cooking time. Put the lid on and bring to a medium simmer.

**4**  After 10 minutes, add the red lentils, stir, and simmer over a medium heat for a further 20 minutes until the lentils are soft and the squash is tender. You might need to add the extra bone broth during cooking – depending on how thick you'd like your curry.

**5**  In the last few minutes, add the sliced cabbage or greens, if using, and stir through. If using spinach, just add when you turn off the heat so it wilts.

**6**  Turn off the heat, add some sea salt and pepper, the juice of the lime or lemon, and check for seasoning and consistency. Add more bone broth now, if you like.

**7**  Stir through the roughly chopped cilantro and ladle into bowls to serve.

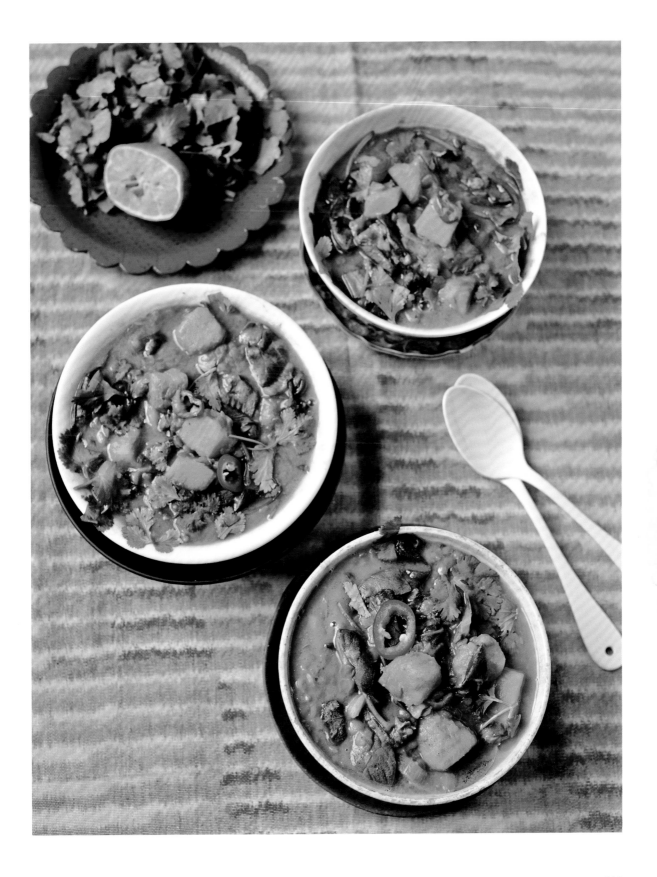

# BEET AND GOATS' CHEESE TERRINE

When we were younger we loved a certain brand of garlic-and-herb cream cheese, which we've recreated here using goats' cheese. It's always good to "vary the dairy" and goats' dairy is one of the easiest to digest. Look for the best-quality goats' cheese you can find – full-fat for flavor and nourishment. We've paired the cheese with layers of colorful beet slices, which are beautiful to behold! Try and get as many colors of beets as you can: golden, purple, and candy-colored Chioggia. We love how every time we make this terrine it looks different. Make this the night before a picnic or dinner party – this dish has the wow factor.

SERVES 6-8

4 purple beets, about
   10 ½ oz
4 golden or any other
   color beets, about
   10 ½ oz (the more colors
   the better)
2 tbsp freshly snipped
   chives
2 tbsp freshly chopped
   parsley
1 tbsp dried oregano
2 garlic cloves, finely grated
14 oz goats' cheese
sea salt and black pepper

**1** Line a 4 x 8 in loaf tin with parchment paper, leaving enough paper hanging over that you can easily cover the terrine when the tin is full.

**2** Scrub the beet, then place in a pan, cover with water, pop on the lid, and cook for about 30–40 minutes until tender. Set aside to cool, then peel.

**3** Meanwhile, mix all the herbs and garlic with the goats'cheese in a bowl and season to taste.

**4** Slice the cooked beets into various thicknesses – some $\frac{1}{8}$ in, some $\frac{1}{4}$ in.

**5** Put a layer of golden or candy-colored beets along the bottom of the tin, followed by a thin layer of the garlic and herb goats' cheese mix. Do this for 6 layers of each, so you have 12 layers in total, and then start on the purple beets and cheese layers until you reach the top. If you have more colors, vary them as you go along.

**6** Pull the parchment paper over so all the terrine is covered. Place a weight on top of the tin and leave in the fridge overnight or for 8 hours to set.

**7** Cover the set terrine with a plate and turn upside down to remove the terrine. Slice and serve or refrigerate the terrine until needed.

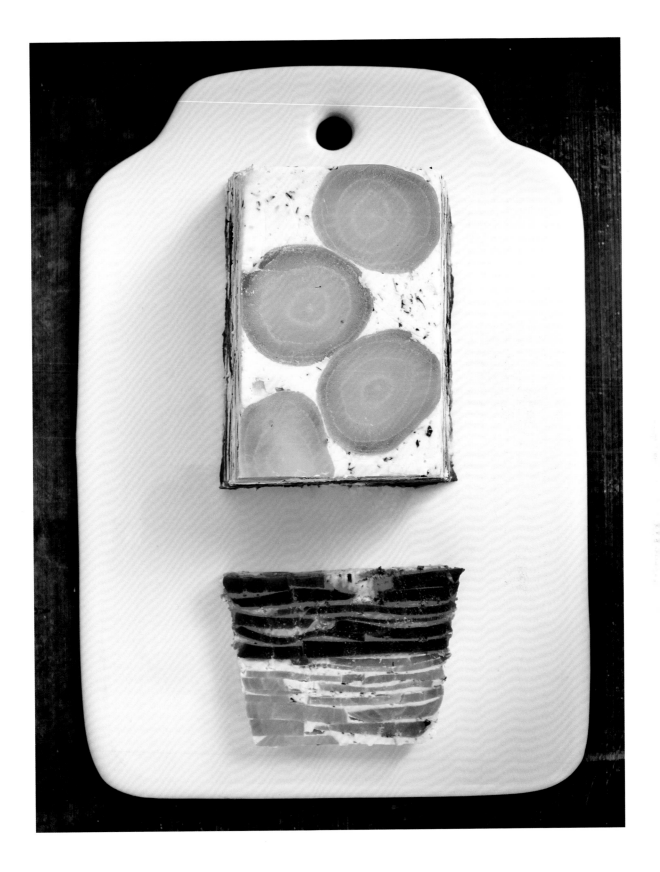

# BUCKWHEAT BURRITOS

These are great for socials – super easy to prep before your guests arrive and everyone can enjoy creating their own. Inspired by the classic French galettes, we've replaced heavy wheat with nutritious, gluten-free buckwheat. For better digestion, make the batter in advance, add a tablespoon of apple cider vinegar and leave to soak overnight on the worktop. This will start breaking down the starch. You can also grind "crispy" buckwheat (page 320) in a blender to make your own flour too.

The thinner the tortilla, the easier it will be to construct the burritos. Fill these tortillas with spiced black beans, guacamole, salsa, cheese, and sour cream. Don't be put off by the long list of ingredients – you can just pick a few fillings. Sometimes, when short of time, we like our tortillas with just guacamole and salsa.

**SERVES 4 (MAKES ABOUT 14 TORTILLAS)**

## FOR THE TORTILLAS

9 oz buckwheat flour

1 egg

½ tsp sea salt

ghee or coconut oil, for frying

## FOR THE FRIED BEANS

1 tsp ghee or coconut oil

1 garlic clove, finely grated

a pinch of ground cumin

a pinch of fresh chili or a little cayenne pepper

2 tins of cooked black or pinto beans (drained weight 18 oz) or 18 oz homecooked beans (dried weight 7 oz, activated overnight see page 300)

sea salt and black pepper

## FOR THE GUACAMOLE

2 large avocados

1 tbsp extra virgin olive oil

juice of 1 lime or ½ lemon

scallion or fresh chives, chopped or snipped

1 garlic clove, finely grated or chopped

sea salt and black pepper

## FOR THE RED PEPPER SALSA

1 large red pepper, diced (or tomatoes if you prefer)

1 tbsp extra virgin olive oil

1 tsp apple cider vinegar

some chopped fresh parsley or cilantro and a little fresh chili

sea salt and black pepper

## FOR MORE FILLINGS, PICK AND MIX ANY OF THE BELOW

4 large tomatoes, sliced or 2 handfuls of cherry tomatoes, sliced

3 handfuls of a crunchy lettuce or red or white cabbage, shredded

a large handful of grated strong cheese

finely chopped jalepeños or any chili of your choice

lime wedges

full-fat probiotic sour cream

a handful of chopped cilantro or parsley

chopped scallions, red onion, or snipped fresh chives

**1** To make the tortillas, whisk together the flour, egg, and salt in a jug with 3 cups water and leave to stand (if you want to get ahead, you can do this the night before).

**2** Bring a lightly greased, well-seasoned cast iron or ceramic pan, about 8 in in diameter, up to a medium-high heat (as with pancakes, you only need the lightest coating of fat, so use a brush to coat the pan or pour out any excess).

**3** Whisk the batter again and use a ladle to add enough batter to cover the bottom of the pan when swirled. (By the third tortilla you will probably have mastered the perfect amount for the size of your pan – they need to be large and thin enough so that you can "wrap" them around a filling.)

**4** Once the underside is lightly browned and lifts off easily from the bottom of the pan (1–2 minutes), it is ready to turn. Flip your tortilla and cook lightly on the other side (too much and the tortilla gets crunchy).

**5** To make the fried beans, gently heat the ghee or coconut oil in a pan and fry the garlic. Add the cumin and the chili and cook for a few minutes. Add the cooked black beans (add a splash of water) and cook for about 5 minutes until they are sticky. Season to taste.

**6** To make the guacamole, scoop out your avocado flesh into a bowl and, using a fork, roughly smash all the ingredients together and season.

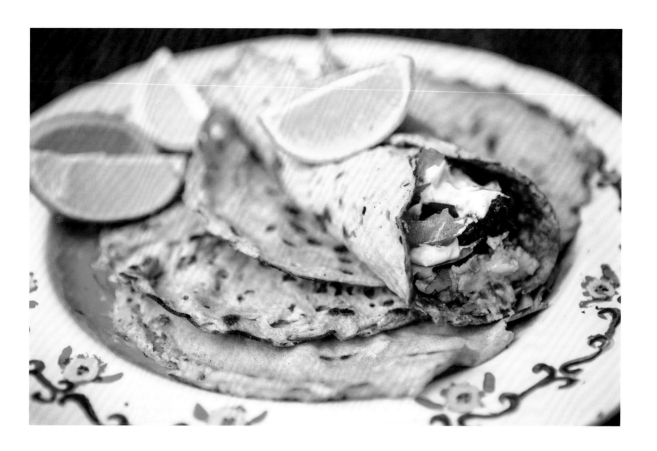

**7** To make the red pepper salsa, mix everything together in a bowl and season.

**8** To serve, pile up the fillings into little individual bowls or arrange over a platter. Warm your tortillas in a pan or the oven just before serving. Smear the tortillas with fried beans, guacamole, and sour cream then sprinkle on the other ingredients. Roll into burritos as best you can and start eating, keeping a napkin close by. If the tortillas are too small or just too messy to eat, then get your knife and fork out and go at it like an open sandwich.

# SOCCA PIZZA

Socca, the speciality of Nice, is a pancake made by stirring chickpea flour into water and olive oil to form a loose batter, which is then baked in an open oven. It makes a great base for homemade pizza. Quick and easy to put together, you just cook as you would a pancake. For best digestion, mix the simple batter the night before with a few tablespoons of probiotic yogurt and leave to soak on the worktop to help break down the complex starches (if this is not possible, be sure to use chickpea flour ground from cooked chickpeas).

Use any of your favorite toppings: roast some peppers, caramelize an onion, and make a tangy tomato sauce as a base. On a hot day, if you want to avoid the oven, you could easily pile up those tasty fillings and eat open-sandwich style. Make soft and flexible socca pancakes by adding a little more water to wrap your favorite grilled vegetables and hummus or to make the perfect substitute for roti or chapati to scoop up spicy curries. Serve warm with antipasti or make them thin and crisp and pour over hot garlic butter for a take on garlic bread.

**SERVES 4 (MAKES 9 SMALL SOCCA PIZZAS)**

**FOR THE SOCCA**

9 oz chickpea flour (also known as gram flour)

2 pinches of sea salt

a pinch of black pepper

a large pinch of fresh herbs (such as rosemary, thyme, or oregano) or 1 small pinch of ground cumin or 1 tbsp grated fresh garlic or 1 tsp garlic powder

coconut oil or ghee, for frying

Choose your favorite toppings from the options on page 220.

For a great tomato base see page 194.

**1** To make the bases, whisk together the socca ingredients with 1 ½ cup water by hand or in a blender.

**2** Leave to stand overnight or for at least 30 minutes at room temperature to allow the chickpea flour to fully absorb the water. Prepare the toppings in the meantime.

**3** Bring a lightly greased, well-seasoned cast-iron or ceramic pan up to a medium-high heat, grease with a touch of coconut oil or ghee, and set over a moderately high heat.

**4** Pour in about 4 tablespoons of the batter, swirl to around 4 ¾ in wide and $1/16 - 1/8$ in thick like a traditional pancake and cook for a few minutes.

**5** Flip the base over (it's ready when it flips over easily) and cook the other side until golden brown. Cook longer for a crisper base. Repeat to make the remaining bases.

*Continued overleaf*

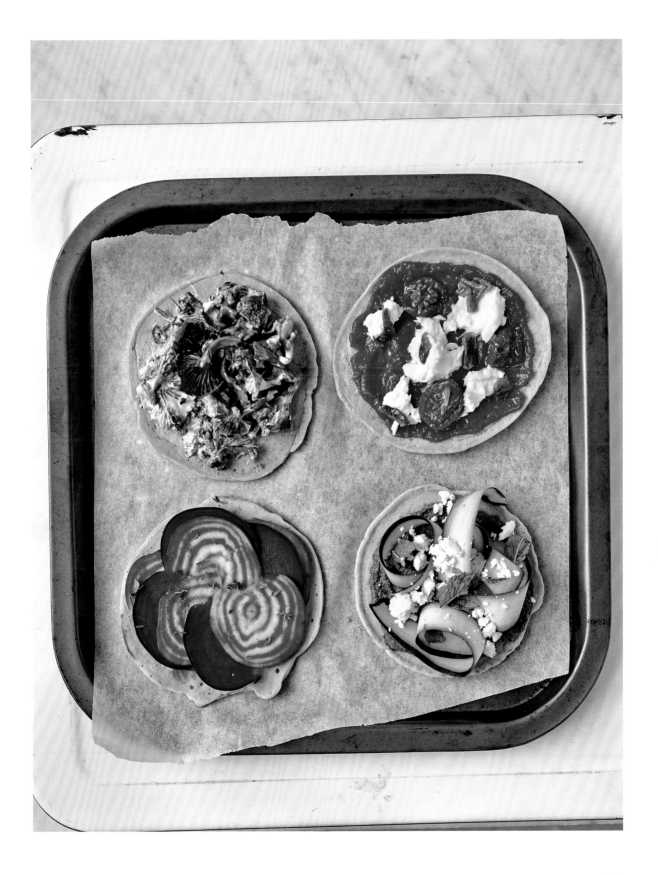

**6** Remove your socca bases and set aside until you are ready to assemble your pizzas. For parties, you can make up the socca pizzas in advance, leave in the fridge until your guests arrive, then throw them in the oven. Alternatively, pour over some garlic-infused extra virgin olive oil or some butter melted with crushed garlic and enjoy straightaway.

**7** To make the pizzas, preheat the oven to fan 390°F.

**8** Make the tomato sauce following the instructions on page 194.

**9** Put your pizza bases onto a wire rack (for a crispy base) or a baking tray, then add your toppings.

**10** Bake the pizzas in the oven for 10 minutes. For a margherita, give the cheese a golden crust with a quick blast in the broiler.

**11** Drizzle with good extra virgin olive oil, scatter on some arugula or fresh herbs, and serve with a salad.

**BEETS AND THYME:** scrub 2 beets well then use a sharp knife or mandolin to cut into thin circles. Spread some gorgonzola or cream cheese on each pizza base, top with a few layers of overlapping beets, and sprinkle over 1 teaspoon of dried thyme leaves or 2 teaspoons of fresh thyme leaves. Season with sea salt and pepper.

**ZUCCHINI, PESTO, AND FETA:** spread 4 tablespoons of Brazil Nut Pesto (page 198) or Kale Pesto (page 233) over the base of each pizza. Use a vegetable peeler to slice 2 small zucchinis lengthways into very wide pappardelle-style ribbons. You might want to cut the long strands in half to make them easier to eat. Top with a small handful of feta and season with a little sea salt and pepper.

**MARGHERITA:** spread tomato sauce (page 194) on the base of each pizza or top with sun-dried tomatoes and 1 small buffalo mozzarella ball torn into pieces. Season with sea salt and pepper.

**MUSHROOMS AND THYME:** fry 4 large handfuls of sliced mushrooms in a hot pan in 1 tablespoon of ghee for a few minutes (wild mushrooms, if you can find them – we like chanterelles, dirt brushed off, not washed, then sliced). Turn down the heat and add 1 finely chopped garlic clove and 1 teaspoon of dried thyme leaves or 2 teaspoons of fresh thyme leaves. Season with sea salt and pepper. Stir through 1 tablespoon of crème fraîche, if desired, then take off the heat.

## SPRING GREENS WITH BLOOD ORANGE DRESSING

This warm salad of greens makes a delicious light supper or easy side. Use tart blood oranges, when they are in season, or lemon and limes for this zingy Asian dressing. Try sunflower and sesame seeds for a variation on poppy seeds and toss through some cooked buckwheat noodles or quinoa to make this stretch to 4 portions.

SERVES 2

### FOR THE SPRING GREENS

1 tsp coconut oil or ghee

7 oz purple sprouting broccoli, stalks trimmed

2 scallions, finely sliced

1 head of spring greens, about 14 oz, stalks removed and roughly sliced or use chard or other cabbages like kale

8 radishes, about 1 ¾ oz, thinly sliced

1 tbsp poppy seeds

1 tbsp fresh mint leaves, torn

### FOR THE DRESSING

just under an ounce fresh root ginger, peeled

½ tsp tamari

½ tsp sea salt

5 tsp blood orange juice or lemon or lime juice

1½ tsp maple syrup

½ tsp toasted sesame oil

6 tbsp sesame oil or extra virgin olive oil

a large pinch of white or black pepper

**1**  First, make the dressing. Grate the ginger onto a plate to catch the juice, then squeeze the grated ginger to release more – to get 3 teaspoons of fresh ginger juice (discard the flesh). Whisk this with the rest of the dressing ingredients in a bowl, or shake in a jam jar, and set aside.

**2**  Heat the coconut oil or ghee in a large frying pan and stir-fry the purple sprouting broccoli until almost tender (about 4 minutes). If you're using kale, add it soon after the broccoli because it needs more time to soften. Then add the scallion and sliced spring greens or chard and fry for 30 seconds.

**3**  Transfer to a serving dish and arrange the sliced radishes on top. Drizzle over the blood orange dressing and finish with the poppy seeds and mint.

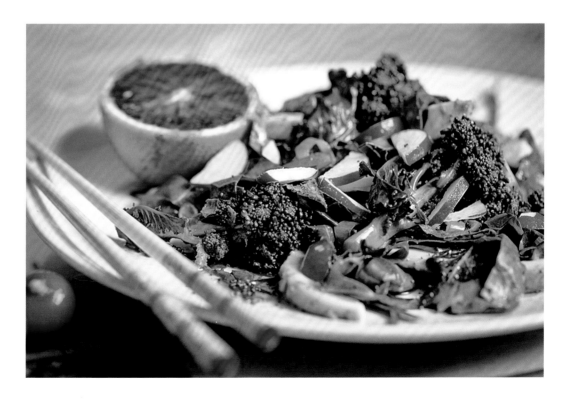

# FETA AND BLACK BEAN BURGERS

These are flavor-packed patties with a jalapeño kick that are crunchy on the outside and soft on the inside. Serve cold, falafel-style in lettuce cups or wraps with our Probiotic Tomato Ketchup (page 306) and our Mung Bean Hummus (page 232) or eat them hot, sandwiched between two slices of Flax Sandwich Bread (page 272) along with avocado, arugula leaves, and our Ginger Poppy Seed Mayonnaise (page 88). Also good with a simple green salad or our Summer Lime Coleslaw (page 80) and a side of Zucchini Fries (page 110).

We like to use black beans in this recipe for their color and because they mash easily but any type would do. Make a big batch of burgers, then freeze them ready to heat in the oven for a simple supper or easy packed lunch.

**MAKES 8 BURGERS**

2 tbsp ghee

1 medium onion, finely chopped

2 garlic cloves, grated

2 tins of black beans (drained weight 18 oz) or 18 oz homecooked beans (dried weight 7 oz, activated overnight see page 300)

3 ½ oz chestnut flour (or buckwheat flour)

1 tsp dried oregano or thyme

about 6 oz sun-dried tomatoes, chopped

a handful of fresh parsley, roughly chopped

1 tbsp chopped jalapeño peppers or fresh chilies

3 ½ oz feta, chopped

sea salt

**1**  Preheat the oven to fan 350°F.

**2**  Heat the ghee in a pan over a medium heat and fry the onion until softened but not colored. Stir in the garlic and cook for a few minutes before adding the drained cooked beans.

**3**  Mash the beans roughly with the back of a wooden spoon so that their excess moisture evaporates in the heat of the pan.

**4**  Transfer the bean mix to a bowl then stir in the flour and mix well to combine everything together.

**5**  Gently fold in the rest of the ingredients and check for seasoning, adding a little salt, if needed, or more jalapeños or chilies, if you like.

**6**  When the mixture is cool enough to handle, form the mixture into 8 burgers using your hands to shape them.

**7**  Lay the burgers on a baking tray lined with parchment paper then flatten each burger so that they are about ¾ in thick.

**8**  Bake the burgers in the oven for about 50 minutes until crisp on the outside and golden brown, turning them over halfway through the cooking time.

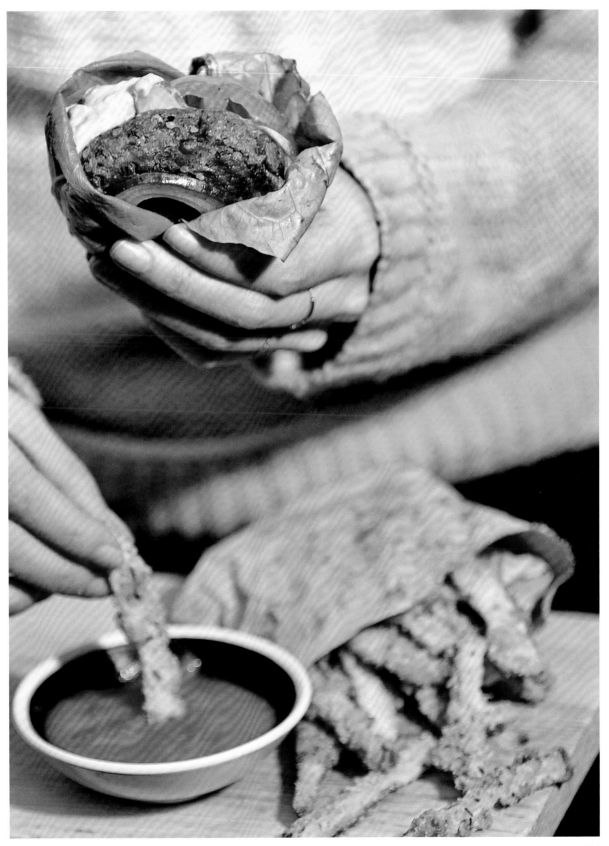

# DRESSINGS AND DIPS

**W**ITH THE RIGHT DIP, DRESSING, OR SAUCE, THE PLAINEST OF FOODS CAN BE TRANSFORMED into mouth-watering dishes, which is why we've dedicated a whole chapter to condiments. Dressings and dips are where we use unrefined, unsaturated plant oils. Choose from our favorite four: extra-virgin olive oil, flaxseed, sesame, and macadamia, or try a mix.

Here you will find recipes that we use time and again; those that are easy to make, keep for a week in the fridge, and instantly pull a meal together. Add antioxidant packed Kale Pesto (page 233) to some leftover quinoa and top with grated carrot for a delicious and speedy plate. The same applies to a bowl of broccoli and buckwheat noodles and our probiotic Miso Carrot Dressing (page 136) or a bunch of watercress and roasted beets is brought to life with our chlorophyll-rich Green Goddess Dressing (page 228) – the mundane becomes magnificent and supercharged.

We make creamy dips using nuts, seeds, beans, lentils, and vegetables; adding roasted veg, such as beets and squash, is a great way of using up leftovers. Season your chosen ingredients with spices and herbs and add an alkalizing zing with a splash of lemon or lime juice, apple cider vinegar, or pomegranate molasses.

A good dressing or dip also adds flair swirled through simple soups, stews, and salads. With the right dip we can happily munch on vegetables all day – try our Bagna Cauda (page 234), which is a delicious way to enjoy more raw veg but also special enough to serve at a party.

Just like soups, dips and dressings do not take much in the way of kitchen skills. Just shake the ingredients together in a jar for a vinaigrette or quickly blitz in a blender along with your chosen unrefined oil and water to achieve your desired consistency. Even our most complicated recipes, such as our Ginger Poppy Seed Mayonnaise (page 88) and Tartar Sauce (page 134), will take you no time at all to master.

As well as the recipes in this chapter, look out for more dips, dressings, and sauces scattered throughout the book – you'll find the Chimichurri Sauce teamed with salmon on page 158, for example, which is just as delicious with duck wraps, stirred through a bowl of soup, or served as a topping for a steak. Thai Sweet Chili Sauce (page 228) is a firm favorite to make any supper shine and keeps well, as will the classic condiment ketchup – but ours comes with a probiotic nutritional twist (see page 306).

Store a selection of dressings and dips in the fridge reusing glass jars. You'll be much more likely to throw together a home-cooked meal at the end of the day if you know you've got a helping hand of flavor ready to go in the fridge. All these recipes are a starting point for you to experiment with and elaborate on, so get creative and make up your own signature dressing or dip.

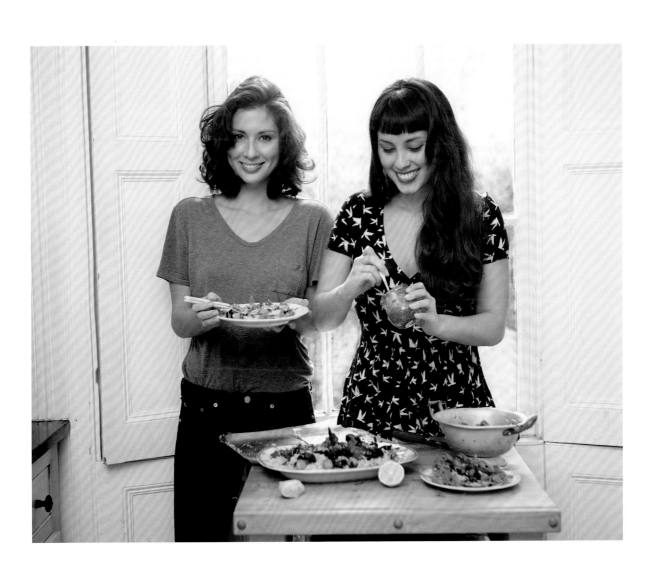

## GREEN GODDESS DRESSING

This luscious dressing is a blend of garlic, scallion, omega-3, protein-rich tahini (sesame seed paste), and plenty of immune-boosting parsley – definitely something you want to be enjoying plenty of. It's punchy and tangy so you could also add an avocado to dilute the flavor and make this dressing thick enough for dipping crudités. We always keep a glass jar of this in the fridge – pour a layer of olive oil over it to keep it fresh for up to a week in your fridge.

MAKES 10 OZ DRESSING

4 tbsp tahini

3 tbsp apple cider vinegar

2 scallions, roughly chopped

1 tbsp lemon juice

1 garlic clove

1½ large handfuls of chopped fresh parsley or 1 large handful of fresh tarragon

¾ cup extra virgin olive oil

sea salt and black pepper

**1** Put everything in a food processor or blender and blend together with 3 oz water until smooth, scraping down the sides as you go.

✚ **FOR A MORE SILKY DRESSING**, blend all the ingredients except the olive oil until smooth, and then blend in the olive oil, stopping when you've reached your desired thickness.

## THAI SWEET CHILI SAUCE

Tastes just like the classic Thai sweet chili sauce, but we've kicked out the refined sugar and used pure maple syrup instead. Fish sauce adds depth and the amount of chili is up to you. If we need the boost we sometimes double the garlic. Drizzle over ribs, serve with a stir-fry or dip your Cucumber Maki Crab Rolls (page 180) into it.

MAKES 5 OZ SAUCE

2 ½ oz maple syrup

1 ¾ oz apple cider vinegar

3 garlic cloves, grated or diced

2 tbsp fish sauce or 1 extra tsp sea salt

1 tbsp chili flakes or 1 fresh red chili, deseeded and finely chopped

1 tsp arrowroot powder

sea salt and black pepper

**1** Mix all the ingredients, except for the arrowroot, together with ¾ cup water in a saucepan.

**2** Simmer over a medium heat for about 5 minutes, until the sauce thickens.

**3** Meanwhile, whisk up the arrowroot with 2 tablespoons water, then add this to the pan and keep stirring.

**4** Simmer for 5 minutes more, stirring occasionally to stop it clumping or catching at the bottom of the pan. It will have reduced by about half to 5 oz. Take off the heat, check for seasoning and leave to cool. Serve at room temperature. Store in the fridge.

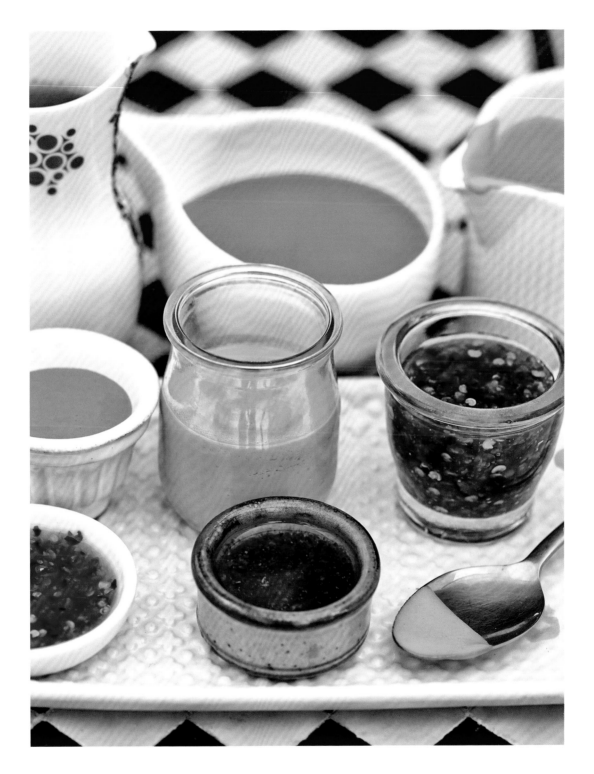

**LEFT TO RIGHT**

Green Goddess Dressing (opposite), Thai Sweet Chili Sauce
(opposite), Pomegranate Molasses Dressing (page 230),
Turmeric Avocado Dressing (page 230).

## TURMERIC AVOCADO DRESSING

MAKES ABOUT 5 OZ
DRESSING

¼ cup extra virgin olive oil

juice of 1 lemon or lime

½ avocado

1 garlic clove

1 tbsp ground turmeric or
½ in piece of fresh
turmeric (unpeeled if
organic), adding more
to taste

1 tsp raw runny honey

sea salt and black pepper

This creamy and punchy dressing is sunshine in a jar. It goes perfectly with big green salads, topped with pink radishes for a riot of color. This is another excellent way to include the super-powers of turmeric in your diet without having to think "curry." As you're not toasting the ground turmeric here, it is really important that your turmeric isn't stale.

**1**  Blend all the ingredients together with ½ cup water in a food processor or blender until smooth, adding more water as you blend for the desired consistency.

## POMEGRANATE MOLASSES DRESSING

MAKES ABOUT 5 OZ
DRESSING

3 oz extra virgin olive oil

2 tbsp pomegranate
molasses

2 tsp ground sumac (if you
can't find this, simply
leave it out)

1 tbsp apple cider vinegar
or lemon juice

1 tsp raw runny honey

1 garlic clove, finely grated
if not being blended

2 tbsp chopped fresh
dill or mint leaves

sea salt and black pepper

**OPTIONAL**

serve with a few fresh
pomegranate seeds

Good-quality pomegranate molasses is made from reduced fresh pomegranate juice. It's sweet yet sharp and adds a depth and richness to sweet and savory foods. It goes perfectly with ground sumac, which comes from the tart and lemony berries of the sumac tree. It's also delicious spooned over a simple soup or stew or try with Papaya, Halloumi, and Watercress Salad on page 78.

**1**  Aside from the fresh herbs and pomegranate seeds, blend or whisk all the ingredients in a bowl.

**2**  Stir in the fresh herbs and serve with a few pomegranate seeds on top, if using.

# SUN-DRIED TOMATO AND JALAPEÑO YOGURT DIP

We were planning on making guacamole one day and then, as often happens, the avocados weren't ripe so we had to come up with another dip – and fast! We always keep sun-dried tomatoes (choose those jarred in extra virgin olive oil) and jalapeños in the fridge as they lend a strong kick to anything that needs perking up, so we created a dip that uses both. We like this with crudités, Baked Zucchini Fries (page 110), and Italian Veg Balls (page 118), spread onto Carrot and Flax Crackers (page 121), or served with some baked fish or grilled steak. It goes beautifully drizzled onto roast squash or beet wedges. Leave the jalapeños and cayenne out for a kid-friendly alternative to ketchup.

MAKES 9 OZ DIP

7 oz full-fat probiotic natural yogurt

6 large sun-dried tomatoes, packed in extra virgin olive oil, drained (keep about 1 ¾ oz of the oil)

8 slices jalapeño pepper (or more depending on how spicy you like it)

1 garlic clove

a pinch of cayenne pepper (more if you like it hotter)

a pinch of sweet smoked paprika, plus extra to serve

extra virgin olive oil, to serve

sea salt and black pepper

**1** Put all the ingredients in a food processor or blender and blend until smooth. Alternatively, chop the ingredients finely and stir through the yogurt in a bowl. Season to taste.

**2** Serve with a drizzle of oil and a sprinkling of smoked paprika.

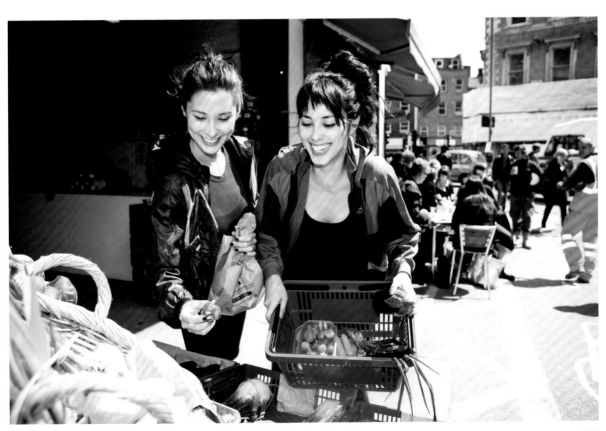

# MUNG BEAN HUMMUS

Hummus is a faithful friend and we always keep a jar on hand. It's perfect for dipping crudités into (see Bagna Cauda, page 234, for our favorite crudités), spreading on sandwiches, and dolloping into spiced stews. We love chickpeas, but you can make a hummus with so much more than just chickpeas. We like sunflower seed hummus, raw zucchini hummus, or this one, our favorite, starring the mung bean, which makes a light and creamy hummus. Mung beans are cheap (especially if you cook your own), high in protein and rich in nutrients, particularly vitamin K, and one of the easiest legumes to digest when prepared properly.

SERVES 4 AS A SNACK
WITH CRUDITÉS

### FOR THE HUMMUS

3 ½ oz green mung beans
   (activated overnight,
   page 300)

3½ tbsp lemon juice

4 tbsp tahini

2 garlic cloves

sea salt and black pepper

### OPTIONAL

fresh red chili or
   chili flakes

### TO SERVE

1 tbsp sesame seeds
   (black or white)

a drizzle of extra virgin
   olive oil

½ tsp ground sumac,
   za'atar, smoked paprika,
   or ground cumin

a small handful of chopped
   fresh herbs, such as dill,
   cilantro, or parsley

**1**  Cook the soaked mung beans in double their volume of water for 30–40 minutes, then drain, rinse under cold water, and leave to cool.

**2**  Gently toast the sesame seeds in a dry pan until fragrant, then set aside.

**3**  Blend the cooked mung beans with 1 tablespoon of water, the lemon juice, tahini, garlic, chili, if using, and some salt and pepper.

**4**  Start adding up to 1 ¾ oz water as it blends, stopping when you get to the desired consistency.

**5**  Pour into a bowl, drizzle over the olive oil, scatter over the sumac, za'atar, smoked paprika or ground cumin, and the toasted sesame seeds, then scatter with herbs.

## KALE PESTO

This is a raw, dairy-free pesto and an excellent way to eat more kale without having to chew through a huge bowl of it. This pesto is delicious with Courgetti (spaghetti made from zucchinis, see page 210), served as a dip, stirred through quinoa or scrambled eggs, drizzled over soups, or whizzed up with more extra virgin olive oil and lemon juice to create a superfood dressing. For bruschetta, we love this spread thickly onto our toasted Multiseed Loaf (page 273) with a little truffle salt or truffle oil. Stir through some buckwheat pasta for a quick packed lunch.

SERVES 4

1 oz cashew nuts
  (preferably activated,
  see step 1)

7 oz kale, stalks removed
  and leaves roughly
  chopped

1 garlic clove

¾ cup extra virgin olive oil

zest and juice of ½
  unwaxed lemon

sea salt and black pepper

**OPTIONAL**

a dash of truffle oil, to serve

or 1 oz parmesan or
  pecorino cheese, grated
  or shavings, to serve

**1** Soak the cashews for 3 hours in double their volume of water with ½ teaspoon sea salt. Be sure to discard the soaking water and rinse before using.

**2** Blend all the pesto ingredients until you get to your desired texture – sometimes we like it smooth and silky, other times with a bit more texture. Add truffle oil or parmesan, if you like.

➕ **NOT A FAN OF RAW KALE?** It can taste a little bitter, so try steaming the kale in a covered pan for 3 minutes in a little water.

## LEMON PARSLEY CASHEW DIP

This dip is great with plenty of fresh raw vegetable crudités or scooped into crisp endive leaves. You can also thin it out with water and extra lemon juice, then drizzle it over baked fish and roast chicken or toss it through salads. Parsley and lemon are rich in antioxidants and vitamins, while raw cashews are creamy and nutritious, especially when soaked in water beforehand.

SERVES 4

2 ¾ oz cashew nuts
  (preferably activated, see
  step 1)

½ cup extra virgin olive oil,
  plus extra for drizzling

2 large handfuls of fresh
  parsley leaves

1 garlic clove

1 tbsp lemon juice

sea salt and black pepper

**1** Soak the cashews for 3 hours in double their volume of water with ½ teaspoon sea salt. Be sure to discard the soaking water and rinse before using.

**2** Blend all the ingredients together with 4 tablespoons water and serve in a bowl topped with a drizzle of extra virgin olive oil.

# BAGNA CAUDA

Bagna Cauda, meaning "hot bath," is a speciality of Piedmont, Italy – a warm, punchy sauce of garlic and anchovy, originally a snack for vine workers. It is eaten by dipping raw, steamed, or roasted vegetables into the warm sauce.

This is a really tasty way to enjoy more raw veg. We especially like endive, celery, and fennel – bitter vegetables that encourage the flow of digestive juices. Delicious as a weekend lunch, we like to follow it with a broth or light soup (to end the meal).

A colorful banquet of crudités, a fondue pot of Bagna Cauda, and plenty of napkins is an excellent way to feed a crowd at a party. Or try this spooned over a plate of roasted veg or as a sauce for meat or fish.

**SERVES 6-8**

8 large handfuls of a selection of raw veg (see note below)

1 ¾ oz butter or ghee

10 anchovy fillets, packed in extra virgin olive oil, drained (keep the oil)

1 tbsp chopped fresh parsley

a tiny pinch of cayenne pepper, or to taste

8 ½ oz crème fraîche

6 large garlic cloves

**1**  Wash and prepare the vegetables. Break the endive down into individual leaves and slice the fennel and celery into crudités. Make sure that they are nice and dry by patting with a clean towel. Keep them somewhere cool until ready to serve.

**2**  Melt the butter or ghee in a saucepan, add the anchovies, parsley, and cayenne and cook gently until the anchovies dissolve into the butter.

**3**  Add the crème fraîche, 8 ½ oz water, and the garlic and slowly bring to boil. Lower the heat and gently simmer for 15 minutes, stirring frequently, until reduced by half, then blend.

**4**  Test a crudité in the mixture to check the consistency. If the flavor isn't intense enough, then simmer a little longer to reduce and thicken.

**5**  Serve in a warm dish over a candle or in a fondue pot, swirling through the extra virgin olive oil kept earlier from the anchovies. If the sauce begins to separate, give it a little whisk.

**6**  Dip the vegetables into the Bagna Cauda and enjoy!

+ **THE SAUCE CAN BE MADE IN ADVANCE** and kept refrigerated. To reheat, warm very gently in a small saucepan, stirring occasionally.

+ **TRY DIPPING** carrots, celery, fennel, cucumber, endive, and radishes, as well as peppers, cooked artichokes, and cauliflower florets.

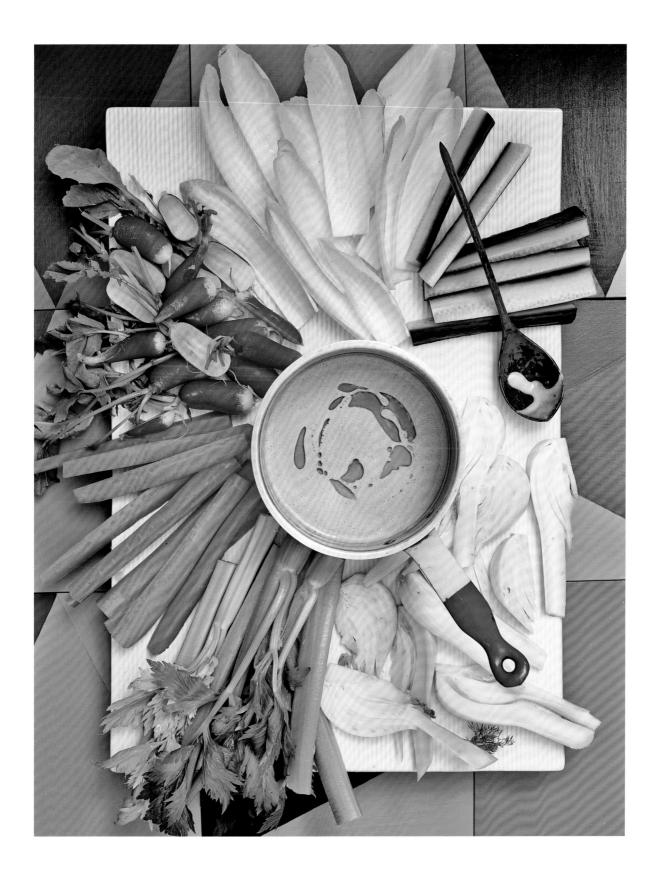

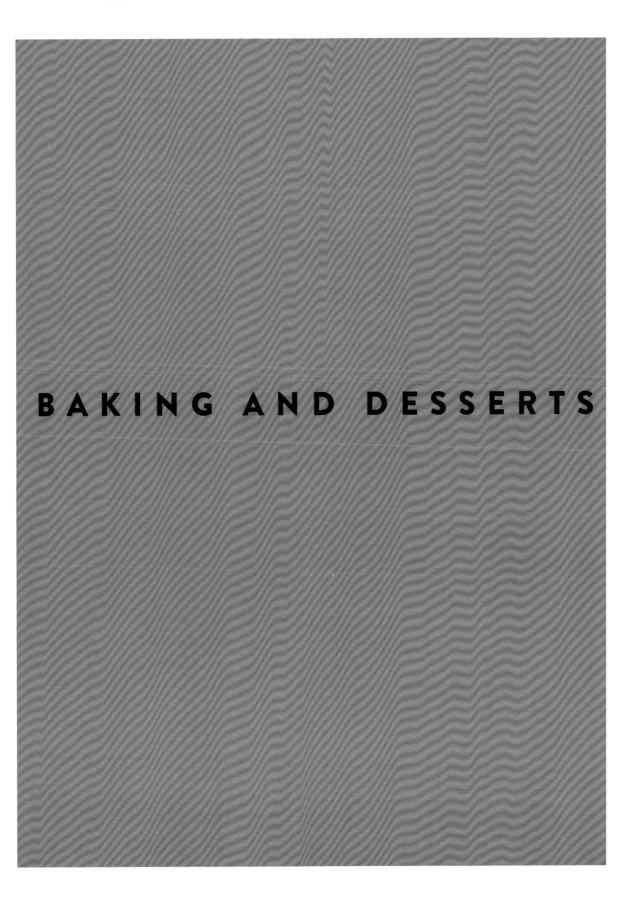

# BAKING AND DESSERTS

**R**EADILY AVAILABLE, LOW-COST COMMERCIAL SWEETS AND SNACKS HAVE CREPT INTO DAILY LIFE. These nutritionally poor, unbalanced foods, often packed with refined sugars, chemical sweeteners, and hydrogenated fats have a negative impact on our health.

The HEMSLEY + HEMSLEY philosophy embraces the pleasure of eating, so we absolutely do not deprive ourselves of desserts and even have a bespoke celebration-cake service. We've enjoyed developing our range of healthy baked goods and sweets over the years all free from grain, gluten, refined sugar, hydrogenated fats, refined vegetable oils, and artificial flavorings.

Instead, our recipes use whole foods like beans, avocado, eggs, coconut, butter, and small quantities of natural sugars such as raw honey, pure maple syrup, molasses, stevia, and fresh and dried fruits. Unlike chemical sweeteners, glucose syrups and refined sugar, these sweet ingredients are less processed and closer to their whole food state. This helps to keep them mineral-rich and ensures more nutrients in every mouthful, which is, after all, the first purpose of food.

We balance these natural sweeteners with fats and proteins such as coconut oil, butter, nuts, and seeds. This not only adds nutrition, but slows down the absorption of sugars, helping to prevent blood sugar spikes and the inevitable energy dips that follow. The fat also gives you a satisfying "mouthfeel" and a luxurious taste. You'll notice that, when you eat real fats, your body will recognize when it is full and feel satisfied more quickly and with smaller portions.

Remember though, that even natural sweeteners with their health benefits should be eaten in moderation. The body is hard-wired to crave sweet things as they are so easily converted into a source of energy, so don't let your sweet tooth get out of hand or be fooled into thinking that a healthy treat is a good alternative to a proper meal. Aim to slowly reduce the amount of natural sweetener you use so that you can reset your taste buds, diminish cravings and learn to enjoy the natural sweetness in food.

As with all our recipes, good-quality ingredients are key to sweet treats too. Compared to refined flours, oil, and sugars, some of our ingredients can seem expensive, but by controlling the quality of the ingredients, you control what goes into your body – a much better way to treat yourself.

If you are still not sold, remember this: when using real and minimally processed ingredients that your body recognizes as food, it won't be as easy to overeat – one or two of our cookies will satisfy you and your body will simply say "thank you, I'm done." So you really can have your cake and eat it!

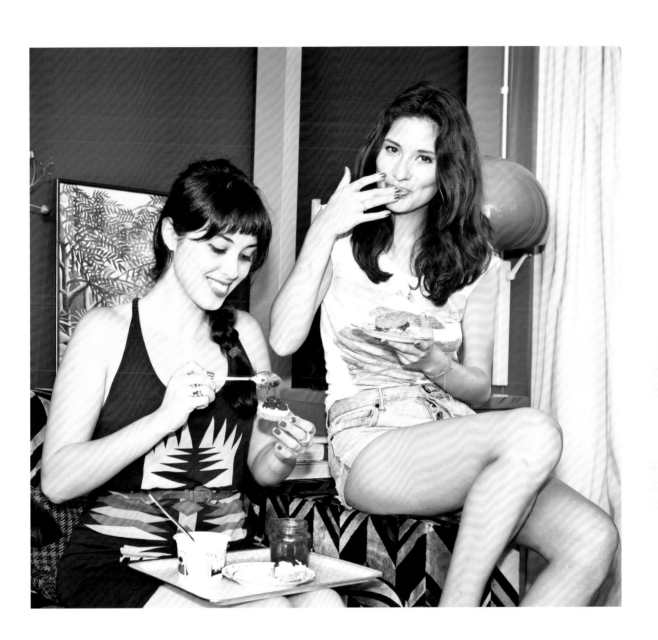

## BB BROWNIES

These chocolate brownies, made from black beans and maple syrup, are proof that grain- and gluten-free baking tastes amazing. You can replace the walnuts with dried cranberries if you have a nut allergy.

Play around with the sweetness – less maple syrup is better for you and gives a slightly more crumbly texture – we don't add extra sweetness if we don't need it. If you have a sweet tooth, start with ¾ cup and gradually decrease whenever you make it, adding a few drops of stevia for added sweetness until your taste buds adjust.

**MAKES 12 BROWNIES**

2 tins of cooked black beans (drained weight 18 oz) or 18 oz homecooked beans (dried weight 7 oz, soaked overnight, see page 300)

8 oz butter or coconut oil at room temperature, plus extra for greasing

4 eggs

3 oz unsweetened cacao powder

⅔ - ¾ cup maple syrup

1½ tbsp vanilla extract

1 tsp coffee extract or use extra vanilla extract

sea salt

4 ½ oz chopped walnuts (preferably "crispy" activated, page 300)

**OPTIONAL**

a few drops of stevia, to sweeten

**1**  Preheat the oven to fan 325°F. Grease the inside of a 9 ½ x 8 in china or glass baking dish. Rinse the black beans and leave to drain. Melt the butter/oil in a saucepan over a gentle heat, then set it aside.

**2**  Place the drained beans, eggs, cacao powder, ⅔ cup of the maple syrup, the vanilla extract, and coffee extract, if using, into a food processor with a pinch of salt. Pulse a few times, then blend until smooth.

**3**  Add the melted butter/oil, very slowly so as not to cook the eggs, while the machine is running. Taste the batter, adding more maple syrup or a few drops of stevia if need be, then stir in most of the chopped walnuts, reserving a handful.

**4**  Pour the brownie mixture into the prepared dish and gently tap the baking dish on a kitchen counter to even out the mixture. Sprinkle the remaining walnuts on top and bake for 40–45 minutes, until the brownie feels firm but springy and its surface is cracked.

**5**  Leave to cool completely before cutting into squares. Refrigerating the brownies makes them wonderfully fudgy.

✛ **FOR A MOCHA-FLAVORED VARIATION THAT'S CAFFEINE FREE** use ⅔ cup of maple syrup and 2 ⅔ oz of carob instead of cacao powder (see page 21). Carob is sweeter that cacoa and not bitter so you don't need as much maple syrup.

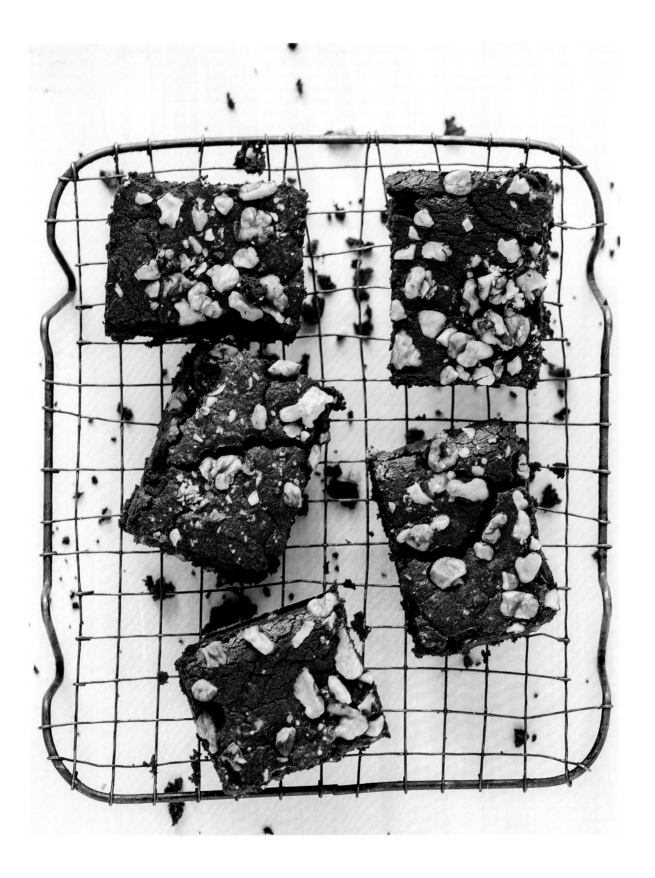

# MINI ALMOND, STRAWBERRY, AND CUSTARD TARTS

**MAKES 4-6 TARTS**

Strawberries are synonymous with summer and for us, only British will do. We've used an almond-based pastry to make crisp, gluten-free tart cases and filled them with strawberries and rich custard. We've taken our custard right back to basics here – just whole eggs, vanilla, and butter with a touch of honey whisked in at the end. The result is a subtly sweet tart, rich in both slow-burning protein and fats, which help to prevent that usual post-dessert crash.

**FOR THE PASTRY**

1 ¾ oz butter at room temperature, plus extra for greasing

5 ⅔ oz ground almonds or Sun Flour (pages 302–303)

a pinch of sea salt

a pinch of baking soda

1½ tbsp maple syrup

½ tsp vanilla extract

**FOR THE TART FILLING**

just under an ounce butter

3 eggs

¼ tsp vanilla extract

1–1½ tbsp raw honey

a container of strawberries, about 9 oz (wiped if organic or washed, dried, and hulled)

a few drops of stevia, to sweeten (optional)

**1** Preheat the oven to fan 350°F. Lightly grease 4 mini tart tins, about 4 in in diameter, with a little butter.

**2** Mix the pastry ingredients together in a food processor – or use the traditional pastry making technique and rub the butter into the dry ingredients using your finger tips, and then mix in the maple syrup and vanilla extract – then press them together to make a smooth ball of pastry. If the pastry feels too warm to work with, chill for 10 minutes in the fridge.

**3** Cut the dough into 4 equal sections. Use the palm of your hand to flatten each ball of pastry before placing each one in the base of a greased tart tin. Use your fingers to spread and smooth the pastry thinly and evenly around the tin, pressing it up the sides. Take a knife and trim the excess pastry to leave a clean edge. Prick the base of the tarts with a fork – this will stop them puffing up.

**4** Chill the tart cases for at least 20 minutes before baking, for a crisper finish.

**5** Place the chilled tarts on a tray and bake for about 12 minutes, depending on the thickness of the tart cases. The edges should be golden, but beware that nut or seed-based pastry can turn dark very quickly.

**6** Remove from the oven and place to one side – the cases will be soft, but will crisp up as they cool. Leave them to harden up slightly, then gently turn out onto a wire rack to cool. Store them in a sealed container in the fridge until needed.

**7** To make the tart filling, place a glass bowl over a small saucepan of hot water, without allowing the base of the bowl to touch the water. Add the butter to the bowl and while it melts, whisk together the eggs in a separate bowl with the vanilla extract.

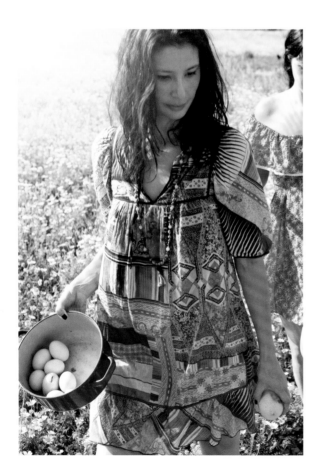

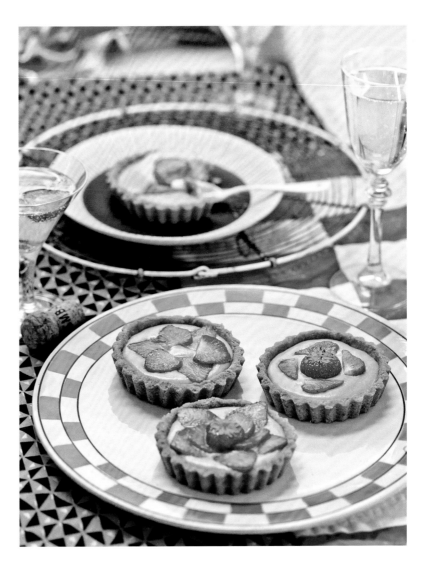

**+ YOU CAN SKIP THE CUSTARD STAGE** – just pile in some strawberries and finish with a drizzle of raw honey.

Also try kiwis, cherries, figs, and other seasonal red berries – they will all taste great.

**8** Bring the pan of water to a gentle simmer and slowly add the beaten eggs to the butter whilst continually whisking using a balloon whisk. Continue to whisk the egg mixture for about 10 minutes. Be patient and don't be tempted to turn up the heat here – you don't want scrambled eggs! When the mixture starts to thicken, watch it carefully and keep stirring to avoid lumps forming. If you get a lump, quickly remove the bowl from the heat and beat furiously until it's smooth.

**9** When the custard is about the thickness of double cream and leaves trail marks from the whisk, remove the bowl from the heat and continue whisking until it cools. Once it is cool enough to touch, whisk in the honey and add a few drops of stevia, if you like.

**10** The tart cases can be made ahead of time, but you need to assemble the tarts just before serving. Spoon a layer of custard into each tart, then slice the strawberries and arrange as you fancy on top. If you think that your tart cases are quite thick, then balance the taste and texture by adding plenty of custard and piling the strawberries high. These are best enjoyed within a few hours of making.

# AVOCADO LIME CHEESECAKE

Our take on a New York-style cheesecake and it's packed full of goodness. Free from refined sugar, flour, and dairy, this cheesecake will leave everyone wondering how anything this tasty can be so nutritious.

The creamy, lime-flavored dessert sits on top of a nutty, chocolate base made from toasted pecans, coconut, and cacao nibs bound together and sweetened with dates — the base is good enough to eat on its own.

Unlike most raw and dairy-free cheesecakes, the topping is completely free from nuts. For anyone with a nut allergy, just swap the pecans in the base for sunflower seeds.

SERVES 12

## FOR THE BASE

- 4 oz pecans (preferably "crispy" activated, pages 300–302)
- 1 ½ oz shredded coconut
- 2 ½ oz cacao nibs
- 6 ½ oz pitted dates
- 3 tbsp coconut oil, melted and at room temperature

## FOR THE FILLING

- 1 ¼ lb avocado flesh (from about 5 medium-large avocados)
- ¾ cup lime juice (roughly 8–10 limes)
- 1 tsp lime zest (avoid the bitter white pith)
- 6 ¾ oz raw honey
- ¾ cup coconut oil, melted and at room temperature
- a few drops of stevia, to sweeten (optional)

**1** Preheat the oven to fan 300°F. Line the base and sides of a springform or loose-bottomed 7 in round cake tin with baking paper.

**2** Toast the pecans and shredded coconut on a lined baking tray in the oven for 7–8 minutes, until golden.

**3** Transfer the pecans and coconut to a food processor and add the rest of the base ingredients. Blend until the mixture is crumbly and holds together when pinched (don't let it go completely smooth).

**4** Tip the base mixture into the prepared tin. Press it down firmly and evenly with the back of a spoon, ensuring it is neat and flat where it meets the sides of tin. Transfer to the fridge while you prepare the filling.

**5** Place all of the ingredients for the filling into a food processor and blend until the mixture is completely smooth and silky. Check for taste and add more lime juice, zest, or sweeten with a little more honey or stevia according to preference, but it's best to keep this deliciously tangy.

**6** Remove the cake tin from the fridge and pour the filling over the base. Cover the tin, using a plate, and return it to the fridge for a couple of hours or overnight, if possible, to set.

**7** To serve, run a knife around the inner edge of the tin and carefully push the base up from the bottom. Transfer to a plate and serve immediately.

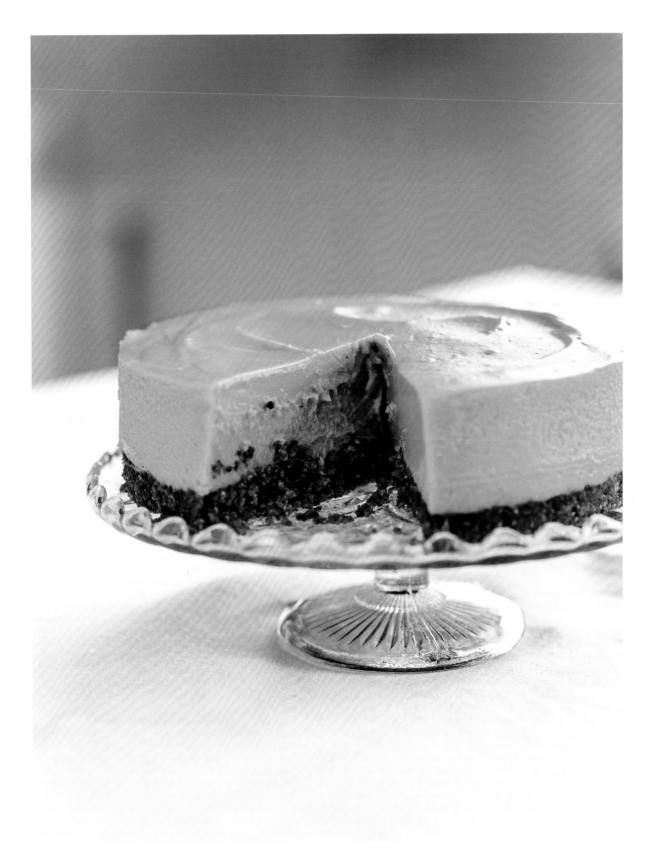

# STICKY TOFFEE PUDDING

This is Jasmine's favorite dessert – she is the sticky toffee pudding monster! Our version takes out everything that's wrong with the traditional recipe – gluten, wheat, and refined sugar – and replaces them with delicious, satisfying, unprocessed ingredients. Dried dates are still simple sugars, so we shouldn't overindulge in them, but because they are unrefined they come with a myriad of other benefits: iron, potassium, fiber, antioxidant flavonoids, and essential minerals.

We first came up with this recipe a few years ago, but over time we've tweaked it to make it even better. This new-and-improved version uses chestnut flour and the result is a deliciously chewy, fluffy cake. If you don't have chestnut flour, use coconut flour but you'll need to use a lot less.

This pudding is so nutrient-dense that you'll be satisfied with a much smaller portion than your usual serving of pud. This is a great dish to make in advance and freeze ready for dinner parties. Or after baking, cut it up so that you can help yourself to a square whenever you feel like it – eat it like a cake or heat and serve with cream and sauce.

SERVES 10

**FOR THE PUDDING**

3 ½ oz butter at room temperature, plus extra for greasing

9 oz pitted dates

7 oz ground almonds

3 eggs

1 ¾ oz chestnut flour or ¾ oz coconut flour

1¼ tsp baking soda

sea salt

a pinch of ground cloves (optional)

crème fraîche, to serve

**FOR THE SAUCE**

3 ½ oz pitted dates, roughly chopped

1 ¾ oz butter

**1**  Preheat the oven to fan 325°F. Grease a ceramic, glass, or enamel baking dish with butter or line with baking parchment.

**2**  Make the sauce first. Soak the dates in 1 ⅓ cup boiling water for 10 minutes. Drain, reserving the soaking liquid. Put the soaked dates and the butter in a food processor and blend until smooth. Slowly add the soaking water until your sauce is as smooth as possible (you can thin it with a touch more water). Set the sauce aside.

**3**  To make the pudding, soak the dates in ¾ cup boiling water for 10 minutes. Drain the dates and put their liquid into a food processor (don't bother rinsing the food processor) along with the butter and ground almonds and process until smooth.

**4**  Add the eggs, a tiny pinch of salt, and ground cloves, if using. Sift in the chestnut or coconut flour and baking soda and process again until creamy.

**5**  Chop the soaked dates and stir through the cake mixture until they are evenly distributed.

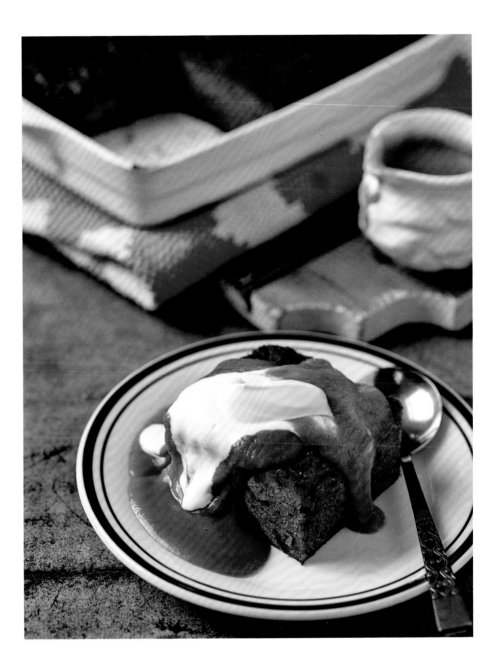

**6** Pour the mixture into the prepared dish and bake for 35 minutes, then cover the top of the cake with baking parchment (this will prevent the cake going too dark). Bake for a further 20 minutes. The pudding will slump slightly when it comes out of the oven.

**7** To serve, heat up the sauce, if desired, in a saucepan. Dish up the hot pudding, pour over the sauce and, for extra extravagance, add some crème fraîche if you like.

**NO FOOD PROCESSOR? THIS CAKE IS REALLY EASY TO MAKE BY HAND TOO.** To make the sauce, substitute the dates for ¹/₂ cup maple syrup and heat in a pan with 2 ¾ oz of butter. Mix in 2 tsp of arrowroot powder with 1 ¾ oz water and add to the pan. Heat gently, stirring, to make a thick sauce.

To make the cake, soak the dates as before then chop into small pieces with a sharp knife. Whisk the eggs, then add all the other cake ingredients, including the soaking liquid from the dates, and mix together with a large spoon. Bake as per step 6 instructions.

# BANANA BREAD

This delicious banana bread needn't be just an occasional treat. Nutritious and satisfying, it's great for breakfast and as an on-the-road snack that will keep your energy levels steady. Rather than a filler of glutenous flour, we use ground almonds and flaxseed. Use a coffee grinder or powerful blender to grind your own flaxseed, if you can, otherwise buy ground flax which is available in most health food stores. We like the flavor of real, grass-fed butter in our bread but you could use coconut oil instead – anything but processed vegetable oils please.

You know your bananas are ripe when the skins turn a deep shade of yellow and are covered in brown speckles. You can also try making the bread without any maple syrup, just adding a dash more vanilla and a few drops of stevia to the mix. Add a small handful of goji berries, roughly chopped walnuts, or cacao nibs for variaton.

**MAKES 1 BREAD OR 15 MUFFINS**

10 ½ oz ripe bananas (roughly 3 bananas)

1 oz butter, at room temperature

2 tbsp maple syrup (adjust to suit your taste buds)

1 tsp ground cinnamon

1 tsp vanilla extract

3 large eggs

½ tsp baking soda

1 tbsp lemon juice

7 ¾ oz ground almonds

1 oz ground flaxseed (also known as linseed)

1 tablespoon whole flax, for sprinkling

sea salt

**1** Preheat the oven to fan 325°F. Line a 9 x 5 in loaf tin with enough baking parchment to double as a wrap for storing the banana bread (if it lasts).

**2** Mash the bananas and butter in a mixing bowl to a pulp with a fork. Add the maple syrup, cinnamon, vanilla, eggs, baking soda, lemon juice, and a small pinch of salt. Mix well with a whisk.

**3** Add the ground almonds and ground flaxseed and mix well. Or, even speedier, you can throw all the ingredients into a blender or food processor and blitz together.

**4** Pour the mixture into the prepared tin, sprinkle with the whole flax and bake for 1–1¼ hours. It's ready when a skewer inserted into the center comes out dry. If your bread starts to look quite brown after the first 30 minutes, then cover the top with baking parchment until it has finished baking.

**5** Remove from the oven and leave to cool a little. Serve warm or at room temperature with some lightly salted butter and a cup of tea. Store the bread, covered, in the fridge (remember there is no sugar or preservatives) for up to a week or slice and freeze (that way you can enjoy a slice at a time reheated in the broiler).

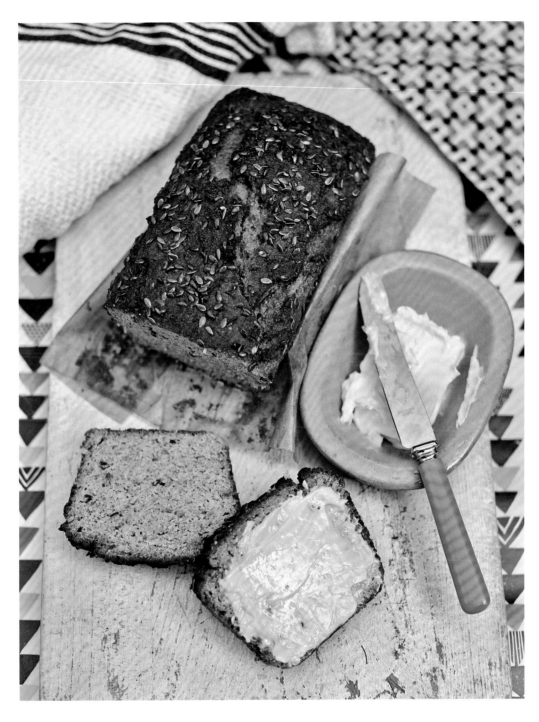

✚ **YOU CAN ALSO BAKE THIS BREAD INTO HANDY SNACK-SIZE MUFFINS.** Line a cupcake tray with paper cases to make 15 small muffins from the mixture and bake for 20 minutes in the oven.

# PEAR AND FIVE-SPICE CRUMBLE WITH GINGER CRÈME FRAÎCHE

SERVES 6

A quick crumble topping of ground almonds and butter or coconut oil is sweetened with the minimum amount of maple syrup – only 1½ tablespoons for the whole pudding.

Chinese five-spice powder is usually associated with savory dishes, but its blend of star anise, cloves, Sichuan pepper, and fennel seeds works really well with sweet pears too. Just be sure to check there's no garlic in your five-spice mix and remember the strength of spice will depend on the freshness and quality of your spices, so adjust accordingly.

## FOR THE CRUMBLE

1 ¾ oz butter or coconut oil at room temperature

6 ½ oz ground almonds

1½ tsp vanilla extract

1½ tbsp maple syrup

1 ¾ oz flaked almonds (or use another 1 ¾ oz ground almonds)

a tiny pinch of sea salt

## FOR THE PEARS

2 tsp five-spice powder

2 ¼ lb pears (about 8 pears) peeled if the skins are tough, cored, and chopped

½ tsp grated orange zest or orange extract

## FOR THE GINGER CRÈME FRAÎCHE

10 ½ oz crème fraîche or full-fat probiotic natural yogurt

1 tbsp grated fresh root ginger (unpeeled if organic)

1–2 tsp raw honey

a few drops of stevia, to sweeten (optional)

**1** Combine all the crumble ingredients, except the flaked almonds, in a bowl using your hands or a fork, until they are a crumbly consistency. Gently mix in the flaked almonds once combined.

**2** Chill or freeze the crumble mixture while you cook the pears (this makes for a crisper topping). Preheat the oven to fan 350°F.

**3** Toast the five-spice powder in a dry saucepan, over a medium high heat for about 30 seconds or until fragrant (the spices can burn easily so stir continuously).

**4** Place the chopped pear and 1 tablespoon water into the saucepan with the spices, cover, and cook gently over a medium heat for 10 minutes until softened, but still retaining color and bite.

**5** Mix in the orange zest or extract, then fill the bottom of a 8 in square ovenproof dish with the cooked pears.

**6** Evenly crumble the topping mixture over the pear (there's no need to press it down) and bake for about 25 minutes or until golden.

**7** Meanwhile, mix together the ingredients for the ginger crème fraîche, adding a few drops of stevia to sweeten if needed. Keep cool and serve with the hot crumble.

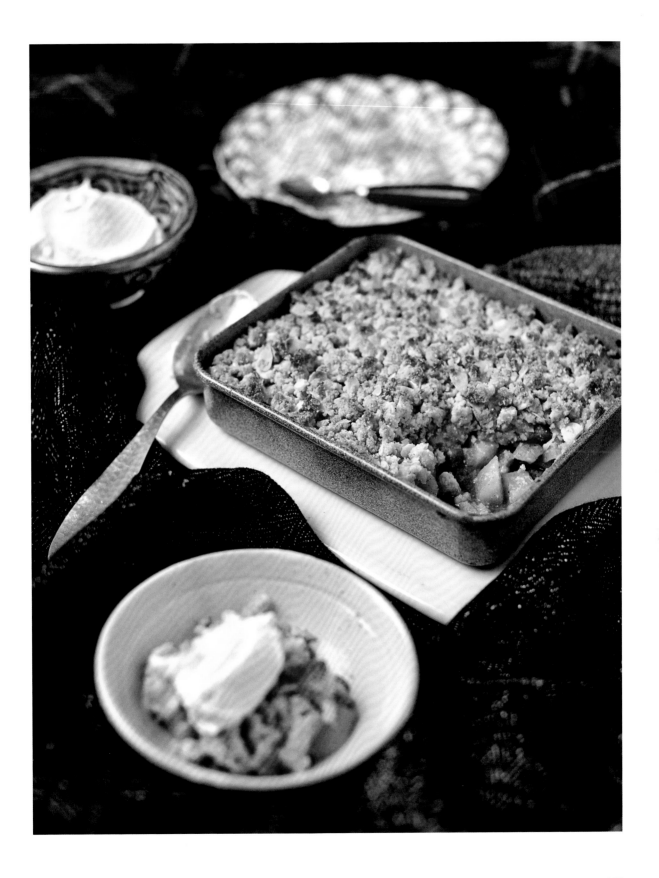

# CHOCOLATE MOLTEN POTS AND CHOCOLATE FIG PUDDING

MAKES 5-6 MOLTEN POTS
AND THE PUDDING
SERVES 6-8

**FOR THE MOLTEN POTS**

2 ⅔ oz coconut oil

4 tbsp cacao powder

4 tbsp date syrup or
   3 ½ tbsp maple syrup

1 tsp vanilla extract

¼ tsp baking soda

3 eggs

sea salt

**OPTIONAL**

a few drops of stevia, to
   sweeten

**FOR THE CHOCOLATE FIG
PUDDING**

7–8 fresh figs (we love
   Bursa figs)

These pots of molten chocolate are gooey in the middle, fluffy on the outside, and so simple to make. Mix them up in 5 minutes, pop into the oven for 10, and by the time you have finished licking the spoon and mixing bowl, there won't be much left to wash up.

Alternatively, you can double the mixture to make one big Chocolate Fig Pudding. The rich chocolate and gooey baked figs are a heavenly combination, particularly when served with a dollop of Mango Cashew Cream (page 30).

**1** Preheat the oven to fan 350°F.

**2 To make Chocolate Molten Pots**, melt the coconut oil in a small saucepan over a medium heat, then set aside.

**3** Add the cacao powder, a tiny pinch of salt, date or maple syrup, vanilla, and baking soda and mix well.

**4** Beat the eggs in a separate bowl, then whisk in the chocolate mixture. It will thicken from the residual heat to a gloopy custard. Taste and add a few drops of stevia, if needed.

**5** Spoon or pour the chocolate mixture into five 2 ¾ in-round ceramic or glass ramekins, leaving at least ¼ in clear from the top.

**6** Place the ramekins on a tray and bake in the oven for about 10 minutes. It's important to keep an eye on them as they approach the 10-minute mark (don't open the oven but look through the glass of the oven door).

**7** The chocolate pots are ready when they have just risen to a dome, but are still very wobbly when you shake the tray. They will continue to cook, so serve them immediately!

**8** You can make these in advance. Just chill them, then cook from cold, remembering to allow extra time in the oven, or freeze them individually and cook for about 20 minutes from frozen for a quick pudding.

**9  To make Chocolate Fig Pudding**, make double the quantity of Chocolate Molten Pot batter, following steps 1−4.

**10** Cut the stalks from the figs, then cut a shallow cross about 1 ¼ in deep in the cut side of each fig. Gently squeeze the figs so that the cross opens then arrange them evenly across the bottom of a 9 ½ in round oven dish, with the cut side facing upwards.

**11** Pour the chocolate batter around the figs, making sure the batter only reaches halfway up the sides of the figs. (If you have too much mixture for the dish, pour the rest into ramekins and bake as Chocolate Molten Pots.)

**12** Bake the pudding for about 20 minutes or until the top has risen and is set, but slighlty wobbles in the middle. Serve hot with Mango Cashew Cream (page 30).

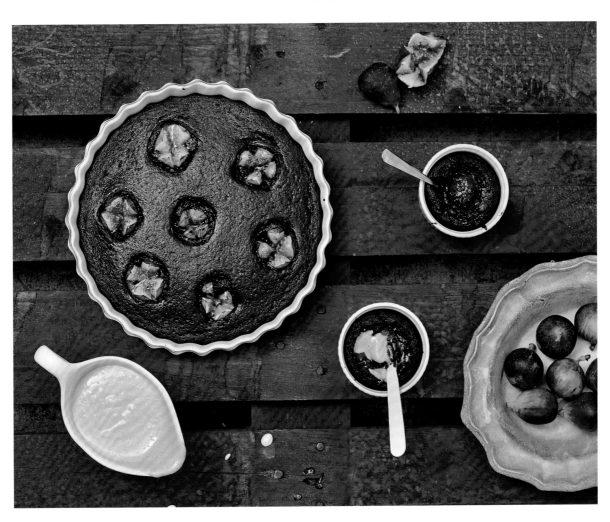

## PISTACHIO, FIG, AND GOATS' CHEESE TRIFLE

This beautiful and luxurious dessert comes together very quickly and can be made in advance, kept cool, then topped with hot toasted pistachios to serve.

This is one of our favorite desserts to serve to friends and, since it's so rich and nutritious, we keep the main course easy to digest (go for one of our soups or Malaysian Lentil and Squash Curry, page 212, and leave some time between courses). The flavors are intense, so use small serving dishes and keep portions small.

Seek out perfectly ripe fresh figs. If you can't find any then rehydrate some dried ones in a little hot water. For a flavor boost, add a splash of Calvados to the yogurt and cheese mix and, if you don't have any pomegranate molasses, just use a little more raw honey or date syrup. Soft goats' cheese can be very fresh and light tasting, but we also like one that is a little more aged for a grown up way to end a meal.

SERVES 4

a handful of pistachios, hazelnuts, or sesame seeds (hazelnuts, or sesame seeds preferably "crispy" activated, pages 300–302)

4 ¼ oz soft goats' cheese

5 oz full-fat probiotic natural yogurt or thick Coconut Yogurt (pages 305–306)

8 fresh figs or use dried ones

pomegranate molasses

runny raw honey or date syrup

**OPTIONAL**

1 tbsp Calvados or brandy

**1**  Toast the nuts or seeds in the oven at fan 325°F for 8–10 minutes until fragrant. Crush with the back of a knife and set aside

**2**  Blend the goats' cheese with the yogurt and a splash of Calvados, if using, by hand (or in a blender if the cheese is quite thick) until smooth.

**3**  How you build this dessert is up to you. You can slice, chop, half, or quarter the figs. We like to arrange 2 halved figs in the bottom of each dessert or cocktail glass then spoon over 2 heaped teaspoons of the goats' cheese/yogurt mixture followed by a tiny drizzle of pomegranate molasses. Repeat, building up the layers.

**4**  Sprinkle the crushed toasted nuts over the top of the trifle and finish with a drizzle of honey or date syrup.

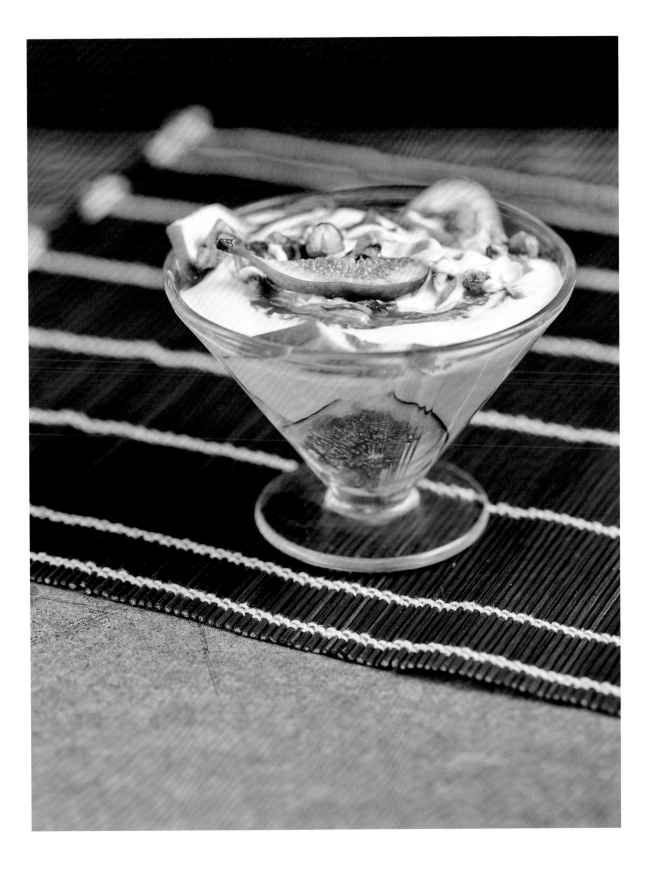

# PINEAPPLE CARPACCIO WITH CHILI, MINT, AND LIME

Fruit makes a delicious and refreshing dessert but not one that digests easily straight after a meal. However we find that pineapple seems to sit well even after a feast – thanks to its enzyme bromelain it can aid digestion rather than delay it and, partnered with mint, it makes a wonderful palate cleanser. This light and refreshing no-cook dish is perfect for making in advance as the pineapple happily marinates in the chili, mint, and lime. Slice it up, throw on the other ingredients, cover, and leave somewhere cool until needed.

SERVES 4-6

1 large ripe pineapple

2 tbsp grated zest and juice of 1 unwaxed lime (avoid the bitter white pith)

6 fresh mint leaves, finely sliced into ribbons

1 tsp finely chopped red chili

1 tbsp raw runny honey, for drizzling

✚ **TO CHECK IF YOUR PINEAPPLE IS RIPE**, give it a good sniff – it should smell sweet. Pull at one of the center leaves in its crown and, if it comes away easily, it's ready to be eaten.

**1** Slice the top and bottom off the pineapple, sit it upright on a board and slice away the skin and all the little brown "eyes." Using an apple corer, remove the core or cut the pineapple in half lengthways and remove the core using a serrated knife.

**2** Slice the pineapple crosswise using a sharp knife to make the slices as thin as possible.

**3** Arrange the pineapple slices on a serving plate, starting on the outer circle and layering inwards.

**4** Squeeze over the lime juice, scatter over the mint ribbons, lime zest, and red chili and finish with a drizzle of honey.

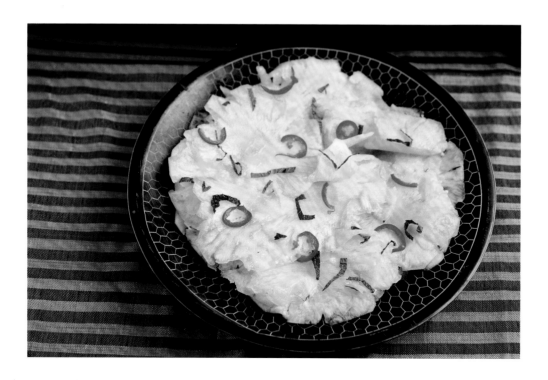

# LEMON POPPY SEED MUFFINS

What's the difference between a muffin and a cupcake? We like to think of a muffin as a less sweet cake but the best description we found was that a cupcake thrown against a wall goes "poof" and a muffin goes "thud."

Nutrient-dense foods tend to go "thud," but don't despair, by making these small we've kept them moist and fluffy like cupcakes. Be sure to follow the instructions carefully as coconut flour has its own set of rules. Keep in the fridge for a week or freeze and heat through in the oven to serve.

MAKES 5 MUFFINS OR
10 MINI MUFFINS

2 ¼ oz butter

1 tbsp unwaxed grated lemon zest (from about 5 small lemons, avoid the bitter white pith) or 1½ tsp lemon extract

3 eggs

4 tbsp maple syrup

1 tbsp poppy seeds or black chia seeds, plus extra to sprinkle

¼ tsp baking soda

2 pinches of ground turmeric

1 ½ oz coconut flour

a tiny pinch of sea salt

**1**  Preheat the oven to fan 325°F. Line a 6-hole cupcake tin with 5 cupcake cases or 12-hole mini muffin tin with 10 mini-muffin cases.

**2**  Gently melt the butter with the lemon zest in a saucepan to release the oils.

**3**  Whisk the eggs together with the cooled melted butter, then the rest of the ingredients. Taste the batter and add more zest or extract, if needed. Leave to cool.

**4**  Divide the mixture among the muffin cases (roughly 3 tablespoons for the larger ones or 1 tablespoon for the mini ones).

**5**  Bake the muffins for 15–20 minutes, depending on their size. They are ready when they're still a little wet inside as they continue to cook as they cool. Remove from the tray immediately and cool on a wire rack.

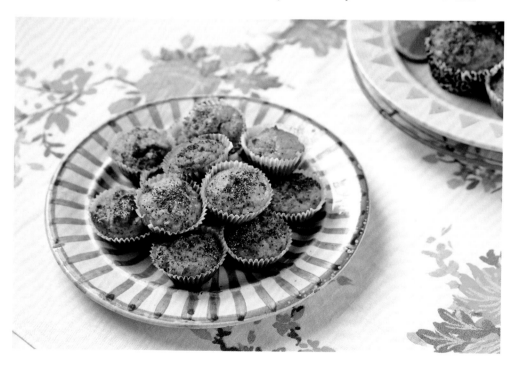

# SALTED APRICOT CARAMELS

Our version of a chocolate salted caramel, utilising both the chewy texture of dried apricots as well as their natural sugars to create the wonderful soft centers. Since organic apricots are not dried with sulphur, they not only have a deep sweet flavor, but a rich dark color that looks like caramel. Be sure to use these dried apricots and not the light orange-colored apricots or those that are soft.

We've covered the apricots in a thick dark chocolate shell for a crisp crunch and to balance the sweetness. Serve them straight from the fridge for the best fudgy texture.

MAKES ABOUT 50
CARAMELS

## FOR THE SALTED APRICOT CARAMELS

9 oz organic unsulphured dried apricots (not orange or soft), chopped

1¼ tsp sea salt

2 ¾ oz butter or coconut oil

2 tbsp hot water

1 tsp vanilla bean paste or vanilla extract

4-7 oz (85 % cocoa solids) dark chocolate (or use our homemade chocolate)

## FOR THE HOMEMADE CHOCOLATE

(makes 7 oz)

7 oz cocoa butter

¾ cup cacao powder

3 tbsp maple syrup

2 tsp vanilla extract

**1** Add the chopped apricots, salt, butter or coconut oil, hot water, and vanilla to a food processor, pulse a few times, then blend until completely smooth.

**2** Use a teaspoon to scoop out enough apricot mixture to make ⅔ in diameter balls. Roll the mixture between the palms of your hands and place each caramel onto a baking tray lined with baking parchment (if you are struggling, pop the mixture in the freezer for 10 minutes or longer then try again).

**3** Freeze the balls for 20 minutes or until needed.

**4** If you're making Homemade Chocolate, melt the cocoa butter very slowly in a glass or metal bowl over a pan of warm water, leaving out a couple of small pieces – make sure the water doesn't touch the bottom of the bowl and don't let the water boil. When the cocoa butter is almost completely melted, take it off the heat and stir in the remaining small pieces of cocoa butter. Once all the cocoa butter is completely melted, stir in the rest of the ingredients, then leave to cool and thicken.

**5** If you're using ready-made chocolate, melt the dark chocolate the same way as above, then allow to cool and thicken.

**6** Take a frozen caramel (they tend to stick to the paper) and give it a quick roll between the palms of your hands to smooth. Use 2 teaspoons to dip the caramels, one at a time, into the chocolate. Lift them out and let any excess run off, then place them back onto the same tray, leaving plenty of room for the other balls. They will set quickly on the cold tray. Re-dip in chocolate for a thicker coating/shell.

**7** Keep the caramels in an airtight container in the fridge until needed.

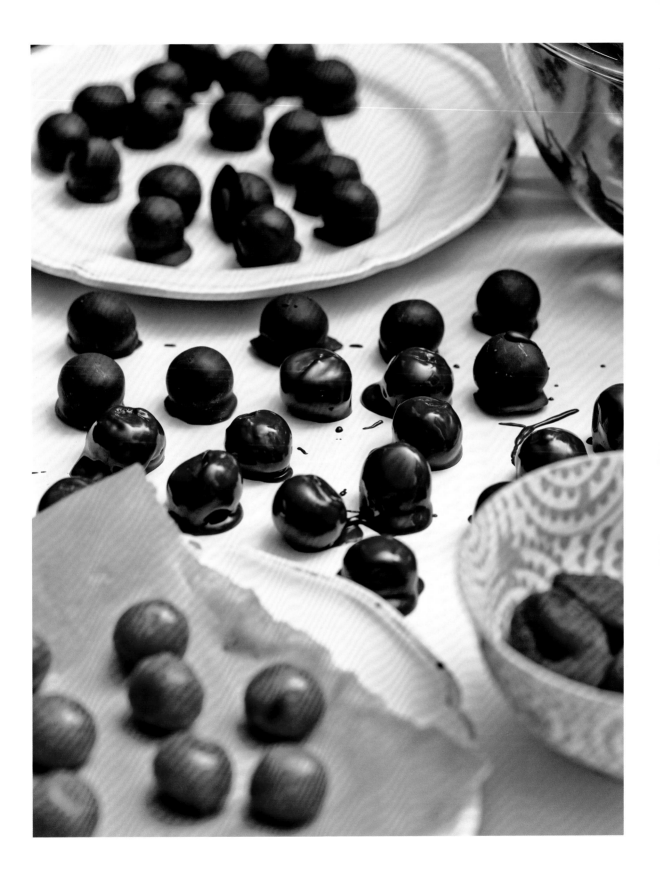

# GINGERNUTS AND CINNAMON AND RAISIN COOKIES

We make a lot of cookies in many flavor variations, but this time we came up with two combinations that made us especially happy. Our gingernuts are really simple and a great way to enjoy ginger, a lovely warming spice. Cook these cookies for a little less time than stated, or make them larger, to get a chewier texture. Our cinnamon and raisin cookies are reminiscent of oaty flapjacks. They're perfect for children and go down very easily with a cup of tea at breakfast. Cinnamon is a hard-working spice that not only enhances the existing sweetness of foods but also regulates your blood sugar levels.

Just a little maple or date syrup is needed to make these (date syrup gives a rich, malty flavor). The high levels of protein and good fat in ground almonds helps to balance the natural sugars and will leave you feeling satisfied. We also use homemade Sun Flour to make cookies (pages 302–303). It works particularly well in the Cinnamon and Raisin Cookies, enhancing their oaty flavor, but it can tinge the cookies green – don't be put off, it's just the Sun Flour reacting with the baking soda.

MAKES 10 COOKIES

**FOR GINGERNUTS**

9 oz ground almonds or Sun Flour (pages 302)

1 tsp baking soda

3 tbsp ground ginger (or less if you don't like the burn!)

grated zest of 1 unwaxed lemon (avoid the bitter white pith)

4 tbsp date syrup or a little less of maple syrup

a small pinch of sea salt

**FOR CINNAMON AND RAISIN COOKIES**

9 oz ground almonds or Sun Flour (pages 302)

1 tsp baking soda

2 tsp ground cinnamon

4½ tbsp butter or coconut oil at room temperature

2 tsp vanilla extract

2 tbsp maple or date syrup for a darker cookie

1 ¾ oz raisins

a small pinch of sea salt

**1**  Preheat the oven to fan 350°F.

**2**  In a bowl or food processor, combine the ground almonds or Sun Flour with the baking soda before adding the rest of the ingredients for either the Gingernuts or Cinnamon and Raisin Cookies. Stir in the raisins using a spoon after all the other ingredients are well mixed.

**3**  Roll 2 tablespoons of the mixture into balls, press slightly to flatten and place on a baking tray lined with baking parchment, leaving plenty of space between each cookie.

**4**  Use your hand to flatten each biscuit further, so that they are all about ¼ in thick – if you want a chewier cookie, make them a little thicker.

**5**  Bake for 10–12 minutes until browned on the edges, then leave to cool on the tray. They will still be soft in the middle, but as they cool they will crisp up. We make a big batch so we can freeze some cookies and store the rest in an airtight container in the fridge.

✚ **IF YOU'RE MAKING CINNAMON AND RAISIN COOKIES WITH COCONUT OIL**, reduce the oven temperature to fan 300°F. They may need less baking time too, so keep an eye on them.

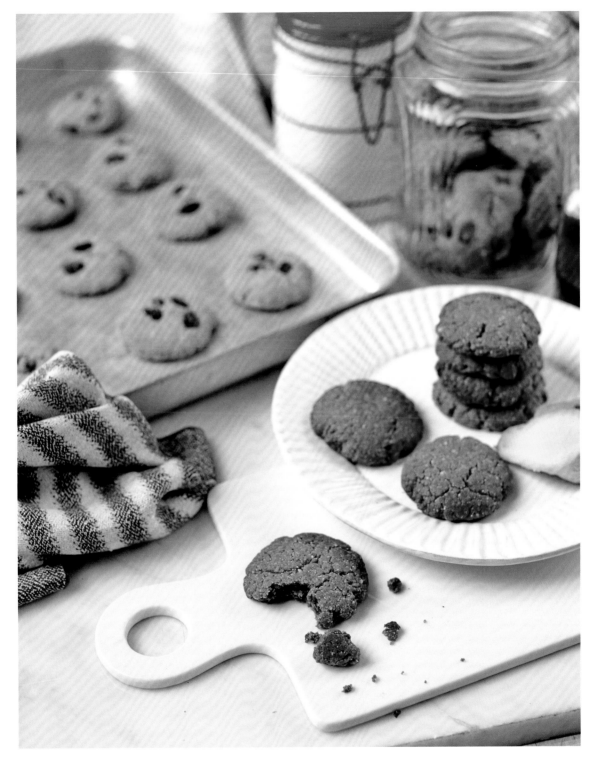

**LEFT TO RIGHT**

Cinnamon and Raisin Cookies
(opposite), Gingernuts (opposite).

## PEA AND MINT ICE CREAM OR LOLLIES WITH CHOCOLATE

A refreshing treat for the summer that's very easy to make. Instead of sugar and pasteurized milk, this ice cream uses coconut milk, probiotic yogurt, and plenty of sweet little peas.

The frozen peas blend with the rest of the ingredients to make a smooth ice cream base in minutes. If you have a high-powered blender, then you can throw some fresh mint in there too – although you'll always need to add a dash of mint extract as well, to get that super refreshing taste.

We pour the mix into our ice cream maker and, an hour later, the ice cream is ready to go. For those without an ice cream maker, try our trick using an ice cube mold or half the recipe to make these cute lollies.

MAKES ABOUT 1 QUART ICE CREAM

**FOR THE PEA AND MINT ICE CREAM BASE**

12 oz frozen petits pois

1 tin of full-fat coconut milk

5 oz full-fat probiotic natural yogurt

4 tbsp raw runny honey

1 tsp peppermint extract or 1 ¾ oz fresh mint leaves and a little peppermint extract too

a pinch of sea salt

a handful of cacao nibs, optional

**FOR THE CHOCOLATE SAUCE**

1 ¾ oz cacao powder

2 ¾ oz raw runny honey

1 tbsp coconut oil

**1** To make the pea and mint ice cream base, blend all the ingredients except for the cacao nibs together until very smooth.

**2** To make the chocolate sauce, measure out all the ingredients into a jug or small bowl and stir together, along with ⅔ cup hot water.

**3 To make ice cream**, place the pea and mint base into an ice cream maker and, following the manufacturer's instructions, churn until you have ice cream. When it is ready, scoop the ice cream into bowls and sprinkle with cacao nibs and drizzle with chocolate sauce to serve.

If you don't have an ice cream maker, pour the pea and mint mixture into ice cube molds and freeze. Pulse the frozen cubes in a food processor for a soft serve ice cream.

**4 To make 6 lollies**, make up half the quantity of pea and mint base and add about 4 teaspoons into the bottom of tall shot glasses or lolly molds and pop into the freezer. After 20 minutes or more, insert a lolly stick into the pea mixture and pour some of the chocolate sauce around it. Repeat with the pea and mint base and finish with the chocolate sauce, freezing for 10 minutes between layers. Freeze the finished lollies for a further 2 hours, then enjoy.

**5** Alternatively, mix the half-quantity of pea and mint base for the lollies with the chocolate sauce and pour into shot glasses. Insert the lolly sticks and freeze for at least 2 hours before serving.

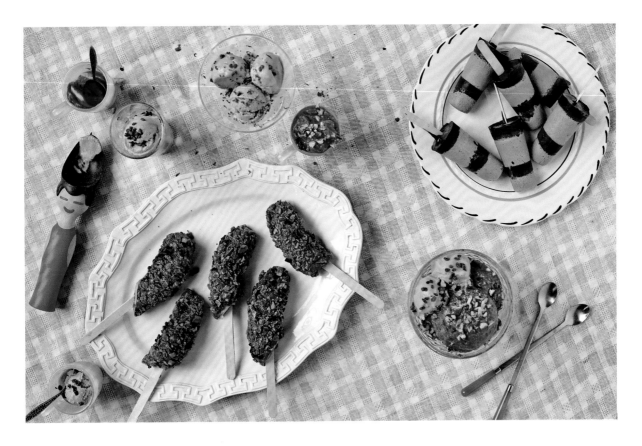

LEFT TO RIGHT: Banutty Choc Ices (page 265),
Pea and Mint Ice Cream (opposite),
Instant Berry and Coconut Ice Cream (page 264),
Pea and Mint Lollies with Chocolate (opposite).

# INSTANT BERRY AND COCONUT ICE CREAM

Perfect for a heatwave, this instant soft scoop ice cream with its chewy dates and chunks of berry is a summer dream. With 2 tins of full-fat coconut milk and a bag of frozen berries, you can have a bowl of ice cream ready in minutes.

Usually, there is a very high sugar content in ice cream, which is fantastic for helping the ice cream freeze to a fine texture, but not so good for our bodies. We add natural sweetness with just a few dates and some tart berries, instead. You could always drizzle over a little raw honey or date syrup to serve, if you want a bit more sweetness.

Work quickly as you don't want the chilled coconut milk and frozen berries to lose their cool – essential for an instant ice cream! Use a food processor rather than a powerful blender or it will heat up too quickly and don't overblend, or you'll end up with a smoothie. If you have an ice cream maker, then you can throw these ingredients in and churn.

**SERVES 3-4**

6 pitted dates, finely chopped, to garnish

1 tbsp of your favorite chopped nuts, such as pecans, hazelnuts, or walnuts (preferably activated page 300)

the solid top part of cream from 2 chilled tins of full-fat coconut milk (save the rest for a smoothie)

1 tsp vanilla extract

7 ¾ oz frozen mixed berries

**OPTIONAL**

a drizzle of raw runny honey or date syrup, to serve

**1** Before removing the berries from the freezer or the coconut milk from the fridge, chop the dates and prepare the chopped nuts.

**2** Working quickly, carefully scoop out the coconut cream from the chilled cans and measure out 7 oz. Place the coconut cream, vanilla extract, and berries in a food processor and blend for a few seconds. Scrape down the sides with a spatula and blend again for a few seconds. Repeat until the berries and the coconut cream start to form a stiff ball, adding a spoonful of coconut water if you feel it needs some to get moving.

**3** When the berries and coconut cream are almost incorporated (chunks of berries are fine), throw in the chopped dates and pulse once to mix.

**4** Serve immediately in chilled glasses or bowls or leave in the freezer for up to an hour. Top with the chopped nuts and a drizzle of honey or date syrup. Any leftover ice cream can be drunk as a smoothie.

➕ **IF YOU OVERBLEND AND GET A SMOOTHIE,** you can pop it back into the freezer for 60–90 minutes, taking it out every 30 minutes to stir vigorously and break up the icy sections that build up round the edges.

# BANUTTY CHOC ICES

Salty peanuts, dark chocolate, and frozen, creamy sweet banana. This is a super easy crowd-pleaser for children and adults alike. We like to add cacao nibs in and amongst our crushed peanuts for extra crunch and a sprinkling of flaky sea salt brings out the flavors. Since bananas are naturally sweet, we don't use any additional sweetness, even in the chocolate sauce. Remember to savor each mouthful, allowing it to warm in your mouth for maximum flavor.

**MAKES 8 CHOC ICES**

4 bananas

5 oz peanuts (preferably "crispy" activated, pages 300)

a handful of cacao nibs (optional)

sea salt, for sprinkling (optional)

**FOR THE SAUCE**

2 tbsp smooth peanut butter (chunky also works)

1 tbsp cacao powder

1 tsp vanilla extract

a pinch of chili

1 tsp ground cinnamon

a small pinch of sea salt

1 tbsp raw honey (optional)

**1** Preheat the oven to fan 350°F.

**2** Peel the bananas and slice each in half widthways. Insert a wooden lolly stick into each of the banana halves then freeze on a baking tray lined with parchment paper.

**3** Spread the peanuts out in a single layer on a baking tray. Roast for 10 minutes until lightly toasted, stirring halfway through cooking. Remove from the oven and leave to cool slightly before rubbing the peanuts together to remove the skins. Roughly chop the nuts and mix with cacao nibs, if using, then set aside.

**4** Combine all the sauce ingredients, except for the honey, with ¾ cup water in a saucepan, whisking until smooth. Remove from the heat and add the honey, if using.

**5** Take a frozen banana half and carefully coat in the sauce, then gently roll the dipped banana in the crushed peanuts. Lay the banana back on the lined baking tray and repeat with each banana half. Finish with a sprinkling of sea salt – the flakier the better!

**6** Freeze the bananas for a further 30 minutes or up to an hour, depending on how hard you want the choc ices to be (we like to eat these lollies half frozen because it gives them a creamy texture). These are also good chilled but not frozen (freeze for at least 2 hours if transporting to a picnic).

# CHOCOLATE AVOCADO MOUSSE

This chocolate concoction has a delicious dinner party feel. We take antioxidant-rich cacao (one of our favorite superfoods) and blend it with the very Brazilian combination of avocado and banana for a smooth, velvety finish – ideal for anyone avoiding dairy. Make sure your avocados and bananas are ripe for maximum flavor and texture and remember, most unripe fruit is not kind to the stomach. Since this is not heated, it's a perfect way to enjoy the powerful antibacterial and antifungal properties of raw honey.

To make this dessert extra special, we add a good splash of amaretto as well as vanilla extract to spice it up. Rum works here too and for those who avoid alcohol, you can use almond extract, which also happens to turn it into a delicious breakfast option (add some malty maca for an extra superfood start to the day). For those who are sensitive to caffeine, you can substitute half or all of the cacao with carob powder (page 21).

If you are using a hand blender, use unfrozen bananas, blend, then pop each serving into the freezer for 1–2 hours, removing 15–20 minutes before eating. If you have a food processor, keep a stock of sliced bananas in your freezer so you can make this dessert at a moment's notice.

**MAKES 4 ESPRESSO CUP/ SHOT GLASS SERVINGS**

1 frozen ripe banana, peeled

3 tbsp cacao powder

1 chilled avocado

2 tbsp raw honey

1 tsp lemon juice

1 tsp vanilla extract

2 tbsp chilled water

a tiny pinch of sea salt

**OPTIONAL**

1–2 tsp amaretto or a few drops of stevia, to sweeten

a sprinkle of cacao powder or cacao nibs, to decorate

**1**   Blend all the mousse ingredients together in your food processor until smooth. (Add the cacao powder first and, as you blend, have all the ingredients on hand in order to adjust the ratios slightly as the size of avocados and bananas varies so much. The perfect ratio in order to avoid the dish tasting too much of either is to use almost equal amounts of both.)

**2**   Taste and add a few drops of stevia if you feel you need more sweetness.

**3**   Fill little cups or shot glasses with the mousse, sprinkle with the cacao powder or nibs and serve.

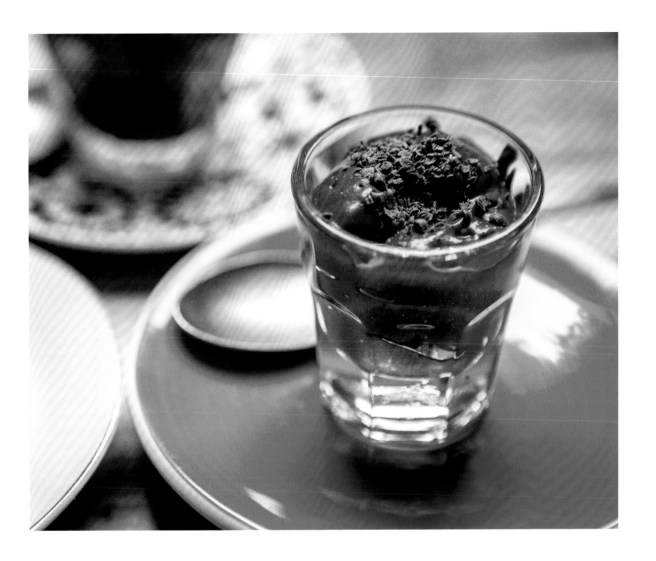

# PARADISE BARS

This is a client favorite so, after much arm twisting, we're finally revealing the special recipe. If we find ourselves stuck somewhere and hungry, these bars do the job without sending our blood sugar levels flying sky high. We prefer them without the additional water, but every now and then we find someone who likes them a little softer in the middle, so add water to the mix if that's you.

To make your own chocolate see page 270 or if you use ready-made chocolate bars, just treat the chocolate gently when melting.

**MAKES 24 BARS**

7 oz bar of creamed coconut

6 tbsp coconut oil

3 tbsp raw honey

1½ tsp vanilla extract

a pinch of sea salt

5 oz shredded coconut

7 oz (85% cocoa solids) dark chocolate (or make up our Homemade Chocolate page 270)

**1** Line a 8 in square tin with baking parchment. In cold weather, place the unopened packet of creamed coconut in a bowl of warm water to melt it through (you can massage the packet to help it along). In warm weather, the creamed coconut will already be fluid enough.

**2** When it's soft all the way through, pour into a bowl and mix in the coconut oil (it will melt if it's hard), raw honey, vanilla, salt, and 2–4 tablespoons water if you like a softer center.

**3** Stir in the shredded coconut evenly to create a doughy consistency.

**4** Pour the dough into the prepared tin. Press the mixture down with the back of a spoon to make it level and set in the fridge for 15 minutes until hard.

**5** Turn the tin of coconut mixture out onto a chopping board and slice into 6 horizontal slices by 4 vertical. Place them onto a baking tray lined with baking parchment and keep in the freezer while you prep the chocolate.

**6** Melt the chocolate in a glass or metal bowl over a pan of warm water – make sure the water does not touch the bottom of the bowl and do not allow the water to boil or simmer – you may have to keep removing from the heat. This should take about 30 minutes.

**7** When the chocolate has almost melted, take the bowl off the heat and place on a tea towel to avoid slipping. Leave it to cool as much as possible without it hardening to give a thicker coating to the paradise bars – stir occasionally.

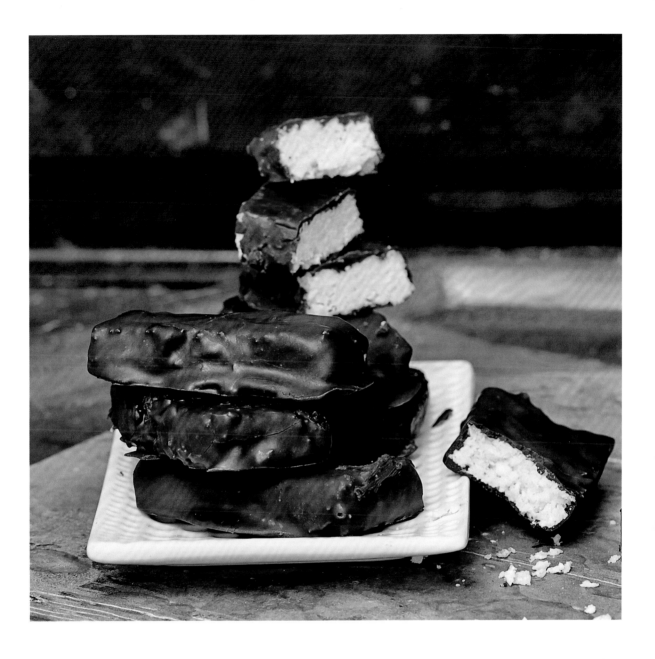

**8** Dip the frozen coconut bars into the chocolate using two forks, letting the excess drop off, and carefully place back onto the cold baking tray, leaving space between each bar. If the chocolate mixture becomes too cold, you may need to put it back over the simmering water again.

**9** When you've finished dipping all the bars, place the tray back in the fridge until set. Once set, seal in a glass or ceramic container in the fridge or freezer until required. If they are kept sealed in the fridge, they will keep for a month – or longer in the freezer.

# DARK CHOCOLATE THINS AND CHOCOLATE WHEELS

We love our chocolate really dark, eaten super slowly – wafer-thin pieces of cold dark chocolate or slices cut from thicker chocolate wheels make a delicious end to a meal.

We avoided making real chocolate for years since it all seemed so technical. Chocolate with a high cocoa butter content needs tempering to give a shiny, smooth chocolate with a pleasing snap. If you heat this type of chocolate too quickly or overheat, then you can end up with a waxy product, a grainy texture and a white bloom. It's not "off," but it's not nice! You can use a thermometer, but we have found the easiest way is to go slowly when melting the chocolate and use the teaspoon technique to test (see below).

MAKES 3 1/2 OZ
CHOCOLATE

**FOR THE HOMEMADE CHOCOLATE**

3 ½ oz cocoa butter

6 tbsp cacao powder

1½ tbsp maple syrup

1 tsp vanilla extract

Choose your favorite flavors from the options opposite.

**1**  Line a baking tray with baking parchment, making sure to fold it into the corners and up the sides for a neat edge.

**2**  Melt the cocoa butter in a glass or metal bowl over a pan of warm water, leaving out a couple of smaller pieces. Make sure the water does not touch the bottom of the bowl and do not allow the water to boil or simmer – you may have to keep removing from the heat. This should take about 30 minutes.

**3**  When the cocoa butter has almost melted, take the bowl off the heat and place on a tea towel to avoid slipping. Stir in the rest of the cocoa butter.

**4**  Once the cocoa butter is fully melted, stir in the rest of the ingredients and any additional flavors (see opposite) and warm again in the glass or metal bowl over the pan of warm water for about 10 minutes. If you have a thermometer on hand, you want to warm to a temperature of 90°F. If you don't, not to worry, just coat the back of a teaspoon with the chocolate and put in the fridge for a couple of minutes to test. It is ready if it sets with a glossy, smooth surface.

**5**  Pour the chocolate into the lined tray and put in the fridge to set (or freezer if you are in a rush). It will take up to an hour in the fridge.

**6**  When completely hardened, snap your chocolate thins into big shards and store in a glass container in the fridge or somewhere cool.

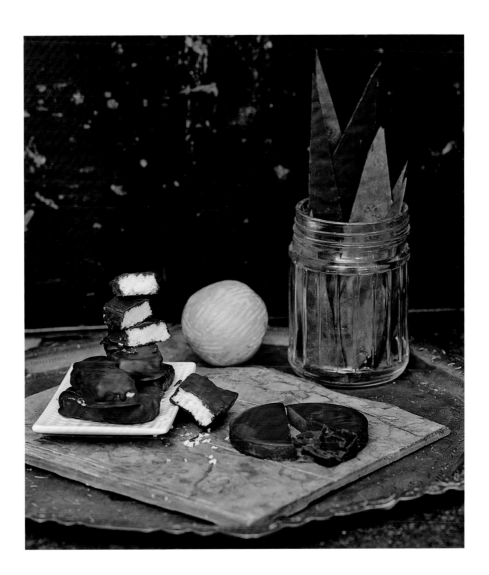

**LEFT TO RIGHT**

Paradise Bars (page 268),
Chocolate Wheels, and
Chocolate Thins (opposite).

### SALTED DARK CHOCOLATE

Add ¼ tsp sea salt flakes or more to the chocolate.

### ROSE AND LUCUMA

More subtle than Turkish delight, but with enough floral fragrance to turn a very dark chocolate into a light summer's day. Lucuma adds a sweet and complex taste taking it closer to a milk chocolate, but don't add too much or it will ruin the texture.

Add just under ½ tsp rose extract and 2½ tbsp lucuma.

### CAYENNE AND ORANGE

The superfood cayenne is delicious with a little orange extract – you get the sweet chocolate orange and a little burn at the end.

Add 1 tsp orange extract then stir in a tiny pinch of cayenne pepper.

### OTHER ADDED EXTRAS TO TRY

We love a few drops of peppermint extract, ground ginger, lemon extract and crushed rosemary leaves, or shredded coconut and lime zest.

# FLAX SANDWICH BREAD

Bread, bread substitutes, and baked goods can all too easily form the basis of what people eat, so we always highlight the importance of meat and vegetables, nature's most unprocessed foods, taking center stage. But bread is a convenient food – sandwiches are an easy food on the go and one of the most popular packed lunches – so with this in mind we've perfected our own bread recipe.

Instead of imitating fluffy white breads that contain gums and refined flours, we're about whole foods, free from grains, so this gluten- and grain-free bread is just made of the good stuff: butter, flax, almonds, and eggs.

We bake this bread focaccia style to get the perfect texture throughout. Split it lengthways and it makes a delicious vehicle for all your favorite toppings. We love it with butter and cheese or topped with Mung Bean Hummus (page 232) or Lemon Parsley Cashew Dip (page 233) and some arugula or try it with our Sardine Butter (page 142), Baked Chicken Liver Mousse (page 168), or our most popular client request, beef and horseradish.

If you fancy a more rustic-style bread then this can also be made with whole flaxseed (as we discovered by happy accident!). Just leave the batter to stand for 15 minutes before baking and remember to chew each and every seed to get the best out of this nutritious food.

**MAKES ENOUGH FOR 4 SANDWICHES**

This makes enough for 4 sandwiches so freeze portions and warm them in the oven whenever you need a sandwich fix.

2 ¾ oz ground almonds

9 oz ground or whole flaxseeds

4 eggs

1 ¾ oz butter at room temperature

1½ tsp baking soda

2 tbsp lemon juice

1 tsp sea salt

**OPTIONAL**

1 tsp oregano, caraway, or fennel seeds

black pepper, to taste

**1**  Preheat the oven to fan 325°F. Line a 9 in square tin with baking parchment.

**2**  Add all the ingredients to a food processor with ½ cup water and blend until smooth.

**3**  Leave to sit for a few minutes to allow the mixture to thicken up, then blend again.

**4**  Put the dough in the prepared tin and smooth the top with the back of a wet spoon or spatula. Bake the bread for 45 minutes until golden brown and springy to touch.

**5**  Leave the bread to cool on a wire rack, then turn it out and slice through lengthways to make a flat sandwich bread.

# MULTISEED LOAF

One of our triumphs. This gluten-free, nutrient-dense bread looks just like a rustic loaf. Packed with a variety of seeds, chewy raisins, and a dough of sweet potatoes or squash and buckwheat (preferably crispy activated), it's a dense, flavorsome bread, which toasts nicely and smells incredible.

The loaf can be portioned up and frozen so that you can grab slices as and when you need them – just toast in the oven, in the broiler, or gently in a toaster for an excellent crunch. It's great for sweet and savory toppings or just plain old salted butter, and small as it is, just two slices will fill you up nicely. It's especially good bruschetta style, topped with Kale Pesto (page 233) or Pea, Mint, and Broccoli Mash (page 115).

**MAKES 1 LOAF
(ABOUT 15 SLICES)**

### FOR THE DOUGH

1 large sweet potato (orange flesh variety works best) or ½ squash

just under 4 oz buckwheat flour

4 tbsp arrowroot (or substitute with buckwheat flour)

¼ tsp baking soda

½ tsp sea salt

1 tbsp ground flaxseed (also known as linseed)

2 tbsp lemon juice

### FOR THE SEED MIX

2 oz pumpkin seeds (preferably "crispy" activated, page 300)

2 oz sunflower seeds (preferably "crispy" activated, page 300)

2 oz sesame seeds (preferably "crispy" activated, page 300)

2 ½ - 3 oz raisins (optional)

**1** Preheat the oven to fan 350°F.

**2** Slice the sweet potato or squash in half and bake for 45–60 minutes until tender. Remove the skin, weigh out 7 oz and blend in a food processor.

**3** Mix in the rest of the dough ingredients until smooth, then knead in the seeds and raisins until completely combined.

**4** Shape into a loaf using lightly floured hands and make shallow slices along the top and bake for 40 minutes until nicely golden. Leave to cool slightly before slicing.

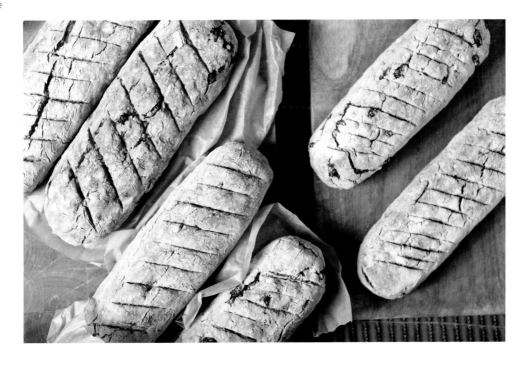

# DRINKS

**W**HAT YOU DRINK IS AS IMPORTANT AS WHAT YOU EAT. Some people aim to eat well, but overlook the importance of hydration. Staying hydrated is absolutely essential for good health; it will boost your energy, keep you alert, and improve your overall body function. Drinking water is one of the best ways to keep hydrated and two to three quarts per day is recommended for adults (depending on body size, climate, and levels of activity). Use citrus fruits, cucumber, ginger, lemongrass, or fresh mint to flavor your water. Make it taste more interesting and you're more likely to drink more without feeling like it's a chore.

Unless you are lucky enough to have access to your own mountain spring, we would recommend getting a good-quality water filter. Your average tap water is safe to drink, but can contain chloride, flouride, traces of heavy metals (like lead and mercury), nitrates, pesticides, and hormones – things we prefer to avoid. A worktop filter jug is a good starting point and, if buying bottled water, we recommend glass over plastic bottles because plastics leach chemicals into the water (and even more so if left in direct sunlight).

It will have been hard not to notice the boom in coconut water in the last few years. We have long been fans and can remember when, if we wanted some, we had to actually order coconuts. Often referred to as the "fluid of life," coconut water contains naturally occurring essential electrolytes in almost the same profile as the human body. We don't drink it as a water substitute because it contains natural sugars but we do use it as an energy boost in place of coffee and it's a favorite pre- or post-workout drink. (It is also pretty helpful if you have a hangover!) Be sure to only drink pure coconut water and not the flavored, sugar-loaded varieties masquerading as health drinks.

Herbal teas, that are naturally caffeine free, come in a great variety of flavors and numerous combinations. You can make your own infusions with fresh herbs and spices: lemongrass and ginger for a boost; cardamom and fennel or peppermint and lemon verbena after a meal; elderflower and rosemary or thyme if you're feeling a bit run down; and chamomile and lavender before bed. Antioxidant-rich green tea is a boost of caffeine if you feel you need it (Matcha green tea is especially good) and makes a refreshing drink, hot or cold, in the morning but is best avoided in the afternoon so as not to affect your sleep.

Juices are a great way to get the goodness of vegetables into fussy eaters while smoothies are a clever way to sneak plenty of raw greens such as spinach and celery into your diet. Always rotate the produce for your smoothies and juices – this keeps them different so you don't get bored and it varies the nutrients. If you're not used to drinking homemade smoothies and juices, start out with a higher ratio of fruit to vegetables and gradually decrease the fruit intake as your taste buds adjust. Remember it's always best to eat ripe fruit and to thoroughly wash and/or peel non-organic produce (for more info on organic see page 12).

Avoid ice cold drinks and drinking too quickly – remember to taste and savor these liquid foods, so as not to shock your system.

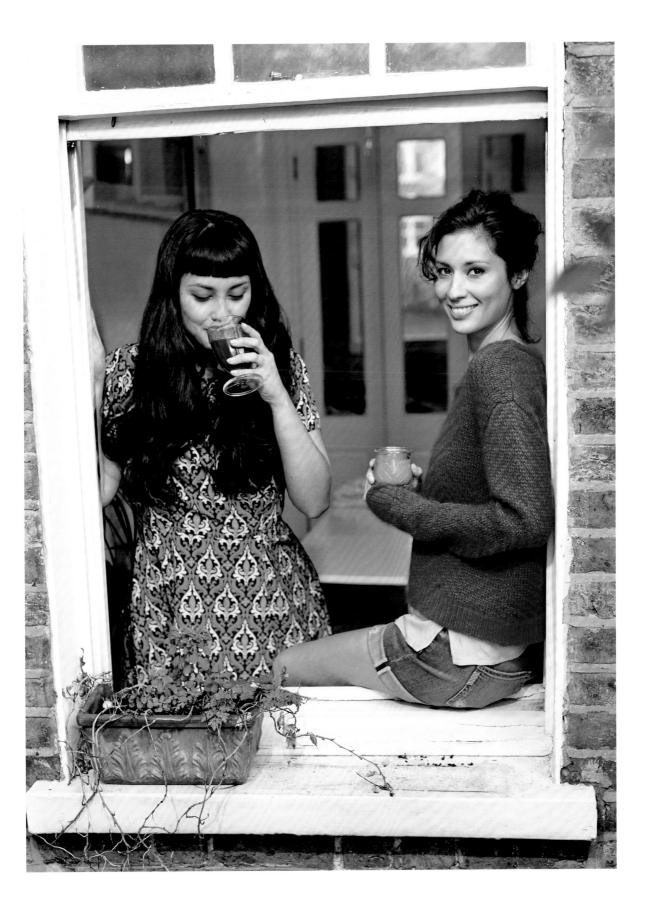

## FENNEL AND MINT JUICE

Fennel has a deliciously mild licorice flavor and is great for cleansing and digestion. It goes perfectly with fresh mint and lime and the ginger gives an extra kick. Super refreshing, this is a great one to enjoy on a hot day with friends. It's also a perfect palate cleanser between meals if you serve in little shot glasses.

SERVES 2 (8 ½ OZ EACH)

2 handfuls of kale (stalks removed) or spinach or dandelion leaves

1 large fennel bulb, about 10 ½ oz

2 small green apples

½ large cucumber, about 7 oz

a thumb-sized piece of fresh root ginger (about 1 ½ oz) – unpeeled if organic

½ large lime or lemon

a handful of fresh mint leaves

**1** Wash the vegetables and fruit well, then chop them to fit your juicer.

**2** Juice all the ingredients and stir well. Drink immediately or pour into a glass jar or stainless steel flask and keep in the fridge for up to 48 hours.

## BROCCOLI AND GINGER JUICE

Broccoli and ginger, one of our favorite soup flavor combinations, is reworked into a green juice. We like juicing most fresh vegetables. People used to be nervous about kale and spinach, but now they're all the rage while broccoli is full of vitamin C and one of the most nutrient-dense foods out there. Give it a try, but unless you have a hardcore palate, remember to pair the vegetables with a little sweetness from apples, pears, or pineapple. We never throw away a broccoli stem as it's where a lot of the nutrients are found. Juicing it is a great way of using it up.

SERVES 2 (8 ½ OZ EACH)

2 handfuls of broccoli, about 9 oz (including stems)

1 large green apple or pear

2 thumb-sized pieces of fresh root ginger (about 2 ¾ oz) – unpeeled if organic

½ large cucumber, about 7 oz

1 small lemon or lime

a handful of fresh mint leaves

**1** Wash the vegetables and fruit well, then chop them to fit your juicer.

**2** Juice all the ingredients and stir well. Drink immediately or pour into a glass jar or stainless steel flask and keep in the fridge for up to 48 hours.

## CLASSIC GREEN CLEANSING JUICE

Cleansing doesn't have to mean embarking on a three-day juice fast. Our bodies naturally cleanse every night if you get a good night's sleep! You can help kick-start your body daily by making a juice full of fresh nourishing ingredients. Celery, fennel, and parsley are known detoxifiers and lemons and limes, although acidic in the mouth, are alkaline-forming in the body and aid digestion

SERVES 2 (8 ½ OZ EACH)

3 celery sticks

1 small fennel bulb, about 3 ½ oz

a handful of kale (stalks removed), spinach, dandelion, or lettuce leaves

2 small green apples

1 small lemon or lime

2 handfuls of fresh parsley leaves and stalks

**1** Wash the vegetables, fruit, and herbs well, then chop them to fit your juicer.

**2** Juice all the ingredients and stir well. Drink immediately or pour into a glass jar or stainless steel flask and keep in the fridge for up to 48 hours.

## CARROT AND CAYENNE BOOST JUICE

How about our Pep-up Turmeric Tea (page 296) in juice form to give you a real lift? This is a boost in a juice, packed full of ginger, turmeric, lemon, and cayenne, plus the goodness of celery and sweet carrots. This plant-based drink will certainly perk you up and refresh, while delivering a touch of heat to warm you and fire up the immune system. Leave out the cayenne for the children and serve in smaller quantities.

SERVES 2 (8 ½ OZ EACH)

a small piece of fresh root ginger (about ⅓ oz) – unpeeled if organic

3 large carrots

1 small lemon or lime

2 celery sticks

½ tsp ground turmeric

a pinch of cayenne pepper

**1** Wash the vegetables and fruit well, then chop them to fit your juicer.

**2** Juice, then stir through the ground turmeric and cayenne.

**3** Drink immediately or pour into a glass jar or stainless steel flask and keep in the fridge for up to 48 hours.

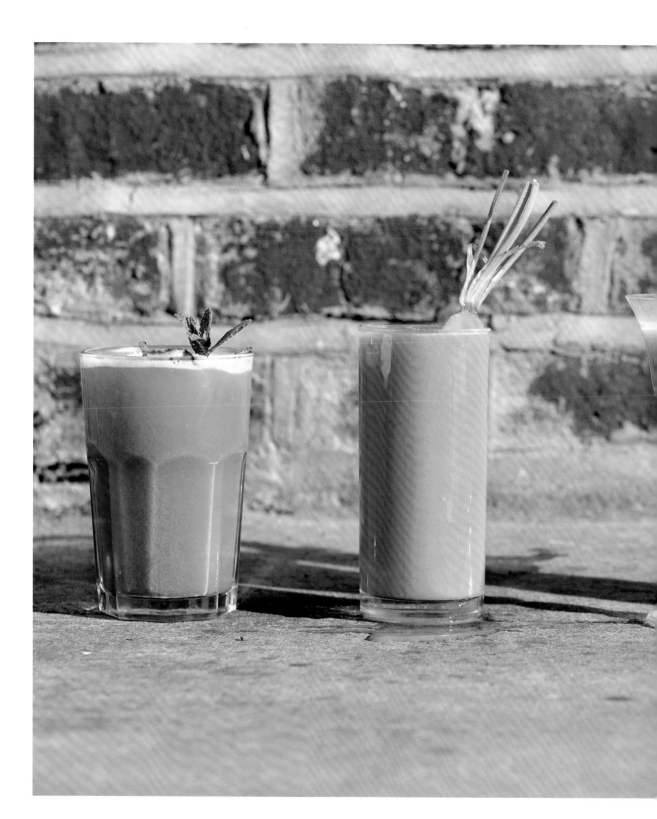

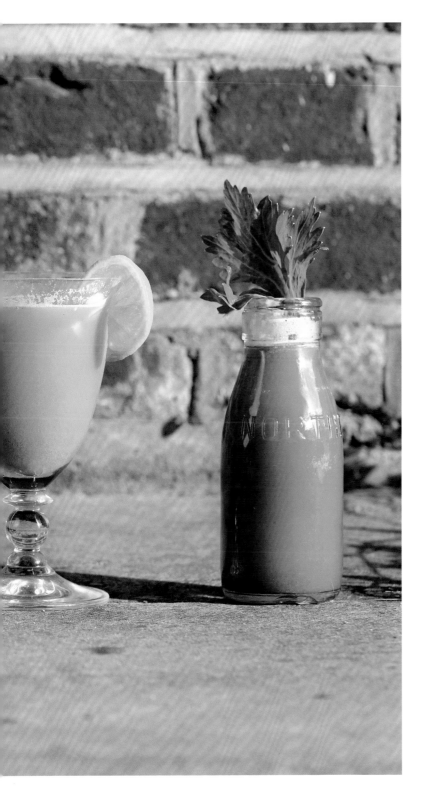

# STRAWBERRY, MINT, AND CUCUMBER SMOOTHIE

Bright summer mornings call for a sweet, creamy glass of something delicious and we've got just the thing. Cucumber and mint make this smoothie light and refreshing – the cucumber provides a cleansing, alkalizing, and hydrating base, packed with antioxidants, while the mint is calming on the stomach. The creamy texture comes from the avocado, almonds, and coconut, whose wonderful fats will help to keep you feeling full – and they're good for you and your brain!

If you like to snack on almonds or spread almond butter on Apple Rings (page 128), leave them out as you don't want too much of a good thing.

SERVES 3 (10 OZ EACH)

a container of ripe strawberries, about 14 oz

½ large avocado, peeled, about 3 ½ oz

½ small cucumber, about 3 ½ oz

½ tin of full-fat coconut milk, about ¾ cup, or 1 tablespoon coconut oil and ¾ cup water

12 almonds (preferably activated, page 300) or 1½ tbsp almond butter

1 tbsp fresh mint leaves

**OPTIONAL**

2 pitted dates or a dash of raw honey, to sweeten

**1**  Wash the vegetables and fruit well, then chop them to fit your blender.

**2**  Blend everything together until smooth, adding water, if needed, to create your desired consistency.

**3**  Drink immediately or pour into a glass jar or stainless steel flask and keep in the fridge for up to 48 hours.

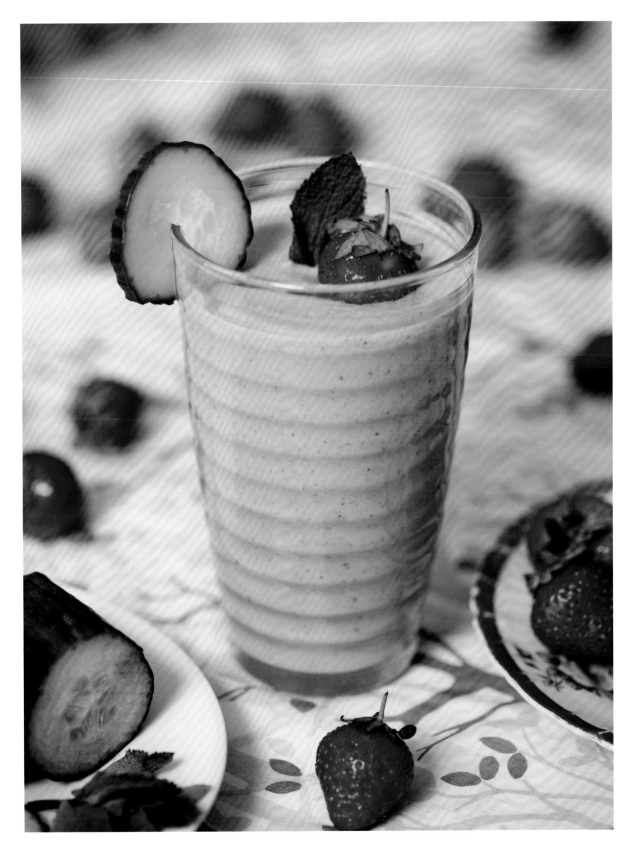

# GO-TO GREEN SMOOTHIE AND GO-TO GREEN RAW SOUP

This is our go-to smoothie for those times when we've been deprived of raw green food or when we need to balance the effects of a rich meal. This drink is alkalizing, hydrating, cleansing, antioxidant-rich, and easy to digest – not to mention it has minimal prep time. Plus, with a few simple tweaks, it can be transformed from a green smoothie to a raw green soup.

Dulse is a sweet, tasty seaweed (sea vegetable) that is packed with nutrients so it's really worth seeking out (see page 23 for more on the benefits of seaweeds).

If you're just transitioning over to the idea of drinking vegetables, or if you have a sweet tooth, then you might want to use two apples, especially if you're using kale as it's a little more bitter than young spinach leaves.

**SERVES 3 (10 OZ EACH)**

### FOR THE SMOOTHIE

a few pieces of dried dulse, about ⅙ oz

½ large cucumber, about 7 oz

1–2 green apples, cored

2 celery sticks

2 ½ oz spinach or kale, stalks removed

½ large avocado, peeled, about 3 ½ oz

a large handful of watercress

a small piece of fresh root ginger (about ¾ oz) – unpeeled if organic

a small handful of fresh parsley

3 tbsp lemon juice

1 tsp powdered chlorella or spirulina (page 24)

### FOR THE RAW SOUP

2 scallions, roughly chopped

1 medium-large garlic clove

a tiny pinch of cayenne pepper

a pinch of sea salt

diced cucumber or chopped parsley and a drizzle of olive oil and some black pepper, to garnish (optional)

**1** Place the dried dulse in a blender with 1 ⅓ cup water to soak while you prepare the other ingredients.

**2** Thoroughly wash the fruit, vegetables and herbs, then chop them to fit your blender.

**3** Add the rest of the ingredients for the smoothie, pulse a few times, then blend until smooth. Add more water, if needed, to achieve the desired consistency.

**4** To make the raw soup, include the soup ingredients when you blend in the previous step and serve at room temperature.

**5** Drink or eat immediately or pour into a glass jar or stainless steel flask and keep in the fridge for up to 48 hours.

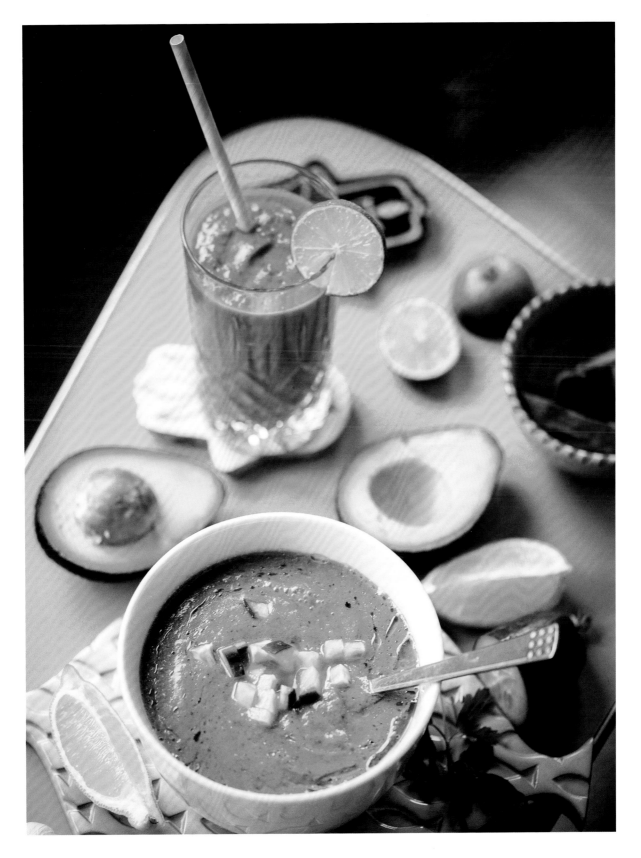

## PAPAYA SMOOTHIE

A breakfast remedy for any overindulgences from the night before or post stomach upsets. If you're feeling sluggish, bloated, or just low on energy, it's time to blend up this smoothie.

The enzymes in papaya are anti-inflammatory and promote healthy digestion, as does ginger. Adding some papaya seeds will help support your body against parasites, but you'll probably need to increase the quantity of seeds slowly as you get used to their peppery taste.

SERVES 2 (12 OZ)

½ large, ripe papaya, peeled and seeds removed, flesh scooped out, about 13 ¼ oz

½ large ripe banana, peeled, about 3 ½ oz

a small piece of fresh root ginger (about ⅓ oz) – unpeeled if organic

juice of 1 lime

1½ tbsp coconut oil

OPTIONAL

1 tsp raw honey if the papaya is not very sweet

1 tsp of saved papaya seeds

1  Wash the fruit well, then chop them to fit your blender.

2  Blend all the ingredients together with about 7 ½ oz water, adding more water if necessary to get the desired consistency.

3  Drink immediately or pour into a glass jar or stainless steel flask and keep in the fridge for up to 48 hours.


## CHOCOLATE, PEANUT BUTTER, AND MACA SMOOTHIE

This is Nick's workout recovery smoothie that hits the sweet spot too. The addition of superfood kale adds valuable nutrition in the form of calcium, iron, and vitamins A, C, and K. Flaxseeds provide essential fatty acids and further antioxidants to help the body repair, whilst you get a good protein hit from the nuts. Using coconut water will help replace electrolytes to speed up rehydration.

Make your own adjustments to the smoothie, perhaps by blending in a raw egg yolk or some hemp seeds for additional protein. If you've been eating the H+H way for a while, try reducing the sweetness, cutting out the honey or dates, and use plenty of cinnamon powder. If you're using spinach, you can get away with packing in much more because it's not as bitter as kale.

SERVES 1 (12 OZ)

1 ripe banana, peeled, about 3 ½ oz

a handful of kale, stalks removed (or use baby spinach as a variation)

2 tbsp cacao powder or cacao nibs

2 tbsp peanut or almond butter

1 tsp ground cinnamon

1–2 tsp maca powder

1 tsp whole flaxseed

OPTIONAL

coconut water, to replace the water if preferred

1 tsp raw honey or 2 pitted dates

1  Wash the kale well, then blend all the ingredients together with about ¾ cup water or coconut water until smooth, adding more liquid if necessary.

2  Drink immediately or pour into a glass jar or stainless steel flask and keep in the fridge for up to 48 hours.

# BLUEBERRY, SPINACH, AND VANILLA SMOOTHIE

SERVES 1 (12 OZ)

A fresh-tasting, antioxidant-rich smoothie hit. The good fats from the avocado, almonds, and coconut oil ensure you don't get a sugar spike, so this smoothie keeps you feeling fuller for longer. Blueberries are naturally high in pectin, so don't be surprised if you leave your smoothie in the fridge for a little while and come back to find you have a blueberry mousse – equally tasty, just swap the straw for a spoon.

5 oz blueberries

½ medium avocado, peeled, about 2 oz

a handful of baby spinach

10 almonds (preferably activated, see page 300) or 1½ tbsp almond butter

1 tsp vanilla extract

1–2 tsp maca powder

3 pitted dates or 1 tsp raw honey

1 tsp coconut oil

**OPTIONAL**

½ ripe banana for a sweeter, thicker smoothie, peeled

coconut water, to replace the water if preferred

**1** Wash the blueberries well and chop the avocado and banana to fit your blender.

**2** Blend everything together with ¾ cup water or coconut water until smooth.

**3** Drink immediately or pour into a glass jar or stainless steel flask and keep in the fridge for up to 48 hours.

# PIÑA COLADA SMOOTHIE

SERVES 2 (12 OZ EACH)

We love this for breakfast. Sunshine in a glass, this is an enzyme-rich meal thanks to papaya, and it is full of vitamin C. The delicious piña colada flavors of coconut and pineapple envelop the anti-inflammatory turmeric, so you don't have to rely on curries to enjoy this spice.

Add a raw egg yolk if you need more oomph and a little honey if you have a sweet tooth. Full of antioxidants, baobab powder is also a great addition (see page 24), adding a delicate sherbert flavor. Grate a little fresh nutmeg over for a true piña colada taste!

½ large pineapple, peeled and cut into blendable chunks, about 10 ½ oz

¾ cup full-fat coconut milk

½ large avocado, peeled, about 3 ½ oz

1 tsp vanilla extract

½ tsp ground turmeric

**OPTIONAL**

1½ tsp baobab powder

1½ tsp raw honey

1 egg yolk

coconut water, to replace the water if preferred

**1** Blend everything together with ⅔ cup water or coconut water until smooth, adding more liquid if necessary.

**2** Drink immediately or pour into a glass jar or stainless steel flask and keep in the fridge for up to 48 hours.

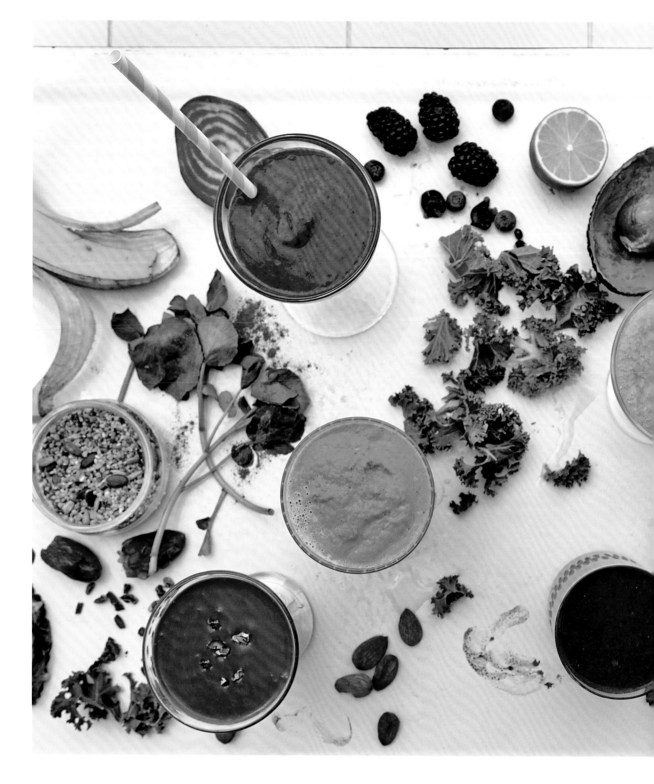

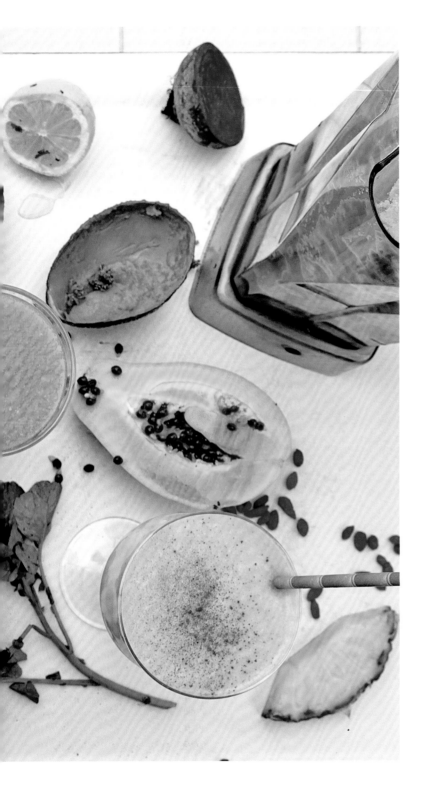

**LEFT TO RIGHT**

Chocolate, Peanut Butter, and Maca
Smoothie (page 286),
Beet Maca Smoothie (page 290),
Go-to-green Smoothie (page 284),
Blueberry, Spinach, and Vanilla Smoothie
(page 287),
Papaya Smoothie (page 286),
Piña Colada Smoothie (page 287).

# BEET MACA SMOOTHIE

Look for beets that come with their leaves intact (this gives you an indication to how fresh your beets are) and don't waste them, they are full of nutrients and great chopped up and added to stews.

Beets are earthy and sweet to taste, so don't pair them with too much fruit otherwise you'll have a sugar overload. This pink smoothie with circulation-boosting ginger, antioxidant-rich acai, goji and blueberries, plus the addition of spinach and maca powder, will give you a powerful jump start in the morning. Great if you have overindulged the night before as beets are also great liver cleansers and blood purifiers.

**SERVES 2**
(8 ½ OZ EACH)

1½ tbsp goji berries

1 tbsp coconut oil

5 oz blueberries

1 raw medium beet, well scrubbed (unpeeled if organic), about 3 ½ oz

a handful of spinach

2 tsp maca powder

a small piece of fresh root ginger (about ⅓ oz) – unpeeled if organic

1 tsp acai powder

**OPTIONAL**

a handful of strawberries, to sweeten

coconut water, to replace the water if preferred

**1** Wash the fruit and vegetables well, then chop the beets into smallish chunks to fit your blender.

**2** Blend everything together with ¾ cup water or coconut water until smooth, adding more liquid if necessary.

**3** Drink immediately or pour into a glass jar or stainless steel flask and keep in the fridge for up to 48 hours.

# VANILLA MALTSHAKE WITH A CHOCOLATE SWIRL

It's all very well having a feast of vegetables and greens in your power-hitting smoothie, but every now and then we fancy something simple, creamy, and sweet. This delicious vanilla milkshake with a hint of malt reminds us of our childhood. Malt is actually fermented grain used to flavor milk powder, so we've used a mix of carob and maca to capture this flavor. A ripe banana adds all the sweetness needed and we balance it with home-made Almond Milk (page 304) or full-fat coconut milk – all healthy fats (or do a cheat's version and blend some whole soaked almonds).

Children love this, especially when you decorate the glass with a simple chocolate swirl. Use the chocolate swirl mixture to drizzle onto the Pea and Mint Ice Cream (page 262).

SERVES 2 CHILDREN

(8 ½ OZ EACH)

If you haven't got time to make the chocolate sauce, then simply scatter over some cacao nibs or try crushed hazelnuts instead.

### FOR THE VANILLA MALTSHAKE

1 ½ cup Almond Milk (page 304) or full-fat coconut milk or 1 tbsp almond butter or 6 almonds (preferably activated, see page 300)

1 ripe banana, peeled

2 tsp vanilla extract

1 tsp carob powder

½ tsp maca powder

½ avocado, for extra creaminess and goodness (optional)

### FOR THE CHOCOLATE SWIRL

2 tbsp cacao powder

1 tbsp raw runny honey

2½ tsp hot water

**1**  Blend the maltshake ingredients together until smooth. (If you are using whole almonds or almond butter, you will need to add an additional 1 ½ cup water for blending.)

**2**  For the chocolate sauce, stir the ingredients together in a mug or small bowl until smooth, then, using a spoon, drizzle the sauce into the glasses while you rotate the glass. Carefully pour in the smoothie. You should still be able to see the chocolate swirl on the glass.

**+  IF YOU MAKE THESE IN ADVANCE**, pop the chocolate-swirled glasses into the fridge while you make the smoothie to help set them first.

## MEXICAN HOT CHOCOLATE

Rich, aromatic, and totally blissful, this chocolate beverage was created by the ancient Mayan and Aztec civilisations of Mexico and was enjoyed for its health benefits, as well as its flavor. Hot chocolate is usually thought of as a naughty, calorific treat, but with the right ingredients it becomes a superfood beverage. We combine antioxidant rich cacao with ground cinnamon and cayenne pepper to balance blood sugar levels and give your circulatory system a boost.

In the winter, we love our hot chocolate with the richness of coconut milk warmed with maple syrup but in the summer we whisk it up with almond milk and serve it cold, sweetened with raw honey.

This makes two large mugs or you could serve it in 4 espresso cups after supper, instead of dessert.

MAKES 2 MUGS OR 4
ESPRESSO CUPS

1 tin coconut milk or
   1 ½ cup Almond Milk
   (page 304)
3 tbsp cacao powder
1½ tsp vanilla extract
1½ tbsp maple syrup,
   to taste, or raw honey
a pinch of sea salt
1 tsp or more of ground
   cinnamon
a tiny pinch of cayenne
   pepper

**1  For hot chocolate**, whisk everything together (using the coconut milk and maple syrup) and warm gently in a saucepan before pouring into mugs or espresso cups.

**2  For cold chocolate**, whisk everything together (using almond milk and raw honey) and pour into glasses to serve.

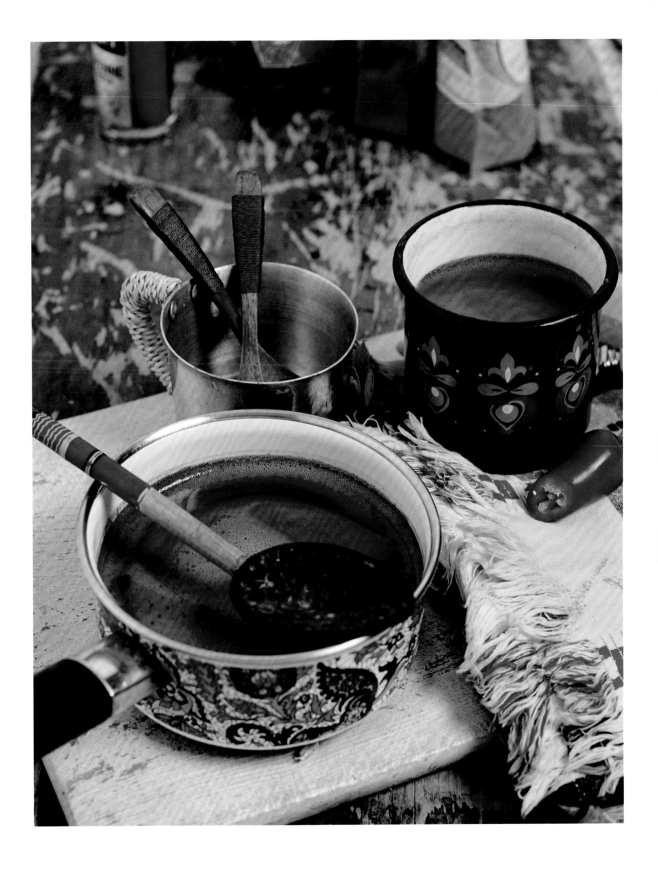

# CHICORY LATTE

You might have come across the delicious, bitter leaves of endive, a member of the dandelion family, in salads or seasoned and fried in butter. The root of the endive plant, once roasted and ground, has a similar flavor to coffee and is sometimes sold as "chicory" – the UK name for endive. Chicory used to be known as "poor man's coffee" and was a popular additive to tea and coffee centuries ago. It is caffeine-free and great for indigestion and constipation.

Chicory replaces coffee in this frothy latte and we've teamed it with homemade Almond Milk (pages 304–305) here. If you haven't got a batch of almond milk on hand, then try our alternative method, which uses 6 activated almonds (crispy or wet) added to the blender with some additional water, instead.

You can make this hot or cold – add maple syrup for a hot latte or sweeten with raw honey for a cool drink.

SERVES 1

8 ½ oz Almond Milk
(pages 304–305) or
1 tbsp almond butter or
6 almonds (preferably
activated, see pages
300–302)

1 tbsp raw honey or
maple syrup

2 tbsp ground chicory

**1** Blend all the ingredients in a blender until smooth. (If you're using almond milk, you can also just shake it all up in a cocktail shaker, flask, or bottle. If you're using whole almonds or almond butter, you will need to add an additional 8 ½ oz water for blending.)

**2** Warm gently in a saucepan, if required, remembering to use maple syrup and not raw honey.

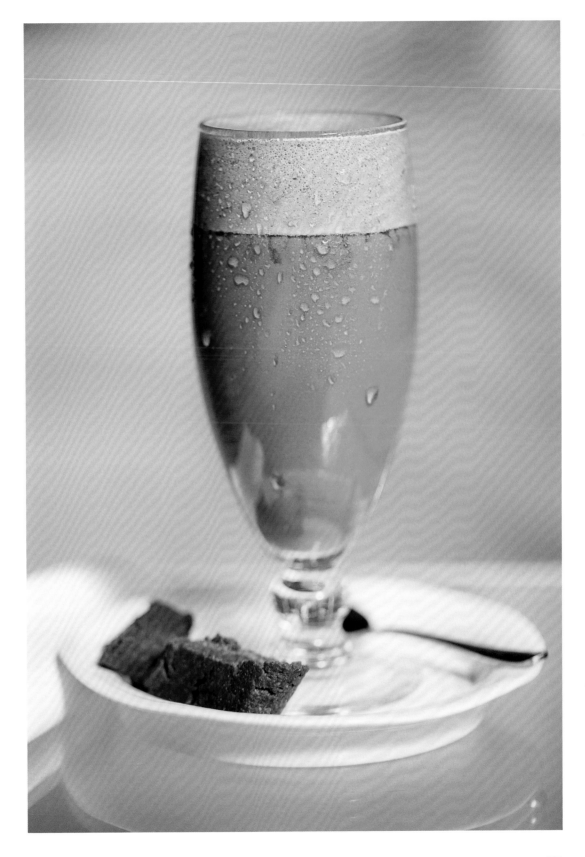

# PEP-UP
# TURMERIC TEA

Ginger, turmeric, lemon, and cayenne – these four ingredients can always be found in our kitchen, but did you know they also form the basis of our medicine chest? We're all aware of just how good lemon and ginger are, but a lemon and ginger tea becomes even more powerful with the addition of bright yellow turmeric (careful it stains!) and spicy red cayenne. Turmeric is detoxifying, anti-inflammatory, and antimicrobial (good for viral and bacterial infections). Cayenne aids digestion, relieves congestion and improves circulation, allowing the healing properties of turmeric to reach the site of infection faster. Blend together for an easy winter pep-up and immune-boosting remedy that can be enjoyed as a caffeine-free brew in the morning or sipped slowly after a meal.

SERVES 2

1 tbsp finely grated fresh root ginger (unpeeled if organic)

½ tsp ground turmeric

a tiny pinch of cayenne pepper (a little more if you like)

2 ½ cup hot water

3 tbsp lemon juice, about ½ lemon

**OPTIONAL**

a little squeeze of raw honey

**1** Boil the kettle and put the grated ginger, turmeric, and cayenne pepper in a teapot.

**2** Fill with hot water (rather than boiling), stir, and leave to brew for 10 minutes.

**3** Strain if you like. Pour into mugs and leave the tea to cool to room temperature before adding the lemon juice and raw honey, if using.

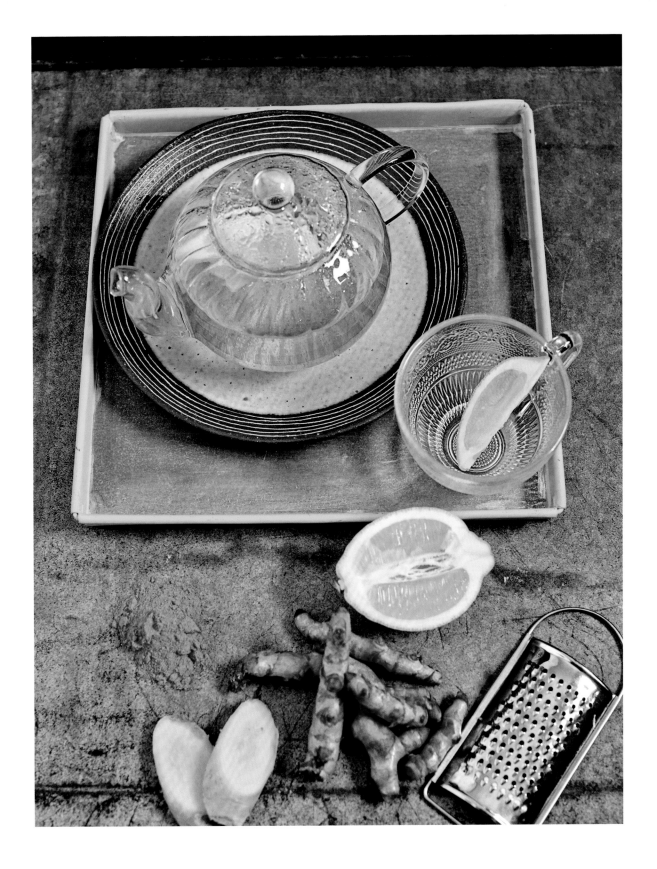

## BLUEBERRY, LIME, AND LAVENDER COCKTAIL

A refreshing pink cocktail with a hint of floral. Raw honey, rather than sugar syrup, lightly sweetens this cocktail. Blueberries, lime juice, and coconut water, help to alkalize this drink and keep you hydrated. If you don't have coconut water or prefer a fizz, then choose a naturally sparkling water.

**MAKES A 1 QUART JUG OF PUNCH (8 GLASSES)**

5 oz fresh blueberries

6 tbsp raw honey (or more to taste)

1½ tsp dried lavender

2 cups coconut water

½ cup lime juice

8 ½ oz vodka

5 oz frozen blueberries, to serve

➕ **USE FROZEN BLUEBERRIES AS ICE CUBES** and let them bob around in this pretty cocktail. Freeze them in a single layer on a baking tray.

**1** Wash the blueberries thoroughly. Pulse them with the honey and lavender in a food processor or blender with 8 ½ oz water to make a lavender infused syrup.

**2** Strain the syrup into a jug using a fine sieve or piece of cheesecloth, making sure you squeeze all the goodness from the blueberry-lavender pulp. Add the coconut water, lime, and vodka and stir thoroughly.

**3** When ready to serve, add the frozen blueberries.

## SPICED APPLE BRANDY PUNCH

This is a great big hearty punch – the perfect winter warmer served hot from the pan, blending whole apples and cranberries with ginger and cinnamon.

Brandy is a grape-based spirit and, just like red wine, it is high in antioxidants, particularly when aged in oak barrels. However, remember that in the case of alcohol, less is more, so enjoy sipping, not gulping on this tummy-warming punch. If you have a very strong blender, then don't worry about peeling the apples.

**MAKES A 1 LITRE JUG OF PUNCH (8 GLASSES)**

6 cored apples

2 oz fresh cranberries or 1 oz dried cranberries

4 thumb-sized pieces of peeled fresh root ginger (about 5 ⅔ oz) – unpeeled if organic

1 cinnamon stick

1 star anise

5 cloves

¾ cup brandy

fresh cranberries or apple slices, to decorate

**OPTIONAL**

add a little raw honey if you need after blending (don't heat the honey)

**1** Chop the apples and add them to a saucepan along with 3 ⅓ cup water, the cranberries, ginger, cinnamon, star anise, and cloves.

**2** Gently simmer the mix over a low heat for about 30 minutes.

**3** When the apples are soft, remove the star anise, cloves, and cinnamon stick and set aside to go into the finished punch. Blitz the apples, cranberries, and ginger together in a blender.

**4** Strain the "smoothie" into a jug using a fine sieve or piece of cheesecloth, pressing as much liquid from the pulp as possible, then add the brandy and rewarm in a pan if serving hot.

**5** Decorate with apple slices or fresh cranberries, the reserved cinnamon stick, star anise, and cloves. Stir in the honey, if using. Serve warm or over ice.

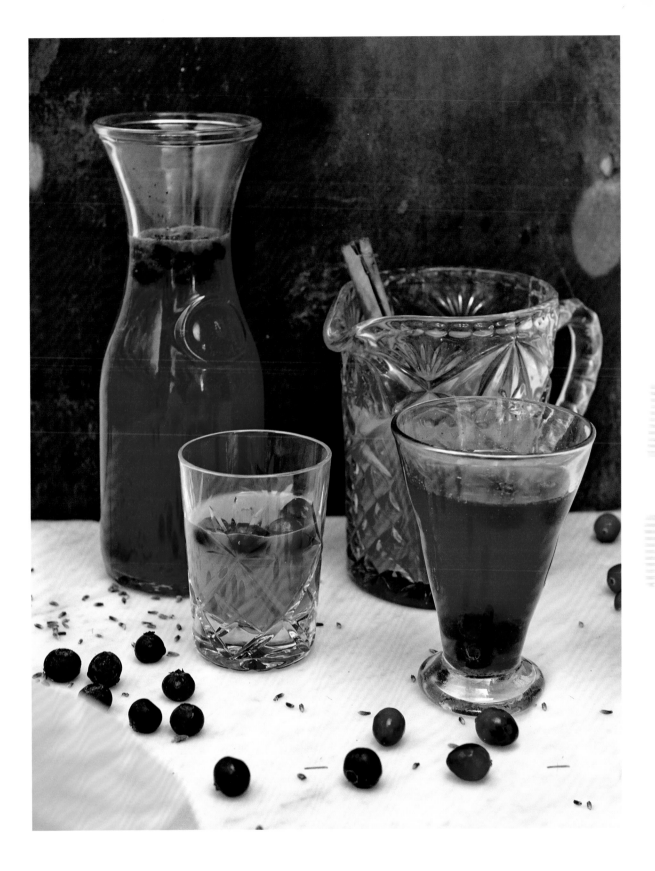

# BASIC RECIPES AND METHODS

Here are our basic recipes and methods for everyday cooking. Some of these processes might be new to you, such as soaking and fermenting, but they bring a wealth of benefits. The extra steps are worth it for great-tasting, real, homemade food that's not just better value for money, but great value for the vitality it will give you. Enjoy these practices – it's empowering to take control of your own food and understand what you are putting into your body.

## MAKING BONE BROTH

Nutrient-rich bone broth is at the heart of all our cooking. It's the first thing we teach new clients and is a kitchen essential. We'd feel lost without it. This nourishing food is simple and cheap to make and makes everything taste amazing. It can be flavored with the addition of onions, carrots, and celery, but if you're frugal like us, you'll be keeping these vegetables for the final dish and throwing in the odds and ends of onions, celery, and carrots instead. Save them up when prepping recipes and stash them in the freezer or fridge, ready to use when you next make a big batch of bone broth.

MAKES 3–4 QUARTS DEPENDING ON YOUR PAN SIZE

4 ½–6 ½ lb beef bones, chicken carcasses, lamb bones (usually free from the butchers), or use the saved bones from a roast, such as chicken, lamb shoulder, or bone marrow bones

OPTIONAL: a generous splash of apple cider vinegar or fresh lemon juice (this can help to extract the minerals from the meat bones)

2 handfuls of any onions, leeks, carrots, or celery ends

1 tbsp black peppercorns

a few dried bay leaves

**1** Place the bones and any optional ingredients into a large stainless steel or ceramic cooking pot and cover with cold water. The water level should cover the bones by 2 in while still leaving room at the top of the pan.

**2** Cover with a lid and bring to boil. Reduce the heat and simmer, lid on, for at least 6 hours for chicken and 12 for beef or lamb, skimming off any foam that rises to the top. The longer the bones simmer, the more nutrients are released. We like to boil the chicken carcass for up to 12 hours until the bones begin to crumble and keep beef bones going for 24 hours until they look as if they were washed up on a beach.

**3** Fresh chicken carcasses from the butcher usually have a fair amount of meat on them. We tend to poach the carcasses for 20 minutes, then pull off the meat (and save it for another meal like a chicken salad or chicken pho) before returning the carcasses to the pot and continuing to simmer to make broth.

**4** Strain the liquid, using a fine mesh strainer for poultry. Use immediately or leave to cool before storing. Bone broth will keep in the fridge for several days or up to a week if you leave it undisturbed, as a layer of fat will form on the surface and keep it sealed from the air.

➕ **YOU CAN ALSO USE A SLOW COOKER.** Just turn to high and cook for 12 hours or more.

➕ **FREEZE IT IN BATCHES FOR USE DURING THE WEEK** – use glass containers and leave a few centimetres at the top for expansion. Small portions are great for cooking up quinoa or braising vegetables and larger containers are great for making batches of soups, curries, and stews.

## ACTIVATING AND COOKING PSEUDOCEREALS, LEGUMES, NUTS, AND SEEDS

We soak most pseudocereals, legumes, nuts, and seeds before eating them. Soaking increases the nutrients available and makes them easier to digest by helping to neutralize the negative effects of too much phytic acid and other anti-nutrients.

This soaking is also known as activating. With a few exceptions, 8 hours or overnight soaking does the job and fits in easily with our routine: putting something on to soak in the morning so that it's ready for supper or soaking something for the next day while cooking the evening meal. It only takes a minute and soon becomes habit – and your body will thank you for it.

As a rough guideline, soak in double the volume of filtered water using a glass or ceramic bowl. Leave at room temperature overnight or for 8 hours, loosely draped with a tea towel if you like. Rinse well and drain. If you are unable to use the activated ingredients straight away, then store, covered, in your fridge, where they will keep for a few days. Rinse again before cooking and/or eating.

You can continue the germination process for a few more days, changing the water regularly, to grow young vegetable shoots to add to salads and stir-fries – we love quinoa, mung, and sunflower seed sprouts.

### Soaking pseudocereals

Remember when planning a recipe, leave at least 8 hours to soak pseudocereals – amaranth,

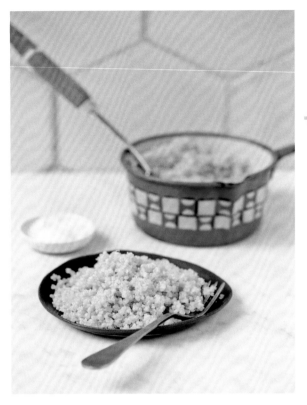

**3** Add the pseudocereal and stir once. Continue to cook on a medium simmer until tender – 12 minutes for quinoa, 15 for buckwheat, and 20 for amaranth.
**4** Take off the heat and leave to stand for 5 minutes. Fluff with a fork before serving.

+ **RED OR BLACK QUINOA** will need an extra 5 minutes cooking time so add an extra 1 oz water.

### Soaking legumes

Legume is a term for dried seeds such as beans, peas, and lentils. Black beans, aduki, butter beans, cannellini beans, chickpeas, navy beans, mung beans, and lentils are some of our favorite legumes. Unlike pseudocereals or nuts and seeds, legumes should not be eaten raw, so after soaking be sure to cook them thoroughly.

Again, most varieties of legumes need around 8 hours soaking time in double the volume of filtered water so we get into the habit of preparing them the night before.

The exceptions are all varieties of beans and red split lentils. Beans need a lot longer soaking, so leave them for 12 hours or overnight. We sometimes sprout by soaking for a few days, rinsing, and replacing with fresh water, until we see a little tail appear on the beans. For those who find beans difficult to digest or gassy, we suggest trying this technique. Red split lentils are hulled and split so don't require soaking at all. They are great for supper in a hurry as they cook in just 20 minutes.

### Cooking legumes

Once soaked, legumes are simple to cook. We like to cook up big batches and freeze in portions ready for use. We'll add handfuls to stews and salads and blend them into dips, sauces, and soups for creaminess. We love baking with them too, making our signature birthday cakes with beans and our BB Brownies (page 240) are unmissable.

Cooking times vary, with beans taking the longest from 1–2 hours (cook up batches and freeze in portions ready to be used) and lentils taking just 20–40 minutes, depending on the variety and what you want to do with them after (cook longer for humus or where legumes need to be very soft; shorter for stews when they will be cooked again; mid time for salads when you still want some 'bite'). Our recipes will guide you on cooking times for each particular kind of bean and lentil, just make sure they are well cooked for easy digestion.

buckwheat, or quinoa – in double the volume of filtered water with the addition of an acidic medium. As a rough guide, use 1 tbsp lemon juice or apple cider vinegar (ACV) for every 8 ½ oz water.

### Cooking pseudocereals

Pseudocereals can be cooked in water, but for savory dishes we like homemade bone broth for extra flavor and nourishment. Resist stirring too much as it can make them stodgy. Serve hot or cold, as a side dish to replace grains, as the base of a salad, or use in our recipes. Cook up big batches and freeze in portions ready to be used.

SERVES 4 PEOPLE AS A SIDE

Beef, chicken, or lamb bone broth (page 300), vegetable
  stock or water
9 oz activated quinoa, buckwheat groats, or amaranth

**1** Using a fine mesh strainer, drain and rinse the soaked quinoa, buckwheat, or amaranth until the water is clear and without foam.
**2** For the quinoa, bring 8 ½ oz bone broth, stock, or water to a medium-high heat. Use 3 cups liquid for the buckwheat or 2 cups for the amaranth.

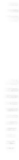

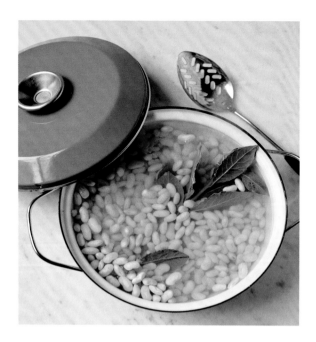

Note: 7 oz of dried uncooked beans makes around 18 oz of cooked beans, which is the equivalent of 2 drained tins of shop-bought, cooked beans.

**1** After soaking, drain and thoroughly rinse the beans. Place in a large pot and cover with three times their volume of water.

**2** Bring to the boil over a high heat (add herbs for flavor if you like), then reduce the heat and simmer without a lid. Skim off any foam from the top with a slotted spoon.

**3** Cook until tender. The times vary according to the variety and how you plan on using them, so check the packet instructions or recipe. Drain.

## Soaking nuts and seeds

Nuts and seeds are used in small amounts in many of our recipes so we like to get ahead and activate them in bulk, soaking whole packets and then drying them thoroughly in a dehydrator, at low temperatures, to keep them raw and preserve the nutrients. Stored in glass jars somewhere cool they will keep for up to 4 months. Once dehydrated, nuts and seeds are ready to sprinkle onto salads, turn into Nut Butter (page 303), or grind into flour (page 302). Drying them out takes time, so if we are using the nuts or seeds in dips and smoothie recipes, we usually soak the required amount fresh and don't dry them, which makes them easier to blend too. Activate a few packets of nuts or seeds a week for the first couple of weeks and you'll soon have a good variety to pick from. We refer to

dehydrated, activated nuts as "crispy nuts" because they have a much crispier texture. For most nuts and seeds, particularly walnuts, you'll find that they also have a much sweeter taste once their bitter coatings have been rinsed away and are more enjoyable to eat.

The soaking times of nuts and seeds vary, but they are mostly around the 8 hour mark, so we tend to leave them overnight with a few exceptions: **Brazil**, **macadamia**, **pine nuts**, **hemp seeds,** and **pistachios** don't require soaking; **Cashews** only need 3 hours – any longer and they go slimy; **Poppy seeds** are used in small amounts and are difficult to drain (and some phytic acid is OK). We don't rinse and drain **chia** and **flax** after soaking as we like to keep their unique thickening and binding properties that occur when they come into contact with water.

### "Crispy" nuts

"Crispy nuts" is the term used for activated (soaked) nuts and seeds that have been dried and returned to their crunchy state. Rinse and drain the soaked nuts or seeds and spread them out on a dehydrator tray. Dehydrate at 115°F for 12–24 hours, depending on the size of the nuts or seeds. Turn them after 12 hours and check for crispness. They need to be completely dehydrated so that mold doesn't develop while in storage. You can also use an oven to dry them at its lowest temperature but they will no longer be raw.

### "Wet" nuts

When nuts and seeds are eaten "wet," as in smoothies, nut milks, dressings, and dips, you can just soak the amount required, rinse, and blend – no need to dry them out first. You can keep soaked, rinsed, and drained (wet) nuts for 2–3 days in the fridge, but after that they will go moldy if not dried out thoroughly.

Whether activated or not, we tend to store all our nuts sealed in the fridge or freezer to make the most of their nutrition, as they can go rancid easily when exposed to light and oxygen.

### MAKING YOUR OWN BASICS

Shop-bought health foods are convenient, but they can be pricey, and though they might avoid gluten and processed sugars, they might not always offer the best nutrition. Give our homemade versions a go and you'll taste the difference.

### Sun flour

Well not flour exactly…this is a fine crumb made from ground sunflower seeds that we use for baking,

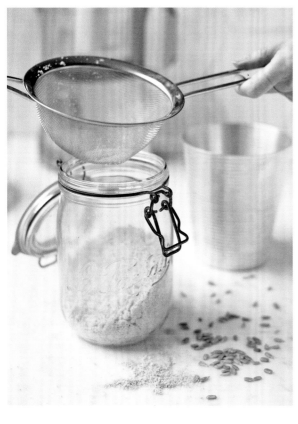

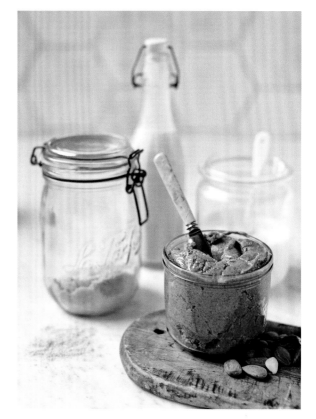

just as we would ground almonds. We use almonds throughout the book, but it is very easy to overdo this super-versatile nut if you are cutting out gluten, grains and sugar from your diet. Sunflower seeds are cheaper than almonds, as well as being delicious and good for you. Best of all, they're suitable for those with a tree-nut allergy.

A powerful blender turns sunflower seeds into a light fluffy flour. A food processor will turn them into a rough crumb that is still nice for baking, but offers a different texture.

✚ **DON'T BE ALARMED** if the chlorophyll in the sunflower seeds reacts with the alkaline baking soda and turns your baking a little green! Nothing to worry about and certainly still good for you, so please don't throw it out. You can counter this with a little lemon or lime juice – the acidity will even it up.

MAKES 18 OZ

18 oz sunflower seeds ("crispy" activated, page 302)

**1** Pour the "crispy" sunflower seeds into a clean and thoroughly dried blender (you can ruin your flour if there's any moisture in your blender). Grind the sunflower seeds in short bursts, keeping the bottom moving so that they don't overheat and release their oil (you'll get "sun butter" otherwise!)

**2** Move the seeds around using the end of a wooden spoon, if necessary, and pulse again.

**3** You are looking for a fine crumb, but won't be able to get this all the way through. When it's nearly done, you can sieve out any hard bits or leave them in. Store the flour in a clean glass jar in the fridge.

**Nut butter**

Nut butter is a tasty and convenient snack and can be spread on anything from toast to apple rings or turned into Bliss Balls (page 124). The most famous nut butter is, of course, peanut butter (though technically a peanut is a bean). The next most popular is almond butter, but you can make butters out of a variety of nuts and seeds – macadamia, pumpkin, and sunflower are some of our favorites—or try a mix of seeds and nuts. They are delicious with a touch of honey, salt, cinnamon, and smoked paprika.

Shop-bought nut butters are either raw or roasted and we've given methods for making both. Using your own activated nuts is more cost effective and nutritionally superior. If you've already started making "crispy" activated nuts, then try whipping up a nut butter. You just need a food processor. You can use a more powerful blender, but for thick pastes like this we don't recommend it – half of your lovely nut butter just gets stuck at the bottom! We like to add coconut oil to give a smoother texture to our nut butter and thin it out a bit, but only add this towards the end otherwise it stops the nut butter fully developing.

Please remember that eating nuts is ridiculously easy to overdo – especially when they taste this good – so please be mindful and eat them in moderation.

We've given the following instructions for almonds, as this is the most popular nut to start with.

MAKES 18 OZ

18 oz almonds (preferably "crispy" activated, page 302)
2 tbsp coconut oil
a pinch of sea salt
**OPTIONAL:** raw honey, to taste
spices, such as cinnamon and ground ginger, to taste
vanilla extract or cacao, to taste

**1** Pour the almonds into a food processor and pulse a few times until the nuts are roughly chopped. For a crunchy nut butter, scoop some out and reserve.
**2** Turn the food processor on again and blend for a few minutes until the almonds become grainy. Use a spatula to collect any that have worked their way up the sides of the processor and then blend again.
**3** After several minutes, the ground almonds will turn into a ball. After several more minutes, the oil in the nuts will start to come out and the mixture will become buttery – this can take 10–20 minutes, depending on the strength of your food processor.
**4** At this point, you can add the oil, salt, and any flavorings you'd like, and then continue to blend until the almond butter becomes smooth.
**5** For crunchy nut butter, add back in the reserved, roughly chopped nuts and pulse a few times to combine.
**6** Scoop into an airtight container and refrigerate. Almond butter will thicken slightly when chilled. Plain or salted nut butter will keep for 2-3 weeks in the fridge. It may not keep as long with other flavors added.

✛ **FOR ROASTED NUT BUTTER**, preheat the oven to fan 350°F and roast the nuts or seeds in a single layer for 10 minutes until fragrant and browned (small seeds will take less time). Set aside for 10 minutes then follow the method above for unroasted nut butter.

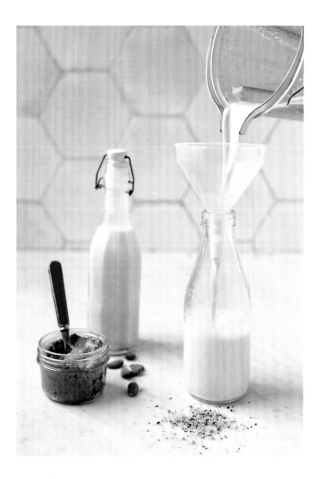

## Nut milk

Quality shop-bought varieties of nut milks, like almond milk, can be expensive for what you're really getting (as little as 6 per cent of nuts blended with water) and they usually contain emulsifiers, thickeners, and sweeteners as well as additives to give them a longer shelf life. If you have a food processor, or even better a powerful blender, making your own nut milk is easy. Try adding a dash of vanilla, cinnamon, honey, or sea salt.

The ratio of nuts or seeds to water will depend on how creamy you like your milk and the longer you soak the nuts – up to 2 days – the creamier it will be (change the water every 12 hours). You can use most nuts and seeds. Our favorites are almond, hemp, sesame, sunflower, and hazelnut. Since the nuts are soaked (and therefore activated) to make them creamy, there is no need to use activated nuts or crispy nuts.

MAKES 16 OZ

3 ½ oz almonds
a tiny pinch of sea salt
**OPTIONAL:** ½ tsp raw honey

**1** Soak the almonds overnight (or longer) in salted water, drain, and rinse.

**2** Combine the almonds and 2 cups water in a powerful blender for 2 minutes or 4 minutes in a food processor.

**3** Add a tiny amount of salt and the honey, if you like, and blend again.

**4** For a smooth milk, strain the "milk" through a nut milk bag or cheesecloth into a bowl, gathering the edges of the cheesecloth and twisting it tightly. Gently squeeze the bag to get the last of the milk out, tightening the cloth as you go. Save the leftover almond pulp for adding to smoothies, curries, and dips.

**5** When making this for ourselves we tend to skip this extra stage, enjoying the pulp at the bottom of our smoothies with a spoon or the extra texture in our granola. Keep the milk in a glass bottle for up to 3 days.

### THE FERMENTED FOUR

The four recipes below are a great introduction into the world of homemade probiotics. Don't be scared to have a go, it's fun, easy, cheaper than shop-bought, and usually more nutritious.

**SOME BASIC RULES FOR FERMENTING:** Use salt that is free of iodine and/or anti-caking agents, which can inhibit fermentation – choose sea salt rather than "table salt."

Chlorinated water can also inhibit fermentation, so use mineral or filtered water if you can.

Don't use metal tools or a metal bowl, or plastic. Traditionally, special ceramic pots are used for making sauerkraut, but glass jars either covered with a muslin cloth and elastic band to keep them sealed tightly or a jar with a tight-fitting, clip-top lid work well.

### Coconut yogurt

Coconut yogurt is a delicious dairy alternative. We first started making this in Australia and then the Philippines using the flesh of young coconuts to make a tangy pudding. Back in England, we experimented with the next best thing – full-fat coconut milk. Coconut yogurt is easy to make and a great way of eating more probiotic food regularly.

This is a "cultured" food because, unlike sauerkraut or kimchi, you have to introduce a culture to get it started. For your culture, you can simply add probiotic full-fat dairy yogurt, the contents from some probiotic capsules, yogurt starter culture, or whey (the liquid part of yogurt) if you want to avoid milk solids. These good bacteria will happily feast on the natural sugars in the coconut. Because of the different strains of bacteria in each of these "cultures," the

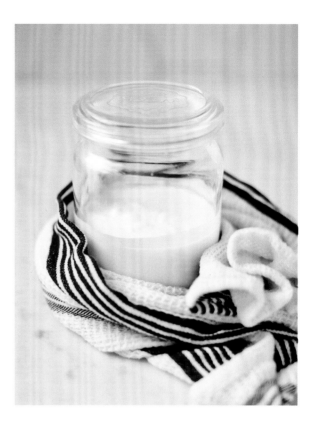

flavor and texture differs and they are all uniquely delicious. Most recipes and shop-bought varieties use thickeners, which we prefer to avoid, so as well as a tangy drinking yogurt that's thin enough to pour over granola, we created an extra-thick version. Both are as easy as each other and have only three ingredients – coconut, water, and probiotic – and each will keep for 1–2 weeks in the fridge.

MAKES A 16 OZ JAR

**FOR THE COCONUT DRINKING YOGURT**

1 ½ cup full-fat coconut milk

**FOR THE THICK COCONUT YOGURT**

7 oz coconut cream (we use a bar of creamed coconut)

1 ½ cups warm water (important to use filtered in order to not affect the good bacteria)

**TO FERMENT BOTH TYPES OF YOGURT**

2 tbsp probiotic yogurt, 2 probiotic capsules, 1 tbsp whey, or ½ tsp powdered starter culture for yogurts

**1** Sterilize a 16 oz jar and lid either by adding hot water for 10 minutes or by popping it through the dishwasher.

**2  To make the coconut drinking yogurt**, shake the coconut milk vigorously. If the temperature of the room is cold and the coconut milk has separated, then warm it gently in a pan and whisk until smooth.

**3**  When it's cool enough to touch, add your chosen culture and stir through. Pour the probiotic coconut mix into a sterilized jar and cover with a lid. Use one of the methods below to incubate the mix: you are ideally looking for a constant temperature of around 115°F.

**IN THE DEHYDRATOR:** 24 hours at 115°F – this is our preferred method.

**IN A YOGURT MAKER:** Follow the manufacturer's instructions.

**IN THE AIRING CUPBOARD:** Place in an airing cupboard for about 24–36 hours.

**IN WARM WEATHER:** Leave in a warm place in the kitchen, but not in direct sunlight, for about 24–48 hours.

**4**  Check the yogurt after 24 hours. If you want a more sour taste, leave it a little longer, otherwise store the yogurt in the fridge until ready to use.

**5  To make the thick coconut yogurt** warm the creamed coconut by placing the unopened bag in a bowl of hot water for 20 minutes, massaging it to help speed up the process. Empty into a bowl and add the hot water, whisking until it's smooth. When it's cool enough to touch, follow steps 3 and 4 above. This yogurt will set in the fridge but will soften at room temperature.

✚ **SAVE SOME OF THE LAST BATCH OF COCONUT YOGURT TO FERMENT YOUR NEXT BATCH** – saving on buying more probiotic capsules or dairy yogurt. We only do this for one ferment as we find the effectiveness starts to reduce.

## Probiotic tomato ketchup

For many people, ketchup is their staple condiment. Make yours work harder by fermenting it for a probiotic boost to any meal. It's also well worth making your own ketchup just to know it's no longer a junk food that you're adding to your burgers or dipping your celery root chips into. We've used a jar of passata here to speed up the process, but if you come across a glut of overly ripe good-quality tomatoes, then they're well worth using. The ketchup can be enjoyed straight away and for up to 5 weeks – fermented or not – if well-sealed and kept in the fridge.

MAKES A 16 OZ BOTTLE OR JAR

1 large onion, chopped

1 tbsp ghee or butter, or more if needed

2 garlic cloves, diced

1 bay leaf

7 tbsp apple cider vinegar

3 cup passata or 2 ⅔ lb fresh tomatoes, roughly chopped

½ cup maple syrup

a pinch of sea salt

**OPTIONAL:** a pinch of cayenne pepper

**TO FERMENT**

1½ tsp Sauerkraut juice (below) or Quick Kimchi juice (opposite) or whey (from dairy yogurt)

**1**  Sterilize a bottle or glass jar with a lid, either by adding hot water for 10 minutes or by popping it through the dishwasher.

**2**  Gently fry the onion in the ghee or butter for 10 minutes until softened, stirring occasionally.

**3**  Add the garlic, bay leaf, and apple cider vinegar and stir for a minute.

**4**  Add the rest of the ingredients and turn up the heat. When it starts to bubble, leave it to simmer gently for about 1 hour, lid off, until you have a thick ketchup (or less if you don't mind it thinner).

**5**  Check for seasoning, adding cayenne, if you like.

**6**  Take off the heat and cool, then blend until smooth. When cool enough to touch, stir through the sauerkraut or kimchi juice or whey, pour into the sterilized bottle or jar, and cover tightly with a muslin cloth. Leave in a warm place on the worktop or in the airing cupboard for 4–5 days, then seal with a tight-fitting lid and transfer to the fridge (it will keep for 2 months).

## Sauerkraut

When you think of fermented foods, sauerkraut is probably the most famous (or infamous). If you have never tried fermented foods before, this is the perfect place to start – very cheap and only two ingredients – cabbage and salt. Cabbage leaves have their own natural bacterial cultures, so all you have to do is create the simple conditions for it to ferment and let it do its thing.

A delicious digestive aid alongside meat, we also love it stuffed into a Flax Sandwich Bread (page 272) sandwich with some mustard and good cheese.

To keep the cabbage submerged in its own juices whilst leaving some room at the top of the jar, we roll up the tough outer leaves of the cabbage and use

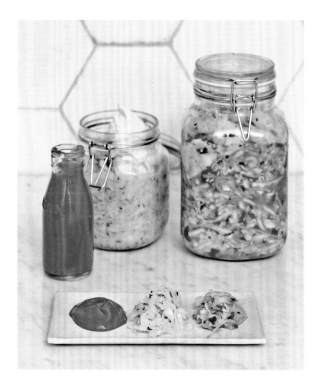

cabbage is completely submerged under the brine making sure you leave at least around an inch of headspace). Seal the jar with its lid, clip top, or tightly cover with a muslin cloth using an elastic band.

**6** Leave the jar to stand at room temperature for 1–5 days to ferment. You may see bubbles inside the jar and brine may seep out of the lid – place a bowl or plate under the jar to help catch any overflow.

**7** Leave it alone for at least 2 days (unless it's high summer, when you should check it after 24 hours). If it's bubbling a bit, it's ready and should be refrigerated, otherwise check every 24 hours until ready. Once it's fermented to your liking, store in the refrigerator for up to a month.

**Quick kimchi**

The Korean version of sauerkraut is far punchier, thanks to pungent sour and spicy flavors, including ginger, garlic, and chili.

Authentic kimchi is time consuming to make so try this quick technique instead – it doesn't keep for as long as traditional kimchi but it's much easier to make. You can eat it straight away as a "fresh" kimchi salad or store it at room temperature for a few days to enjoy fermented kimchi. A fermented kimchi develops a tangy ripe taste as well as a slight fizziness from the ferment – a wonderfully cheap way to jazz up any dish as well as take your probiotics.

Kimchi can be mild or fiery, it's your choice, but don't overdo the ginger and garlic – the flavors get stronger during fermentation so you don't want something too overpowering.

We love kimchi as a digestive aid before dinner or as a delicious remedy for a tummy ache or indigestion. It also makes a great pick me up.

them to wedge the Sauerkraut down. Then cover the whole thing with a tea towel to stop dust getting into any gaps. We have always made this with clip-top jars – no explosions to date – but lift that lid carefully!

MAKES A 16 OZ JAR

1 medium-large head of white, red, or green cabbage
   (about 3 ⅓ lb with the core)
1½ tbsp sea salt
**OPTIONAL:** ½ tbsp caraway seeds

**1** Sterilize a 16 oz glass jar with a lid, either by adding hot water for 10 minutes or by popping it through the dishwasher.

**2** Remove the outer leaves of the cabbage and set to one side, then quarter and remove the core. Shred the cabbage by hand or by using a food processor grating attachment.

**3** Place the cabbage in a mixing bowl and sprinkle with the sea salt and the caraway seeds, if using.

**4** Mix well and then add handfuls to the jar. Use your fist or the back of a rolling pin to pack each handful down tightly – this forces water out of the cabbage to create a brine. Top the sauerkraut with a tablespoon of water, if need be, to keep the cabbage covered.

**5** Take the reserved outer cabbage leaves, roll up and use to wedge the sauerkraut down so that the chopped

MAKES A 1 QUART JAR

1 medium-large head of Chinese cabbage (or try pointed
   or white cabbage)
1 large carrot, chopped or grated
2 ⅔ oz pink radishes or 1 white radish (daikon), sliced
4 garlic cloves
2 red chilies or 2 or more tbsp Korean chili powder
2–3 scallions
a thumb-sized piece of fresh ginger (about 1 ½ oz)
2 tbsp fish sauce (make sure it is free from chemical
   preservatives, which will inhibit a proper ferment. You can
   also try tamari or just more sea salt)

**1** Sterilize a jar with a lid, either by adding hot water for 10 minutes or by popping it through the dishwasher.

**2**  Remove the outer leaves of the cabbage and set to one side, then quarter and remove the core. Coarsely chop the cabbage – larger pieces are more authentic, but we tend to slice into ribbons or grate in a food processor as it's much easier to eat that way.

**3**  Place the cabbage, carrot, and radish into a large glass or ceramic mixing bowl and pour over enough brine to cover – we find 3 cups water mixed with 3 tbsp sea salt does the trick. Cover the top of the vegetables with a smaller plate and weigh it down with a heavy bowl on top. Leave to stand for 5 hours or overnight and then drain the veg, reserving the brine water.

**4**  Use the small bowl of a food processor to pulse a coarse, rather than smooth, paste from the rest of the ingredients (or use a sharp knife to finely mince the garlic and fresh chilies, coarsely chop the scallions, and grate the ginger before mixing with the fish sauce). Mix this paste in with the drained vegetables, using two spoons to thoroughly coat them (or wear gloves to avoid chili burn!)

**5**  Enjoy some kimchi straightaway if you like, otherwise pack all the kimchi tightly into the sterilized jar, pressing down on it until the brine rises to cover the vegetables. Take the reserved outer cabbage leaves, roll up, and use to wedge the kimchi down beneath the brine, leaving at least around 1 inch of headspace. Seal the sterilized jar or cover tightly with some muslin cloth using an elastic band.

**6**  Leave the jar to stand at room temperature for 1–5 days to ferment. You may see bubbles inside the jar and brine may seep out of the lid – place a bowl or plate under the jar to help catch any overflow.

**7**  Check the kimchi after the first day or two (in cold weather it will take longer – watch it like a hawk in high summer!) and taste it. If you like the flavor, you can start eating it right away – transfer it to the fridge to slow fermentation. If it needs longer for your tastes, then press down on the vegetables with a clean spoon to keep them submerged and taste again a day or two later. If it's bubbling a bit, it's ready and should be refrigerated. When you open the jar don't lean over it and smell it or you'll inhale the full fizz!

**8**  Once it's fermented to your liking, store in the refrigerator for up to a month. If you want, add a sprinkle of toasted sesame seeds over the kimchi to serve.

### HOMEMADE WASH FOR FRUIT AND VEG

Non-organic fruit and veg often have residual pesticides on their skins. To help reduce the residue, there are three washes you can use.

**1**  Mix 1 tbsp of lemon juice with 2 tbsp of baking soda

**2**  Mix $\frac{1}{4}$ cup vinegar with 2 tbsp of sea salt

**3**  Mix 1 tbsp of lemon juice with 2 tbsp vinegar

**METHOD**: Soak the fruit and veg in a clean sink filled with water and one of the above washes for 20 minutes, then rinse them thoroughly. If you use strong chemicals to clean your sink, consider using a small bucket to soak fruit and veg in instead. Baking soda is a great alternative for cleaning stainless steel sinks, by the way.

## THE SUNDAY COOK OFF

Making interesting meals from real whole foods is always going to take a little time to prepare. Sure you can steam and season some quinoa, fold through a bag of baby spinach leaves and dress with lemon juice and olive oil in the same time it takes to cook pasta and heat a supermarket sauce, but unless you're a kitchen whizz who's well practiced at these foods, then you are going to have to devote a bit more time to being in the kitchen while you master this new way of cooking. The more you do it, the quicker it becomes and with our recipes, you'll see we're fans of one-pot cooking and meals that are fuss-free with easy steps.

Here is how we get ahead to ensure that there is always something delicious and nourishing on hand in the fridge, freezer, at your desk, or in your bag. As you plan your first Cook Off, remember that this isn't about being a culinary genius, this is about being able to feed yourself in a natural and convenient way as much as you can.

Below are the eight things to do at the weekend to make your life so much easier. You certainly don't have to do them all every weekend, but once you get through the list, you'll have a huge selection of food ready to go. A handful of hours and plenty of containers (page 25) is all you need to fill your fridge and freezer with delicious home-cooked food. Get a friend involved and it will take even less time and the more you do it, the more efficient you will become. Roasting veg and simmering broth take care of themselves after the initial prep and you'll save hours of time during the week. We like to think of the Sunday Cook Off as an investment for the working week.

### Use your freezer

We are big fans of freezing one-pot meals, so consider cooking double batches (don't worry, this doesn't mean double the work and it isn't just for families). If you have the freezer space, then you can stockpile individual portions for a freezer full of homemade "ready meals." Be sure to label and date each dish and, over the weeks, you will build up a variety of breakfasts, lunches, dinners, breads and baked goods to pick and choose from.

Defrost large dishes thoroughly before reheating. Pull out what you want from the freezer and pop it into the fridge to defrost overnight or before you leave for work, ready to reheat on your return. For individually portioned soups and stews, you can heat from frozen. We never use microwaves, so to reheat simply pop pies and bakes into the oven to heat through, or bring stews and soups to a boil in a pan, lid on, with a splash of water, and simmer gently. Don't reheat anything more than once or freeze anything twice.

**+ SMALL OR NO FREEZER?** Use your fridge to store a stew, soup, and a big salad that you can eat over 3 days so that you're not stuck in the kitchen every night or reaching for a shop-bought ready meal at the end of a long day. Keeping a couple of dressings or toppings on hand also adds variety.

**1  ROAST** Season a whole chicken or chicken pieces with sea salt and coconut oil or ghee and roast on a bed of vegetables. Turn the vegetables a few times during cooking to baste them in the fat. Once cooked and cooled, shred the chicken ready to add to salads, stews, and stir-fries and freeze the rest for future meals. Enjoy the roasted vegetables in salads topped with watercress or fold them into cooked quinoa and sprinkle with seeds and a dressing. Leftover roasted vegetables are delicious when puréed with garlic, olive oil, and spices to make a dip or blended with broth to make soup.

While the chicken is roasting, add a whole butternut squash to the oven (cutting one in half can often be a tough job so we don't bother). Place in the bottom of the oven and bake until tender when pierced, then chop or scoop out the flesh ready to use in salads, stews, or soups. You can also add it to porridge (page 34), smoothies, or use it to bake bread (Multiseed Loaf page 273).

**2  BONE BROTH** Once you've shredded the cooked chicken, simmer the chicken carcass or bones to make broth for the week and freeze in portions (page 300). Alternatively, use beef or lamb bones (ask your butcher, they are often free). A quick supper is onions, cabbage, and egg poached in the hot broth. For more ideas, try our Chicken Pho (page 66) or Tinola (page 56), which never fails to lift our spirits. Leftover pesto, dips, veg, quinoa, or meat can be stirred into broth to magically transform it into a delicious and warming soupy feast.

Always have red split lentils on hand for last minute dishes – no need to soak. Our Sunday favorite growing up was our mum's leftover soup – a peppery minestrone-esque affair with diced up odds and ends of vegetables that was different every week. Try an exotic version with the spices from our Prawn Laksa (page 178).

**+ DON'T ADD CABBAGE, CAULIFLOWER, OR BROCCOLI (CRUCIFEROUS VEGETABLES)** to stocks, broths, or slow cookers as they don't do well with long cooking. If you want them in your soups or stews, add them in towards the end of the cooking time.

**3  SOAK** When it comes to nuts, seeds, legumes, and pseudocereals, make sure you change them up for variety and get into the habit of soaking them in advance. With a few exceptions, 8 hours or overnight soaking is fine. For more info on soaking and activating, see page 302.

**4  SIMMER** Soaked quinoa can be simmered with water or bone broth and over the course of the next few days it can be turned into quick lunchbox salads or teamed with vegetable stews and curries. Cook soaked legumes (page 301) in water or bone broth until tender and turn into a dip or an easy midweek supper, such as Dahl (page 186) or Smoky Baked Beans (page 208). Stored in the fridge, these dishes will keep for 3–4 days. Beans also bulk out a soup or blend them in to make it extra creamy.

Don't forget about breakfast: batch cook Buckwheat and Amaranth Porridge (page 34) and freeze in portions so you have variety on hand all week.

**5  BAKE** Bake a bread like Multiseed Loaf (page 273) or Banana Bread (page 248), slice, and freeze. Or make some Flax Sandwich Bread (page 272) for the perfect lunch on the go. Bake a batch of muffins or cookies and freeze in portions so that you always have a satisfying sweet ready when you need it.

**6  PREP** Prep smoothie ingredients for easy mornings: chop up apples, pears, banana, spinach, kale, celery, and berries and freeze in individual portions so you can add them straight to the blender every morning for a fresh smoothie. This is a great way to use up fresh fruit and vegetables before they turn or a bulk buy bargain at the farmers' market. Drink at room temperature.

**7  BLEND** Make dressings with fresh herbs, chopped or blended with apple cider vinegar, lemon juice, and flax or olive oil. Take a jar to work on a Monday so that you've got something on hand in the fridge for your packed lunches all week. A good dressing transforms the simplest of meals.

Whip up a thick blend like a nut pesto or veg dip to have as a snack with crudités.

Blend some soaked nuts or seeds with filtered water to make a nut milk (page 304).

Whizz up a smoothie and freeze it in portions – not as good as fresh, but a much better choice than most high street breakfast and snack offerings.

**8 SHOP** Scan your cupboards for anything that you need to stock up on and note anything that you need to buy fresh to accompany your meals. If you want to get really organized, then make a list of all the meals in your freezer and cross off as you eat them – then you can avoid the disappointment of thinking you have a dahl in the freezer for your supper, when actually you ate it on the weekend!

Here's a sample Sunday Cook Off to try:

**ON SUNDAY MORNING: Soak** a batch of quinoa; Check which nuts/seeds you are running low on and soak a bag to activate (page 300).

**DURING SUNDAY EVENING: Roast a chicken**, trays of starch and low-starch veg, and a whole butternut squash. Whilst these are cooking, **drain, rinse, and cook the quinoa** and **whip up a pesto**. Enjoy an early supper of roasted chicken and low-starch veggies (for better food combining), saving a portion for Monday's lunch. **Shred the rest of the chicken and freeze** to add to soups and stews in the week. **Simmer the carcass/bones** until you go to bed or place in a slow cooker overnight. Strain and keep the broth in the fridge for quick soups, risottos, and curries. **Make Monday's supper** – a salad of quinoa and Roasted Vegetables (page 192). Just before serving on Monday night, add a handful of watercress and drizzle with your favorite oil and lemon juice. **Make Tuesday's lunch** – blend the rest of the roasted veg with bone broth from your freezer or miso paste and water and add your favorite herbs or spices, try a pinch of ground cumin and coriander or a tablespoon of garam masala, to make a soup. **Scoop out the butternut and mash**. Use some to make two Multiseed Loaves (page 273) and slice and freeze one. Refrigerate the rest of the butternut squash to make Chia Chai Butternut Breakfast Pudding (page 42) in the week or to add to soups for extra creaminess. **Drain the soaked nuts/seeds** and blend some to **make a nut milk**, if desired, then pop the rest into your dehydrator overnight.

✚ **IF YOU WANT TO ENJOY THE ROAST AS A SUNDAY LUNCH**, then start everything earlier, remembering to soak the pseudocereals on Saturday night.

# MENUS

To start you off, we've categorized some of our most popular recipes into handy menus. It is by no means exhaustive and we encourage you to experiment.

**QUICK MEALS**
Serve any of the below meals with the suggested salad for lunch or, in the evening, team them with lightly steamed green veg, sautéed cabbage, or Cauliflower Rice (page 102) or Cauliflower Mash (page 104).

For a late-night supper, stick to a starch-based recipe (remembering to chew well) and leave out the raw food – a vegetable-based soup is perfect.

Steak with Mustard Leek Sauce and Watercress Salad (page 139)
Sesame Chicken Salad with Cucumber Noodles (page 172)
Salmon with Argentinian Chimichurri Sauce and Quicker-than-toast Zucchini Salad (pages 158 and 84)
Beef Ragu and Courgetti with Kale Caesar Salad (pages 140 and 94)
Hot Buckwheat Noodle Salad (page 200)
Anytime Eggs and Spicy Avocado Dip (pages 32 and 126)
Frittata with Fennel, Cucumber, and Dill Salad (pages 39 and 97)
Papaya, Halloumi, and Watercress Salad (page 78)

If you have bone broth on hand, the following are also super quick to make.

Prawn Laksa with Rainbow Chard and Kelp Noodles (page 178)
Asparagus and Pea Risotto with Mint and Parsley Oil or Mushroom and Stilton Quinoa Risotto (pages 204 and 206) and an arugula side salad
Malaysian Lentil and Squash Curry with Summer Lime Coleslaw (pages 212 and 80)
Watercress Soup (page 54) or Broccoli, Pea, and Basil Soup (page 59)

## PACKED LUNCHES AND SNACKS

Make sure to pack a snack along with your lunch so you aren't tempted by chips and chocolate bars before you get home for dinner. We've added some suggestions to team with your lunch. Remember, leftover stews are easily heated up and transported in a flask, as are soups.

### Cold

Use a glass container and avoid plastic.

Sea Bream Teriyaki, Broccoli Slaw with Ginger Poppy Seed Mayonnaise, and Toasted Coconut Chips (pages 155, 88, and 122)

Mackerel with Miso Carrot Dressing and a Bliss Ball (pages 136 and 124)

Salmon with Argentinian Chimichurri Sauce and a BB Brownie (pages 158 and 240)

Sesame Chicken Salad with Cucumber Noodles and a Paradise Bar (pages 172 and 268)

Quinoa and Roasted Vegetable Salad with Brazil Nut Pesto and a Lemon Poppy Seed Muffin (pages 198 and 257)

Flaxbread Sandwich with Steak and Watercress and a Cinnamon and Raisin Cookie (pages 272 and 260)

Superfood Salad with Miso Tahini Dressing and Baked Broccoli Fritters and Spicy Avocado Dip (pages 76 and 126)

Warm Puy Lentil, Beet, and Apple Salad with Chocolate Avocado Mousse (pages 82 and 266)

Hot Buckwheat Noodle Salad and Southwestern Spiced Nuts (pages 200 and 119)

### Hot

Get yourself a 16 oz stainless steel flask.

Vietnamese Chicken Pho with Zucchini Noodles and a Banana Bread Muffin (pages 66 and 248)

Lamb Meatballs and Cauliflower Tabbouleh with a slice of Avocado Lime Cheesecake (pages 144 and 244)

Broccoli, Ginger, and White Bean Soup with Crudités and Mung Bean Humus (pages 60 and 232)

Sausage and Cider Stew and Dark Chocolate Thins (pages 148 and 270)

Zucchini and Eggplant Curry and a Lemon Poppy Seed Muffin (pages 196 and 257)

Mushroom and Stilton Quinoa Risotto and a BB Brownie (pages 206 and 240)

Kelp Pot Noodle (just add hot water) with Carrot and Flax Crackers (pages 68 and 121)

## EASY ENTERTAINING

It's always nice to spend more time with your guests rather than slaving over the stove. Here's a few of our go-to recipes that are easily prepped in advance, making entertaining much more enjoyable.

### Impressive enough to share

**START WITH:** Veg Balls with Mung Bean Humus or Lemon Parsley Cashew Dip (pages 118, 232, and 233)

**FOLLOWED BY:** Burritos, Socca Pizzas, or Flower Power Pizzas (provide the wraps or bases and everyone can get involved) (pages 216, 218, and 194)

**WITH:** Fennel, Cucumber, and Dill Salad or Kale Caesar Salad (pages 97 and 94)

**AND TO FINISH:** Chocolate Fig Pudding (make it up in advance and pop in the oven to heat through when you're ready) (page 252)

### Light and refreshing

**START WITH:** Cucumber Maki Crab Rolls (page 180)

**FOLLOWED BY:** Duck Tamarind Lettuce Wraps (page 174)

**AND TO FINISH:** Avocado Lime Cheesecake (page 244)

### Something spicy

**START WITH:** Baked Broccoli Fritters and Spicy Avocado Dip (page 126)

**FOLLOWED BY:** Zucchini and Eggplant Curry (page 196)

**WITH:** Cauliflower Rice (page 102)

**AND TO FINISH:** Pistachio, Fig, and Goats' Cheese Trifle (page 254)

### Classic British menu

**START WITH:** Baked Chicken Liver Mousse and Carrot and Flax Crackers (pages 168 and 121)

**FOLLOWED BY:** Fish Pie with Celery Root Mash (page 156)

**WITH:** Garlic Lemon Green Beans (page 113)

**AND TO FINISH:** Instant Berry and Coconut Ice Cream (page 264)

## PICNICS AND SUMMER PARTIES

We love a summer picnic or barbecue, but all too often it means refined grains and bread, and a couple of tomatoes if you're lucky. Here are some colorful salads, satisfying mains, and refreshing desserts to bring to the party.

Summer Lime Coleslaw (page 80)

Pablo's Chicken and Probiotic Tomato Ketchup (pages 166 and 306)

Beet and Goats' Cheese Terrine (page 214)

Feta and Black Bean Burgers with Celery Root Chips and Sun-dried Tomato and Jalapeño Yogurt Dip (pages 222, 134, and 231)

Pea, Peach, and Goats' Cheese Salad (page 90)

Fennel, Cucumber, and Dill Salad (page 97)

Caramelized Garlic Tart with Almond Crust (page 202)

Mini Almond, Strawberry and Custard Tarts (page 242)

Pea and Mint Ice Cream Lollies with Chocolate (page 262)

Chocolate Avocado Mousse (page 266)

Pineapple Carpaccio with Chili, Mint, and Lime (page 256)

## SUNDAY ROAST

Who doesn't love a good Sunday roast? Try our Mushroom Quinoa Nut Roast with a Chestnut Apricot Topping or roast meat on the bone (save the bones to make broth) and serve with plenty of delicious low-starch vegetables. We make Shepherd's Pie with leftover lamb and add any chicken to soup or stews.

**START WITH:** Bagna Cauda with Crudités (page 234)

**FOLLOWED BY:** Slow-roasted Lamb with Anchovies or Mushroom Quinoa Nut Roast with a Chestnut Apricot Topping (pages 146 and 190)

**WITH:** Kale Caesar Salad, Kohlrabi Dauphinoise, and Garlic Lemon Green Beans (pages pages 94, 211, and 113)

**AND TO FINISH:** Pear and Five Spice Crumble with Ginger Crème Fraîche or Chocolate Fig Pudding with Mango Cashew Cream (pages pages 250, 252, and 30)

## FESTIVE SEASON

The holiday season needn't mean complete overindulgence. Follow our meal plan for your special day and we guarantee you will be satisfied without the guilt of seasonal excess.

**START WITH:** Beet and Goats' Cheese Terrine or Bagna Cauda with Crudités (pages 214 and 234)

**FOLLOWED BY:** Mushroom Quinoa Nut Roast with a Chestnut Apricot Topping or Roast Duck with Cranberry and Orange Jam (pages 190 and 152)

**WITH:** Roasted Vegetables with White Wine Miso Gravy (page 192)

**AND ALSO:** Red Cabbage, Bacon, and Apple Salad (page 96)

**AND TO FINISH:** Sticky Toffee Pudding (page 246)

**DRINK:** Spiced Apple Brandy Punch (page 298)

## AFTERNOON TEA

**DRINK:** Fennel and Mint Juice (page 278)
Strawberry, Mint, and Cucumber Smoothies (page 282)
**ENJOY:** Lemon Poppy Seed Muffins (page 257)
Sardine Butter Flax Bread sandwiches (page 142)
Mini Almond, Strawberry, and Custard Tarts (page 242)
Salted Apricot Caramels (page 258)

## DINNER FOR TWO

**START WITH:** Baked Chicken Liver Mousse and toasted Flax Sandwich Bread – cut into rounds with a cookie cutter (save leftovers to make croutons) (pages 168 and 272)
**FOLLOWED BY:** Salmon with Argentinian Chimichurri Sauce (page 158)
**WITH:** Braised Fennel with Lemon and Rosemary and Cauliflower Mash (pages 109 and 104)
**AND TO FINISH:** Chocolate Molten Pots (page 252)
**DRINK:** Blueberry, Lime, and Lavender Cocktail (page 298)

## IF YOU ARE FEELING UNDER THE WEATHER

Pep-up Turmeric Tea (page 296)

Carrot and Cayenne Boost Juice (page 279)

Broccoli, Ginger, and White Bean Soup (page 60)

Chicken Tinola (page 56)

Mung Dahl (page 186)

# A GUIDE TO EATING OUT

How to eat well when you're on the go or away from home is something we get asked a lot. Here are our tips for keeping things simple and stress free. Treat it like everyday life and be flexible.

### RESTAURANTS

Going out to a restaurant should be a relaxing experience. The good news is that the tide has turned and local, natural, ethically sourced food is now fashionable again and restaurants are much more accommodating. Don't fret if this is not the case – be confident in picking a "better than" option to enjoy.

### Before

• Firstly, if you can steer your party to a restaurant with a natural food philosophy and a good ethos in terms of food provenance, then half of the work is done for you.

• Book early and eat your main course around 7 p.m. An early supper is always better for digestion and allows your body time to digest before it switches to sleep (regeneration) mode.

• Don't be tempted to starve yourself leading up to a meal out so that you can have a blowout in the restaurant. Aside from the obvious reasons as to why this is not a good idea, it will play havoc with your energy levels and could spoil your evening.

• Make sure you are well hydrated before you arrive, rather than catching up during a meal – too much water will dilute your digestive enzymes. If you do arrive thirsty, order a still water, no ice, ASAP. When you sit down, try not to gulp the first thing you get hold of (usually wine!). Despite all good intentions, water is generally the last thing to come to the table, so be aware.

### At the restaurant

• Tell the waiter straight away that you don't need that bread basket so that you aren't tempted by it.

• Opt for wild or pasture-fed meat or fish if available and ask your waiter about where the chef sources the ingredients (it is sometimes stated on the menu).

• We tend to choose a protein option for our meal as it is usually easier than trying to find a starch that doesn't include gluten or grains. Couple this with low-starch vegetables – don't be shy of asking your waiter to team one half of a dish with another. We find most restaurants are very happy to help.

• If pasta is on the menu, you could order a vegetable side dish with the sauce of your favorite pasta poured over as a main course. Italian grilled vegetables with a spicy seafood arrabiata is one of our favorites.

• Ask for your food to be grilled, steamed, baked, or fried using butter, ghee, animal fat, or coconut oil.

• Go easy on the alcohol. It can increase your appetite and make you crave simple carbohydrates. It can also affect your sleep if you drink too much in the evening. Instead, savor your drink alongside the meal. We like a glass or two of antioxidant-rich red wine with a meal and a glass of still water to sip at and cleanse the palate.

• Finish your meal with a peppermint or fresh ginger tea, sipped slowly.

### For best digestion

• Squeeze plenty of fresh lemon or lime juice over meat, fish, and seafood to aid the digestion of animal protein.

• Avoid ice cold drinks and too much liquid in general.

• As a rule, avoid too much raw veg in the evening as it is more demanding to digest.

• Eat slowly and savor and enjoy every bite. Go at your own pace and don't feel that you need to eat at the rate of the company you are in.

• Chew thoroughly (remember that there are no teeth in your tummy!).

• Stay tuned to your body and once you feel 80 percent full, stop eating.

• An overly full tummy will disturb sleep. Think of your stomach as being roughly the size of two fists so don't overburden yourself, no matter how much food is being served. Oh, and by the way, we have never been shy of asking for a doggy bag (that's tomorrow's breakfast sorted!).

### TRAVEL

Looking after yourself while you travel can be a stressful experience and being away from your kitchen or routine is where it can all come undone.

However, when you've mastered the H+H way of cooking, preparing food for trips away will become second nature. Develop the knack of throwing together meals: those leftover cooked vegetables, coupled with the salad and herbs that need eating up, will provide the hit of hydration and antioxidant-rich greens that you need for your trip. Be confident and play around with your own variations.

### Tips for travel food

• Choose ingredients that will keep well without refrigeration or get a cool bag and an ice block.

• Make something that is easy to eat. On a plane you can ask for cutlery, but make sure you've packed a spoon or fork if you need it.

• Choose ingredients and make dishes that keep their texture – salad leaves and delicate ingredients are best avoided. Keep cherry tomatoes whole so they don't break down when they're getting jiggled about.

• Opt for thick dips and pestos to fold through your foods – dressings can get a bit messy.

• Remember to chew well to avoid bloating. Travelling on anything other than your own legs is a good time to actually sit, chill, chew, and enjoy your food.

• Keep drinking lots of liquids while travelling, especially on planes, and avoid alcohol and caffeine as they will dehydrate you.

• Before you leave, put some homemade food in the freezer. When you get home from holiday, just take something out and let it start defrosting or heat it while you unpack your suitcase.

### What to pack

• A Green Smoothie (page 284) with coconut water helps you to keep hydrated; lemon juice will help to keep it fresh.

- A lemon to squeeze into water.
- Herbal tea bags – peppermint and chamomile to perk you up or calm you down. And we always carry a Rooibos Earl Grey for a proper brew.
- The client favorite – a Flax Bread sandwich with steak, watercress, and ginger mayo or try Mung Bean Humus, grated carrot, and avocado packed in tightly.
- A lunchbox of Quinoa and Roasted Vegetable Salad with Brazil Nut Pesto or Buckwheat Noodle Salad.
- Flax and Carrot Crackers or crudités and a thick dip like Lemon Parsley Cashew Dip – good for those hours spent waiting around surrounded by temptations.
- An apple – one of the original and best portable snacks. Pack a piece of cheese to eat with it.
- You could even carry a whole gem lettuce or endive. Compact and fresh, they provide the fresh veg that you need. Just bite into the whole thing and team with a mouthful of nuts, cheese, etc.
- A jar of flavored nuts or a small jar of nut butter.
- A handful of goji berries and sunflower seeds or our favorite snack for the road – Bliss Balls!
- Banana Bread, Cranberry Quinoa Breakfast Bars, or an Apple Cheddar Buckwheat Muffin – great for breakfast or a 4 p.m. snack with a cup of tea.

## STOCKISTS

### Useful websites

www.msc.org Marine Stewardship Council – for information on sustainable fish
www.soilassociation.org – the UK's organic association
www.eattheseasons.co.uk – guide to seasonal produce in Britain

We tend to shop at our local healthfood shops and farmers' markets as well as receiving seasonal veg boxes direct from a local farm. Supermarkets stock most of the more specialist ingredients in our book, but for anything you can't find, use online shops, which are often very cost effective, especially when buying in bulk – look out for special offers and stock up your fridge, freezer, and cupboards with your favorite ingredients. Please see www.hemsleyandhemsley.com for a full list of our favorite stockists.

## ACKNOWLEDGEMENTS

Thank you to all our dear clients for constantly inspiring us and for insisting we write this cookbook.

Thank you to Sjaniel Turrell, Nicky Smiles, and Barnaby Smith; our wonderful publisher powerHouse Books, Craig Cohen, Will Luckman, Wes Del Val, our UK editors at Ebury – Lizzy Gray, Laura Higginson, Kay Halsey; the incredible brains of Susie Pearl, Raj Bachu, Nisha Tailor, Geetie Singh, Richard and Lizzie Vines; our agents Cathryn Summerhayes, Andy McNicoll, Jo Rodgers, Simon Clarkson, Gordon Hagan, Isabella Zaltowoski; our designers Colm Roche @ Imagist and David Eldridge; our shooting team – Frankie Unsworth, Imogen Smith, Nathan Chandler, Polly Webb Wilson, Charlie Phillips; our amazing publicists at Becca PR - Becca Parrish, Alexis Altschuler, Helen Medvedovsky, Meghan Sherrill, our UK team Sarah Bennie, Tanya Layzell–Payne and Victoria Slater, Pippa Lord, our recipe testers extraordinaire – Stephanie and Francesca Cura, Chloe, Sasha and Juanita Kerman, Shelley Martin-Light, Steve Ball, Rory Maclean, Jocelyn Cox, Chevi Davis, Liz Taw, Luke Day, Jessica Malik, Emma and Alex Pye, Mellany Robinson, Nicola Sutton, Florence Lefebvre, Daisy Ellison, Sunshine Bertrand, Sima Bibi, Eve Kalinik, Will Francis, Matt Delahunt, Katie Halil, Francesca Burns, Angelo Pennetta and Ian Jeffries, George Lamb, Carine Dauphin, Christina Agnew, Liam Hart, Clare Callan, Lyz Marsden, Jo Boffey, Jackie Passmore, Howie Payne, Nicola Roberts, Elle Hitchens, Nick Brett, Lenie Sanchez, Amanda Sanchez, Katie Felstead, Mark Baverstock, Maud Arrault, Madeleine Smith and all the Smiths, Henry Relph, the Houshmands, official taste testers Dale and Jaden Turrell and our loved ones Dr Ro Hopper, Jack and Evangelina Hemsley.

# INDEX

# HEMSLEY + HEMSLEY  THE ART OF EATING WELL

Text © Melissa and Jasmine Hemsley 2014
Photography by Nick Hopper © Ebury Press 2014

Published in the United States by powerHouse Books, a division of powerHouse Cultural Entertainment, Inc.
37 Main Street, Brooklyn, NY 11201-1021
telephone 212 604 9074, fax 212 366 5247
e-mail: info@powerHouseBooks.com
website: www.powerHouseBooks.com

DISCLAIMER: The information in this book has been compiled by way of general guidance in relation to the specific subjects addressed, but is not a substitute and not to be relied on for medical, healthcare, pharmaceutical, or other professional advice on specific circumstances and in specific locations. So far as the authors are aware the information given is correct and up to date as of June 2014. Practice, laws, and regulations all change, and the reader should obtain up-to-date professional advice on any such issues. The authors and publishers disclaim, as far as the law allows, any liability arising directly or indirectly from the use, or misuse, of the information contained in this book.

The paper used in the production of this book was made from trees grown in independently inspected forests, and certified as meeting the highest standards for environmental, social, and economic responsibility.

First edition, 2014

Library of Congress Control Number: 2014941819

Hardcover ISBN 978-1-57687-727-2

Design: Two Associates
Food stylist: Frankie Unsworth
Stylist: Polly Webb Wilson

Printed and bound through
Asia Pacific Offset

10 9 8 7 6 5 4 3 2 1

Printed and bound in China

## CONVERSIONS

| | |
|---|---|
| Inches to centimeters: | **multiply by 2.54** |
| Fluid ounces to milliters: | **multiply by 29.57** |
| Quarts to liters: | **multiply by .95** |
| Fluid cups to milliters: | **multiply by 236.59** |
| Ounces to grams: | **multiply by 28.35** |
| Pounds to kilograms: | **multiply by .453** |